Breast Oncology: Techniques, Indications, and Interpretation

Samantha L. Heller • Linda Moy
Editors

Breast Oncology: Techniques, Indications, and Interpretation

Springer

Editors
Samantha L. Heller
Department of Radiology
New York University Langone
Medical Center
New York University School of Medicine
New York
USA

Linda Moy
Department of Radiology
New York University Langone
Medical Center
New York University School of Medicine
New York
USA

ISBN 978-3-319-42561-0 ISBN 978-3-319-42563-4 (eBook)
DOI 10.1007/978-3-319-42563-4

Library of Congress Control Number: 2016963641

Printed on acid-free paper

This Springer imprint is published by Springer Nature
The registered company is Springer International Publishing AG
The registered company address is: Gewerbestrasse 11, 6330 Cham, Switzerland

Linda Moy
To my parents, Fee and Helen, who taught me to persevere and pursue my dreams
To my children, Cindy and Ethan, who fill my life with joy and laughter
To my husband, Dale, who is a wonderful partner
To Dan Kopans who nurtured a passion for breast imaging
To Hildegard Toth for her unwavering support

Samantha L. Heller
Thank you to my wonderful colleagues—I am so very lucky to work with you.
Raj, Kannon, and Dashiell, this is for you—with love and a bottle of pie.

Foreword

Magnetic resonance imaging (MRI) has become a standard breast imaging tool. Breast MRI is widely accepted as a suitable screening exam for women at high risk for breast cancer and is often invaluable in the diagnostic setting. Yet despite an overall increase in understanding of the strengths and applications of breast MRI and despite increasingly nuanced and evidence-based guidelines, breast MRI techniques, protocols, and indications are not static and may vary from practice site to practice site. In addition, breast MRI has some limitations: it is an expensive exam with the potential to impact on overall health-care costs. As well, false-positive findings generated through the MRI exam can lead to additional imaging and biopsy.

Because the field of breast MR continues to evolve, we hope to introduce the reader to emerging breast MRI techniques and applications even as we offer a complete and thorough review of current breast MRI practice and guidelines. Because the stakes are high surrounding appropriate MR interpretation, we have also aimed to provide a book presenting practical tips regarding optimal MR technical parameters and pearls regarding study evaluation.

To accomplish these goals, we have organized our book into three themed sections. The first section focuses on MRI techniques with the goal of detailing the parameters of breast MRI from standard sequences to up-to-date, cutting-edge techniques. The second section reviews accepted indications for breast MRI and analyzes the available evidence-based support for these indications. The third section focuses on specific MRI findings, interpretation strategies, and management of breast MRI findings. Throughout this book, the authors contextualize controversies and debates within the field. The chapter authors provide both national and international perspective on these topics.

New York, NY, USA — Samantha L. Heller and Linda Moy

Contents

Part I Techniques

1 **Breast MRI Technique** 3
Habib Rahbar, Roberta M. Strigel, and Savannah C. Partridge

2 **Breast MRI: Standard Terminologies and Reporting** 25
Dipti Gupta, Lilian Wang, and Sarah Friedewald

Part II Indications

3 **MRI and Screening** 49
Sabrina Rajan and Barbara J.G. Dall

4 **MRI and Preoperative Staging in Women Newly Diagnosed with Breast Cancer** 65
Su-Ju Lee and Mary C. Mahoney

5 **Magnetic Resonance Imaging and Neoadjuvant Chemotherapy** 103
H.T. Carisa Le-Petross, Bora Lim, and Nola Hylton

6 **Breast MRI and Implants** 121
Claudia Seuss and Samantha L. Heller

7 **Problem Solving Breast MRI for Mammographic, Sonographic, or Clinical Findings** 141
Eren D. Yeh and Catherine S. Giess

8 **Post-operative Findings/Recurrent Disease** 163
Amy Melsaether and Yiming Gao

Part III MRI Findings, Interpretation, and Management

9 In Situ Disease on Breast MRI 181
Heather I. Greenwood and Bonnie N. Joe

10 MRI appearance of Invasive Breast Cancer 197
Lea Gilliland and Maria Piraner

11 Targeted Ultrasound After MRI 221
Chloe Chhor and Adrienne Newburg

12 Breast Biopsy and Breast MRI Wire Localization 233
Steven Allen

13 Breast MRI and the Benign Breast Biopsy 251
Amy M. Fowler and Wendy B. DeMartini

14 BI-RADS 3 Lesions on MRI 267
Pascal A. Baltzer and Claudio Spick

15 Multiparametric Imaging: Cutting-Edge Sequences and Techniques Including Diffusion-Weighted Imaging, Magnetic Resonance Spectroscopy, and PET/CT or PET/MRI 283
Maria Adele Marino and Katja Pinker-Domenig

16 Abbreviated Breast MRI 321
Victoria Mango and Linda Moy

17 Personalized Medicine, Biomarkers of Risk and Breast MRI 337
Elizabeth J. Sutton, Nina Purvis, Katja Pinker-Domenig, and Elizabeth A. Morris

Index 351

Contributors

Steven Allen, MBBS, MRCS, FRCR Department of Imaging, Royal Marsden Hospital, London, UK

Pascal A. Baltzer, MD Department of Biomedical Imaging and Image-Guided Therapy, Medical University of Vienna, Vienna, Austria

Chloe Chhor, MD Department of Radiology, NYU School of Medicine, New York, NY, USA

Barbara J.G. Dall, MB ChB, FRCR, FRCP Department of Radiology, Leeds Teaching Hospitals NHS Trust, St. James's University Hospital, Leeds, West Yorkshire, UK

Wendy B. DeMartini, MD Department of Radiology, Stanford University School of Medicine, Palo Alto, CA, USA

Amy M. Fowler, MD, PhD Department of Radiology, University of Wisconsin School of Medicine and Public Health, Madison, WI, USA

Sarah Friedewald, MD Department of Radiology, Northwestern Memorial Hospital, Chicago, IL, USA

Yiming Gao, MD Department of Radiology, NYU School of Medicine, New York, NY, USA

Catherine S. Giess, MD Department of Radiology, Section of Breast Imaging, Brigham and Women's Hospital, Boston, MA, USA

Lea Gilliland, MD Department of Radiology, Emory University Hospital, Atlanta, GA, USA

Heather I. Greenwood, MD Department of Radiology and Biomedical Imaging, University of California, San Francisco Medical Center at Mt. Zion, San Francisco, CA, USA

Dipti Gupta, MD Department of Radiology, Feinberg School of Medicine, Northwestern University, Chicago, IL, USA

Samantha L. Heller, PhD, MD Department of Radiology, New York University School of Medicine, New York, NY, USA

Nola Hylton, PhD Department of Radiology, University of California, San Francisco, San Francisco, CA, USA

Bonnie N. Joe, MD, PhD Department of Radiology and Biomedical Imaging, University of California San Francisco at Mt. Zion, San Francisco, CA, USA

Su-Ju Lee, MD, FACR Department of Radiology, University of Cincinnati Medical Center, Cincinnati, OH, USA

H.T. Carisa Le-Petross, MD, FRCP Department of Radiology, University of Texas MD Anderson Cancer Center, Houston, TX, USA

Bora Lim, MD Breast Medical Oncology, The University of Texas MD Anderson Cancer Center, Houston, TX, USA

Mary C. Mahoney, MD, FACR Department of Radiology, University of Cincinnati Medical Center, Cincinnati, OH, USA

Victoria Mango, MD Department of Radiology, Memorial Sloan Kettering Cancer Center, New York, NY, USA

Maria Adele Marino, MD Division of Molecular and Gender Imaging, Department of Biomedical Imaging and Image-Guided Therapy, Medical University of Vienna, Vienna, Austria

Department of Biomedical Sciences and Morphologic and Functional Imaging, Policlinico Universitario G. Martino, University of Messina, Messina, Italy

Amy Melsaether, MD Department of Radiology, NYU School of Medicine, New York, NY, USA

Elizabeth A. Morris, MD, FACR Department of Radiology, Memorial Sloan Kettering Cancer Center, New York, NY, USA

Linda Moy, MD Department of Radiology, New York University School of Medicine, New York University Langone Medical Center, Laura and Isaac Perlmutter Cancer Center, New York, NY, USA

Adrienne Newburg, MD Department of Radiology, University of Massachusetts Medical School, UMass Memorial Medical Center, Worcester, MA, USA

Savannah C. Partridge, PhD Department of Radiology, University of Washington, Seattle Cancer Care Alliance, Seattle, WA, USA

Katja Pinker-Domenig, MD Division of Molecular and Gender Imaging, Department of Biomedical Imaging and Image-Guided Therapy, Medical University of Vienna/General Hospital Vienna, Vienna, Austria

Maria Piraner, MD Department of Radiology and Imaging Sciences, Emory University Hospital, Atlanta, GA, USA

Nina Purvis, MPhys Department of Radiology, Memorial Sloan Kettering Cancer Center, New York, NY, USA

Habib Rahbar, MD Department of Radiology, University of Washington School of Medicine, Seattle Cancer Care Alliance, Seattle, WA, USA

Sabrina Rajan, BMed Sci(Hons), BMBS, MRCP, FRCR MRI Department, Leeds Teaching Hospitals NHS Trust, St. James's University Hospital, Leeds, West Yorkshire, UK

Claudio Spick, MD Department of Biomedical Imaging and Image-Guided Therapy, Medical University of Vienna, Vienna, Austria

Roberta M. Strigel, MD, MS Department of Radiology, University of Wisconsin School of Medicine and Public Health, Madison, WI, USA

Claudia Seuss, MD Department of Radiology, New York University School of Medicine, New York University Langone Medical Center, Laura and Isaac Perlmutter Cancer Center, New York, NY, USA

Elizabeth J. Sutton, MDCM Department of Radiology, Memorial Sloan Kettering Cancer Center, New York, NY, USA

Lilian Wang, MD Department of Radiology, Prentice Women's Hospital, Northwestern Medicine, Chicago, IL, USA

Eren D. Yeh, MD Department of Radiology, Section of Breast Imaging, Brigham and Women's Hospital, Boston, MA, USA

Part I
Techniques

Chapter 1
Breast MRI Technique

Habib Rahbar, Roberta M. Strigel, and Savannah C. Partridge

Abstract Although there is no single standard protocol for breast MRI acquisition, high quality breast MRI generally requires use of a dedicated breast MRI coil and adequate ($\geq$ 1.5 T) magnetic field strength. Currently, breast MRI requires gadolinium contrast agent administration for cancer detection and a dynamic acquisition (dynamic contrast enhanced, or DCE, MRI) using a method that allows for homogenous fat suppression. In order to maximize sensitivity and sensitivity, MRI protocols must balance spatial and temporal resolution so that important morphologic and kinetic enhancement features can be readily identified. In addition, it is important to develop an approach that attains consistency, addresses technical challenges, and minimizes artifacts. Finally, advanced approaches, such as use of higher magnetic field strength (e.g. 3 T) scanners, diffusion weighted imaging, and MR spectroscopy present unique opportunities and challenges that must be considered and addressed prior to adoption in routine clinical practice.

Keywords Breast MRI • Technique • Acquisition • Protocol • Spatial resolution • Temporal resolution • Artifacts • 3 T • Dynamic contrast enhanced • Fat suppression

1.1 Introduction

Breast MRI was initially proposed for breast cancer detection in the 1970s [1] using pre-contrast intrinsic signal properties related to differences in longitudinal (T1) and transverse (T2) relaxation times exhibited by abnormal breast tissue when compared to normal tissue in vitro [2]. However, MRI use did not gain wide clinical acceptance until it was demonstrated that breast cancers exhibit higher signal on

H. Rahbar, MD (✉) • S.C. Partridge
Department of Radiology, University of Washington School of Medicine, Seattle Cancer Care Alliance, 825 Eastlake Avenue E, Room G3-200, Seattle, WA 98019, USA
e-mail: hrahbar@uw.edu

R.M. Strigel
Department of Radiology, University of Wisconsin School of Medicine and Public Health, 600 Highland Avenue, Madison, WI 53792-3252, USA

S.L. Heller, L. Moy (eds.), *Breast Oncology: Techniques, Indications, and Interpretation*, DOI 10.1007/978-3-319-42563-4_1

T1-weighted images after the administration of intravenous gadolinium-based contrast [3]. Breast MRI is now commonly used for a variety of clinical indications, which are covered in greater detail in Section II of clinical indications for breast MRI. In order to maximize the clinical utility of breast MRI, one must carefully balance patient and equipment factors in order to develop a breast MRI program that provides consistent, high quality images with superior sensitivity for breast cancer detection. This chapter discusses the technical considerations that are central to the performance of quality breast MRI for a variety of clinical indications.

1.2 General Breast MRI Technique Considerations

Despite the increasing utilization of breast MRI for a variety of clinical indications, there is currently no single standard protocol for image acquisition. Both the American College of Radiology (ACR) and the European Society of Breast Imaging (EUSOBI) have set minimum standards for acquisition of breast MRI. However, each of these guidelines allow for much flexibility in how images are acquired and what equipment is used. As reflected in these guidelines, there is consensus that high quality breast MRI acquisition should employ a high spatial resolution dynamic contrast-enhanced (DCE) protocol with bilateral acquisition that provides complete coverage of the breasts and axillae using a dedicated breast MRI coil. The clinical images should include key pulse sequences with appropriate spatial and temporal resolution for assessment of lesion morphologic and kinetic information and be free of significant artifacts. Such an approach allows for effective morphologic and semi-quantitative enhancement kinetic feature assessment of breast lesions, as described in the standardized American College of Radiology (ACR) Breast Imaging-Reporting and Data System (BI-RADS) MRI lexicon [4].

1.2.1 Patient Positioning and Comfort

Breast MRI should be performed with the patient positioned prone in the MRI scanner with the breasts pendant in the dedicated breast coils. This allows the breast tissue to be optimally imaged and findings to be accurately localized by stretching out the normal fibroglandular tissue elements away from the chest wall. This approach also has the advantage of increasing the distance of breast tissue from the heart and lungs, which helps to minimize cardiac and respiratory motion artifacts. Most commonly, the patient's arms are raised above her head in order to avoid wrap artifact; however, some coil designs allow the arms to remain at the patient's side yet posterior to the breasts.

Proper positioning with attention to patient comfort and clear communication allows breast MRI to be performed efficiently and without the aid of cardiac or respiratory gating. Maximizing patient comfort can decrease the likelihood of significant intra- and inter-scan motion. Common points of discomfort are the face, ribs, elbows, and sternum, which can be relieved with appropriate placement of vendor-supplied pads to support the sternum, head, and outer edge of the chest and cushions and/or pillows to support the hips, and elbows. It may be preferable to image patients feet first (in the bore of the magnet) rather than head first to decrease claustrophobia. Patients who have limited range of motion at the shoulder joint may require imaging with their arms at their sides (along the torso). In such cases, it may be useful to wrap the arms so that they are fixed in position and increase the field of view to include the arms to minimize the potential for wrap-around artifacts. Finally, specific yet concise instructions and communication allows patients to anticipate what they will experience while in the scanner, which improves compliance.

1.2.2 Magnetic Field Strength

Breast MRI should not be performed at low magnetic field (B_0) strength and ideally should be performed with a 1.5 tesla (T) or greater magnet. Higher field strength allows for increased signal to noise ratio (SNR), which can facilitate acquisition of MR images that meet general spatial and temporal resolution standards. Over the past decade, breast MRI is increasingly being acquired clinically at higher field strength (e.g. 3 and 7 T), which can allow acquisition of high spatiotemporal resolution images with improved contrast resolution that simply cannot be achieved at 1.5 T. Higher field strength imaging also can decrease scan times; however, there are technical, physical, and safety challenges posed by 3 T and higher field strength imaging that need to be addressed. These challenges are discussed further at the end of the chapter (Imaging at Higher Field Strengths).

1.2.3 Coils

In order to maximize signal, breast MRI should be performed using only dedicated breast surface coils, and preferably using coils with a high number of coil elements. Having a high number of coil elements allows for parallel imaging, which is particularly efficient for breast imaging because it can facilitate high spatial resolution acquisitions in less scan time [5]. Newer MRI systems typically support 32 or more simultaneous radiofrequency (RF) channels, with 16-channel phased-array breast coils commercially available [6]. The breasts should be stabilized within the coil in the lateral-to-medial direction (for axial acquisitions) to minimize the effects of motion, such as ghosting artifacts, and degradation of the subtraction images [7].

1.2.4 Contrast Agent

Although non-contrast MRI techniques, such as diffusion weighted imaging and MR spectroscopy, have shown early promise for breast cancer detection and characterization, all clinical breast MRIs performed for cancer detection or characterization currently require the administration of a gadolinium contrast agent. Chelated gadolinium has paramagnetic properties that result in decreased T1, T2, and T2* relaxation times [8]. Thus, fluid-sensitive imaging, such as T2-weighted series, should be acquired prior to the administration of contrast. Since the decrease in relaxation from injection of the gadolinium chelate is greatest for T1-weighted sequences, DCE MRI is performed with T1-weighting. For breast imaging, the gadolinium chelate should be injected intravenously at a dose of 0.1 mmol/kg body weight followed by a 20 mL saline flush at a rate of approximately 2 mL/s using a power injector. This method both ensures contrast quickly reaches the intravascular space and allows for consistency in contrast enhancement timing across examinations.

1.2.5 Primary Imaging Acquisition Plane and Bilateral Imaging

One of the first decisions when building a breast MRI protocol is to decide on the primary acquisition plane, which may be the only image orientation acquired during the exam. Coronal, sagittal, and axial acquisition planes are all acceptable, particularly because high-quality multi-planar reformats can be reconstructed from imaging at or near isotropic resolution. Primary sagittal and axial acquisitions offer more intuitive orientations of the breast when compared to primary coronal acquisitions. Because the breast is organized anatomically into segments that extend anteroposteriorly from the nipple, both sagittal and axial acquisitions allow optimal visualization of these segments since the full anteroposterior span of the breast is presented on each image. Furthermore, the full plane of the sagittal images closely correlates with standard mediolateral oblique (MLO) and medial-lateral (ML) views obtained on x-ray mammography, whereas the full plane of axial images closely correlates with standard craniocaudal (CC) views. An additional benefit of a primary axial acquisition plane when compared to sagittal is that it allows for more natural side-by-side comparison of the breasts on each image. The authors' practices perform a primary axial acquisition plane for this reason, with multi-planar reformats generated in coronal and sagittal planes. Primary coronal acquisition is rarely performed because it provides the least intuitive orientation and thus is not considered further in this chapter.

Regardless of plane of acquisition, bilateral imaging is favored over unilateral imaging for several reasons. First, bilateral imaging is clinically desirable because it allows for evaluation of both breasts at an identical post-contrast injection time point. Bilateral scanning also allows for assessment of symmetry of enhancement, which is useful for discriminating unique foci and non-mass enhancement lesions from normal background parenchymal enhancement (BPE). There are also technical reasons to perform bilateral imaging rather than unilateral imaging for breast MRI. Because the phase-encoding gradient is typically applied in the left—right direction to minimize the effects of cardiac motion, images acquired in the axial plane with unilateral acquisition are more prone to wrap-around artifacts from the non-imaged contralateral breast [7].

1.2.6 Field-of-View

The appropriate field-of-view (FOV) used for breast MRI depends on the primary acquisition plane. In general, the smallest FOV necessary to include the entire breast and both axillae is recommended in order to maximize in-plane spatial resolution for the same matrix size. For a bilateral axial acquisition plane, the FOV must be large enough to cover both breasts and axilla in the right—left direction. The appropriate FOV for a sagittal primary acquisition plane must account for the entire breast and axilla in the superior—inferior direction.

1.3 Key Breast MRI Pulse Sequences

A standard breast MRI examination includes multiple acquired sequences, which typically comprise the following (Fig. 1.1):

(i) Scout or localizer obtained in all three perpendicular planes.
(ii) T2-weighted (bright fluid) sequence, most commonly with fat suppression.
(iii) Non-fat suppressed T1-weighted sequence.
(iv) Multi-phase T1-weighted sequences performed before and multiple times after contrast administration.
(v) Silicone sensitive sequence (if silicone implants are present).

Of the above sequences, the 3-plane localizer, T2-weighted sequence, and T1-weighted multi-phase (DCE) sequences (including a pre-contrast and an early and delayed post-contrast series) are required by the ACR Breast MRI Accreditation Program [9]. Although optional from an ACR accreditation standpoint, most complete breast MR examinations also include a non-fat suppressed T1-weighted sequence. Furthermore, a silicone sensitive sequence should also be obtained in

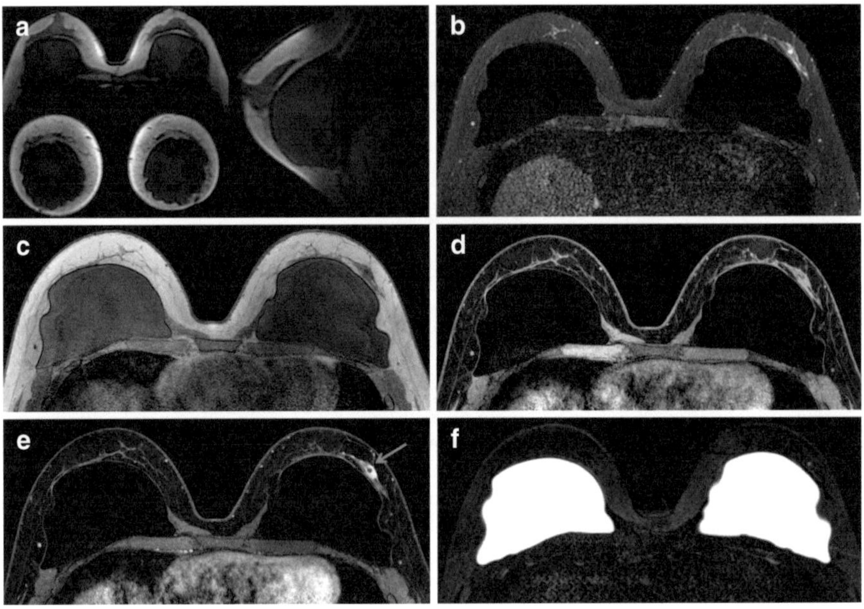

Fig. 1.1 Key breast MRI pulse sequences. Thirty-nine year old woman presents for breast MRI to evaluate extent of disease for known invasive ductal carcinoma of the left breast (*arrow*). Basic sequences include three-plane localizer sequence (**a**), fluid-sensitive sequence (in this case, fast spin echo T2-weighted image with fat saturation) (**b**), non-fat suppressed T1- weighted sequence (**c**), multiphase dynamic contrast-enhanced T1-weighted series with representative pre-contrast (**d**) and first post-contrast (**e**) images presented. Note the enhancing mass (*arrow*), which represents the biopsy-proven invasive ductal carcinoma, with susceptibility artifact within, representing a biopsy marker clip. A silicone-weighted series (**f**) was also obtained in this woman with pre-pectoral silicone implants

women with silicone breast implants. The role and optimization of each individual sequence is discussed in detail below.

For all sequences except the three-plane localizer, the frequency encoding gradient is applied in the anterior-posterior (AP) direction to minimize artifacts due to cardiac motion that would project into the breasts and simulate or obscure suspicious enhancement if the phase encoding direction was AP [10]. Thus, for sagittal acquisition the preferred phase encoding direction is superior—inferior and for axial acquisition the preferred phase encoding direction is left–right.

1.3.1 Three-Plane Localizer

A scout or three-plane localizer is required on all systems to localize the breasts. This allows the technologist to select the appropriate FOV for the patient's anatomy and scan acquisition plane (FOV considerations are discussed in more detail above).

1.3.2 T2-Weighted (Fluid-Sensitive) Sequence

A fluid-sensitive, typically T2-weighted, sequence is important for improved characterization of lesions and benign findings in the breast. For example, simple cysts, lymph nodes, and some fibroadenomas have high signal on the T2-weighted images. There are multiple acceptable sequence types for fluid-sensitive imaging. The most common are spin echo (SE), fast spin echo (FSE), and short tau inversion recovery (STIR) with an inversion time selected to null fat. These sequences are typically acquired as multi-slice 2D acquisitions because of the long repetition times required for T2-weighting and resulting longer acquisition times, which are more prohibitive for three dimensional (3D) imaging [10]. Thus, the T2-weighted images are typically unable to achieve spatial resolution equivalent to the T1-weighted sequences in a reasonable scan time with adequate SNR. Most protocols utilizing SE or FSE technique for T2-weighted imaging also perform fat suppression in order to readily differentiate bright fluid signal from fat. However, others choose to perform T2-weighted images without fat suppression because it can allow for acquisition of higher spatial resolution images and/or decreased scan times.

1.3.3 Non-fat Suppressed T1-Weighted Sequence

If active fat suppression is used for the DCE sequences (discussed below), it is recommended to perform an additional T1-weighted sequence without fat suppression prior to the multi-phase T1-weighted sequences. The sequence is fast, provides an overview of breast anatomy, can aid in assessing the amount of fibroglandular tissue in the breast, and is helpful in distinguishing fat from water-based tissues (such as fibroglandular tissue, breast lesions, etc.). Additionally, this sequence can aid in the identification of fat containing lesions, which is important because lesions containing fat (e.g. fat necrosis) are typically benign. This sequence should be performed with similar parameters and spatial resolution as the multi-phase T1-weighted sequences (as described below), but without active fat suppression, which allows for comparison of lesion characteristics across all the T1-weighted sequences.

1.3.4 Multi-phase T1-Weighted Sequences

The pre-and post-contrast multi-phase T1-weighted MRI images sequences are the most important images for identifying and characterizing lesions. It is imperative that identical scan parameters be used for the multi-phase T1-weighted images so that image registration can be performed, the pre-contrast images can be subtracted from the post-contrast images, and signal differences between sequences can be directly compared. Subtraction images are particularly useful for identifying signal from gadolinium contrast agents and are mandatory if active fat suppression is not utilized so that contrast-enhancement can be readily differentiated from the bright signal of fat (described further below).

The multi-phase T1-weighted images are used for lesion detection, assessment of lesion morphology, and evaluation of lesion contrast enhancement over time. Characterizing lesion morphology, such as shape, margin, and internal enhancement pattern, requires high spatial resolution images with in-plane resolution of ≤1 mm to depict fine features, such as lesion margins. Through-plane slice thickness should be ≤3 mm; however, thinner slices that approach in plane resolution size (i.e. closer to isotropic) decrease volume averaging in the through-plane direction, which can increase the contrast of small lesions compared with background tissue. Additionally, thin slices facilitate higher quality image reformats, eliminating the need to acquire additional images in different planes (discussed further below). Conversely, voxel size should not be so small that SNR suffers.

A 3D GRE pulse sequence is preferred for multi-phase T1-weighted imaging with a short TR. The GRE pulse sequence should be spoiled to avoid any confounding T2 contrast [11]. There are no consensus guidelines for the number of post-contrast acquisitions or total acquisition time for the multi-phase T1-weighted sequences, although at least two post-contrast sequences should be performed in order to allow for the most basic assessment of contrast enhancement kinetic features. Invasive cancers typically enhance early, peaking in enhancement approximately one to two minutes after contrast injection. Although breast cancers more frequently exhibit initial fast enhancement (increase in signal from pre-contrast to first post-contrast series of >100 %) and delayed washout (decrease in signal from first post-contrast to final post-contrast series of >10 %) than benign findings, there remains substantial overlap in the kinetics of malignant and non-malignant lesions of the breast [12]. The multi-phase T1-weighted MRI protocol should be constructed so that one of the early-phase post-contrast sequences will sample the high frequency data at the center of k-space (which defines image contrast) between one and two minutes. This is important to potentially capture the peak enhancement of invasive cancers, but also to differentiate lesions from benign BPE, which typically increases over time (Fig. 1.2). For the majority of Cartesian sequences with rectilinear k-space sampling, the center of the sequence captures the high frequency data. However, Cartesian sequences with elliptical centric k-space sampling and other k-space sampling trajectories, such as radial, may acquire the center of k-space near the beginning of the sequence. Knowledge of the sampling pattern is thus important to properly time the post-contrast sequences.

1.3.5 Silicone Implants

Silicone, like water, has a longer T2 relaxation time than fat. Thus, on a standard T2-weighted sequence without fat suppression, water will be brighter than silicone, which is brighter than fat [13]. For evaluation of silicone implant rupture, it is often

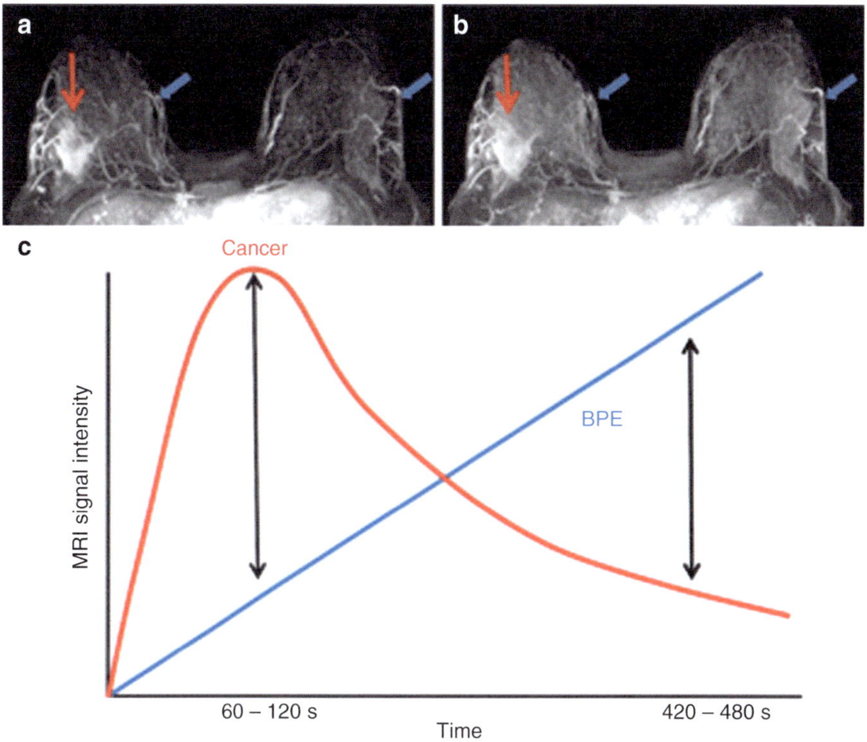

Fig. 1.2 Lesion conspicuity based on dynamic contrast enhanced (DCE) imaging timing. Early-phase 3D subtraction MIP images obtained in the early-phase post-contrast between 60–120 s (s) (**a**) demonstrates the patient's outer posterior right breast cancer (*red arrow*), easily differentiated from the moderate benign background breast parenchymal enhancement (BPE, *blue arrow*). Delayed-phase 3D subtraction MIP image obtained between 420–480 s demonstrates that the cancer (*red arrow*) is less conspicuous because it has begun to washout while BPE (*blue arrows*) has increased in both breasts (**b**). Since in general, cancers tend to washout over time while BPE tends to increase (**c**), it is recommended that early phase DCE images be utilized for breast cancer detection

ideal to have a sequence that suppresses both the water and fat, leaving silicone as the only material remaining bright on imaging. This is possible using a T2-weighted FSE pulse sequence with water suppression and an inversion pulse with an inversion time to null fat [13].

1.4 Balancing Spatial and Temporal Resolution

High spatial resolution and high temporal resolution are typically competing demands of MR acquisition. High spatial resolution imaging results in longer scan times, decreasing the temporal resolution. High spatial resolution is critical for accurate assessment of lesion morphologic features, but high temporal resolution is necessary for accurate depiction of lesion enhancement curves over time. Studies have shown that when forced to compromise, spatial resolution and accurate depiction of lesion morphology is more important to diagnostic accuracy than characterization of the signal enhancement curve. Thus, when creating a breast MRI protocol, spatial resolution is often prioritized over temporal resolution [14].

In general, the compromises between spatial and temporal resolution have decreased with state-of-the art MR systems and breast coils. The ACR Breast MRI Accreditation Program [9] requires that the early-phase post-contrast sequence be completed by four minutes after contrast injection; however, three minutes or less is most desirable [14, 15] and should be achievable without difficulty on modern scanners. Parallel imaging is now standard on modern MRI systems and also helps to shorten scan times [16–19]. There has been much research in recent years to develop novel accelerated MRI acquisition techniques to provide simultaneously high spatial and high temporal resolution scans. These include techniques such as novel k-space sampling schemes and reconstruction using high spatial frequency k-space data from adjacent time frames (view-sharing) [20–23]. Some of these methods are being used to obtain hybrid high spatiotemporal resolution imaging protocols [24, 25], although their exact benefit in the routine clinical setting is not known.

1.5 Methods of Fat Suppression

Either passive (image subtraction) or active removal of fat from the DCE MR images is necessary to ensure detection of contrast-enhancement separate from the bright signal of fat. The benefit of utilizing subtraction for fat suppression is that it allows for higher temporal resolution as well as potentially more complete fat suppression since it does not rely on B_0 homogeneity and shimming. Relying only on image subtraction for detection and characterization of enhancing lesions also has drawbacks—misregistration resulting from interscan motion can result in "pseudoenhancement" and lead to diagnostic errors. Furthermore, subtracted images are prone to degradation of image quality [26]. Thus, it is the authors' preference to perform active fat suppression for the T1-weighted DCE MRI images and additionally perform image subtraction. Using this approach allows an examination to be interpreted solely from the acquired T1-weighted fat suppressed images if the subtraction images are degraded by motion artifact.

Multiple methods exist for active fat suppression, exploiting the small differences in resonant frequency between lipid and water protons and/or the difference in T1 relaxation times between adipose tissue and water to suppress the fat signal. Intermittent fat suppression with a frequency selective fat saturation pulse to eliminate fat signal is commonly employed for T2-weighted SE and FSE sequences and T1-weighted GRE sequences. Inversion pulses and water only excitation pulses are also possibilities. More recently, fat-water separation techniques such as two-point

Dixon based methods [27], including Iterative Decomposition of water and fat with Echo Asymmetry and Least squares estimation (IDEAL) [28], have become more common. These methods acquire multiple echo times (two or more) allowing separation of water and fat and result in water-only and fat-only images. A longer minimum TR is required to acquire the multiple echo times, thus acquisition time is longer. However, uniform suppression of fat signal is challenging in breast MRI due to B_0 inhomogeneity given the complex anatomy and variation in tissue types across the FOV. Dixon methods improve the robustness of fat removal in the presence of B_0 inhomogeneity [29]. Additionally, Dixon methods also provide fat-only images, eliminating the separate non-fat suppressed T1-weighted MRI acquisition and saving overall scan time.

1.6 Image Reformats

Subtraction of post-contrast images from the pre-contrast T1-weighted images is required to remove bright signal from fat (if active fat suppression is not used) so that contrast-enhancing lesions can more easily be seen. However, regardless of the use of active fat suppression for the DCE MR images, the use of image subtraction can be helpful since it removes non-enhancing fibroglandular tissue and other non-enhancing anatomy (besides adipose tissue), enabling easier visualization of potential suspicious areas of contrast enhancement. Subtraction images are most valuable for accentuating enhancing lesions that are evident on the early-phase (for the same reasons described above) DCE images, but can be performed for any of the post-contrast sequences by simply subtracting the pre-contrast images' signal from the desired post-contrast images. One of the most commonly used subtraction reformats is a 3D subtraction maximum intensity projection (MIP) that is created from an individual subtraction series (most frequently the first post-contrast DCE series). The MIP is valuable clinically as an "overview" image that allows for quick assessment of symmetry, BPE, and the presence of suspicious findings.

If the acquired images have sufficient spatial resolution and thin slices, multiplanar reformats (MPRs) can be performed (Fig. 1.3). MPRs allow suspicious findings to be evaluated in multiple planes, aiding detection and characterization, as some lesion types such as non-mass enhancement can be at times easier to detect in a second plane. Also, creation of MPRs eliminates the need to acquire additional sequences in perpendicular planes, saving overall scan time.

1.7 Attaining Consistency and Addressing Challenges

There are inherent challenges to performing breast MRI that must be addressed to obtain consistent high quality breast MR examinations. First and foremost, a quality breast MRI program includes highly trained technologists who regularly perform

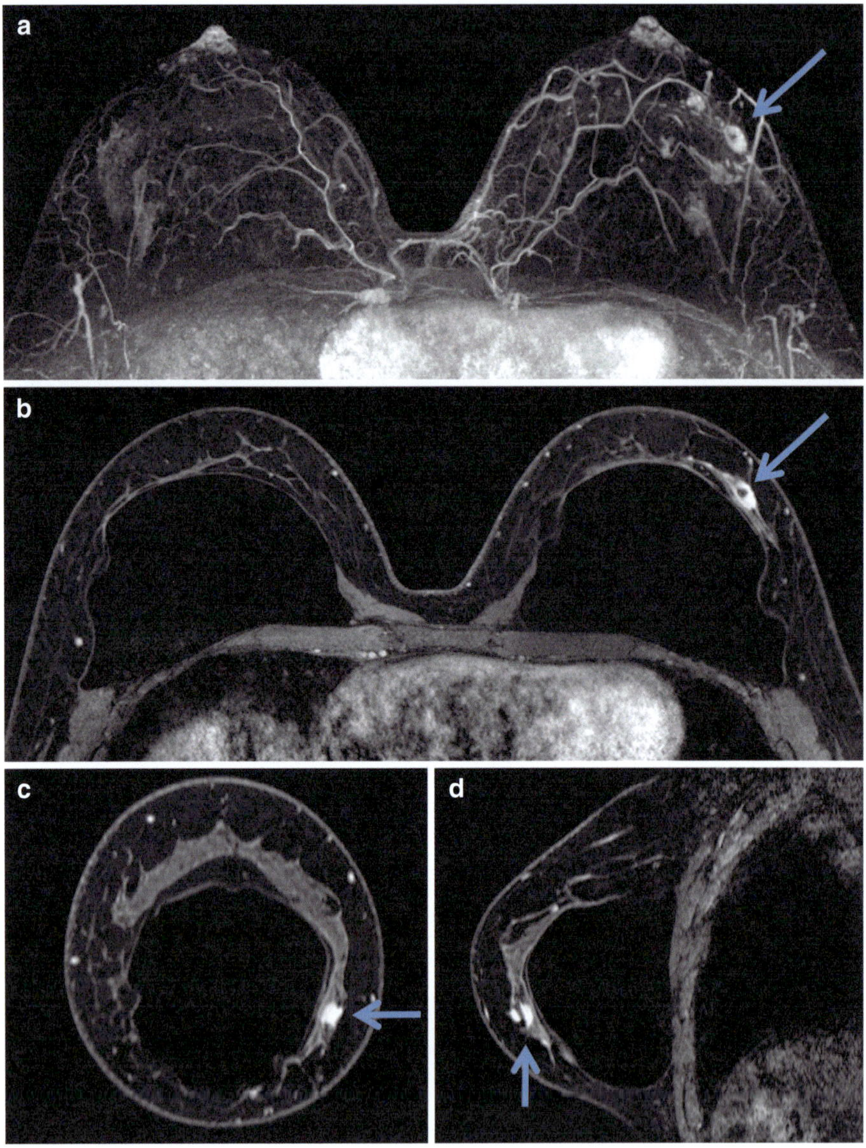

Fig. 1.3 Subtracted maximum intensity projection (MIP) and multi-planar reformats (MPRs) in a 39 year old patient with biopsy proven left invasive ductal carcinoma (*arrows*, same patient as in Fig. 1.1). Patient with biopsy-proven invasive ductal carcinoma (*arrow*) with evidence of multifocal malignancy on MIP (**a**). Known malignancy is evident as a mass (*arrow*) on the source first post-contrast T1-weighted dynamic contrast enhanced (DCE), which was acquired in the axial plane (**b**). Multi-planar coronal (**c**) and sagittal (**d**) reformats from the source first post-contrast DCE image (**a**) provide improved characterization and localization of the known malignancy

breast MRI and are comfortable with appropriate patient positioning and communication. Protocol sequences and sequence timings should be as consistent as possible from patient to patient, regardless of breast size or body habitus. However, the FOV can be adjusted for body habitus for image optimization and reduction of artifact as needed. Finally, there are technical and physical challenges to obtaining high quality breast MRI, some of which are accentuated at higher magnetic field strength, which require attention and are discussed in greater detail below.

1.8 Artifacts

Imaging artifacts can occur in breast MRI scans from a variety of sources. Such artifacts are important to recognize as they can cause misinterpretation by obscuring and/or mimicking pathology. Several of the most common artifacts affecting clinical breast MRI are summarized here.

1.8.1 Motion Artifacts

Both physiologic and non-physiologic movement during image acquisition can cause artifacts. Sources of physiologic motion commonly impacting breast MRI are blood flow and vessel pulsation, respiration, and cardiac motion. Motion artifacts propagate in the phase-encoding direction; therefore, the direction of the phase-encoding gradient must be selected to minimize detrimental effects of such motion on the diagnostic quality of the images. In order to minimize physiologic motion artifacts across the breasts, the phase-encoding gradient should be left—right for axial imaging and superior—inferior for coronal or sagittal imaging (Fig. 1.4).

1.8.2 Misregistration Artifacts

Even slight patient motion during the multi-phase T1-weighted imaging sequences can significantly compromise image subtraction and associated MIP images, reformats, and temporal kinetic evaluation. Resulting image misregistration can create artifacts in subtraction images that simulate suspicious enhancement (i.e. "pseudoenhancement," Fig. 1.5). This issue becomes even more pronounced in protocols with higher spatial resolution. In addition to proper patient positioning and communication, minimizing overall scan time (e.g. by performing multi-planar reformats instead of acquiring alternate scan planes) is important to minimize patient discomfort and motion. Motion correction software may also be helpful to reduce misregistration [26], but cannot be relied upon alone.

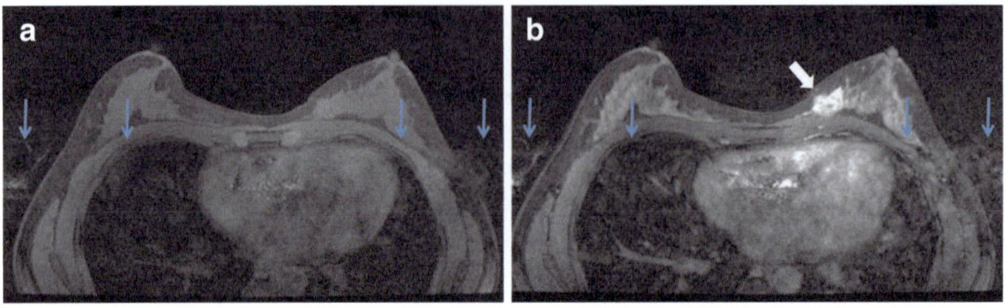

Fig. 1.4 Cardiac motion artifact evident in the phase encoding direction on 1.5 T MR images in a 38 year old woman with a newly diagnosed invasive cancer in the left breast. Pre-contrast (**a**) and initial phase (**b**) post-contrast T1-weighted MR images (axial primary acquisition) demonstrate cardiac motion artifact in the phase encoding (right—left, *vertical blue arrows*) direction in a 44 year old patient with known invasive ductal carcinoma (*angled white arrow*) in the left breast. Note that due to gadolinium concentrating in the heart and great vessels, this effect is accentuated on the post-contrast images (**b**). Alternate selection of anterior-posterior as the phase encoding direction could cause the cardiac motion artifact to overlay and obscure much of the lesion and surrounding area. As a result, it is recommended that the phase encoding direction be left—right for primary axial acquisitions and superior—inferior for primary sagittal or coronal acquisitions

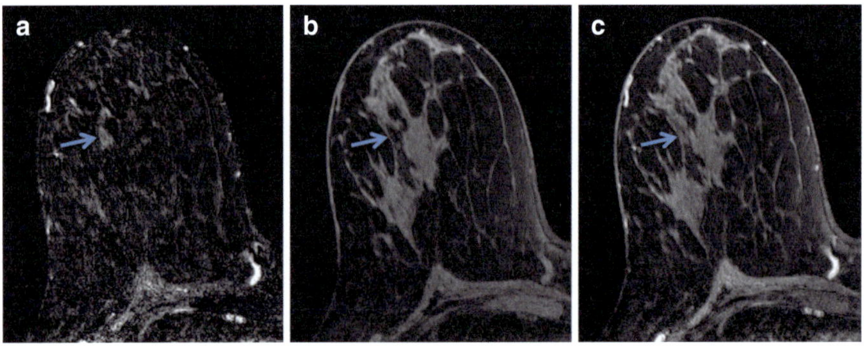

Fig. 1.5 "Pseudoenhancement" on subtraction MR images resulting from interscan patient motion in a 49 year old woman presenting for high risk screening due to personal history of treated breast cancer and BRCA mutation. Subtraction image (**a**) created by subtracting the pre-contrast (**b**) from the initial post-contrast (**c**) 3D T1-weighted fast gradient echo 3 T images demonstrates an apparent rim-enhancing mass in the central right breast (*arrow*). Direct comparison of the anatomic landmarks at the same slice number on the source pre-contrast (**b**) and initial post-contrast (**d**) images demonstrates the apparent enhancement is artifactually created by misregistration of normal non-enhancing signal (*arrows*) on T1-weighted images due to mild inter-scan patient motion

1.8.3 Inhomogeneous Fat Suppression

Uniform fat suppression is important for the detection of breast cancer, as the high signal of fat can hinder detection of enhancing lesions. Inhomogeneous fat suppression is a common problem in breast MRI and can be due to a variety of factors,

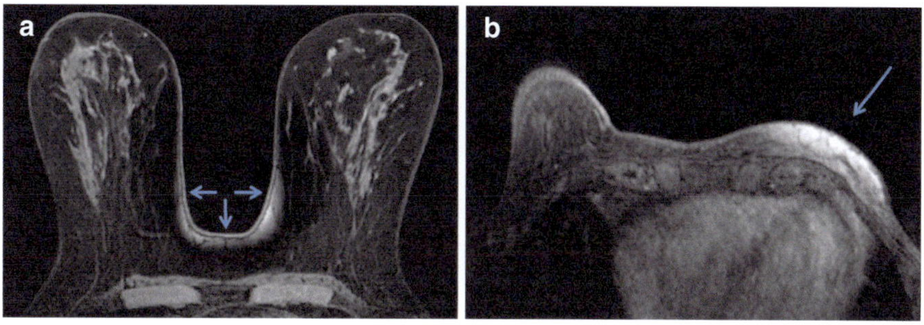

Fig. 1.6 Inhomogeneous fat suppression due to B_0 inhomogeneity secondary to suboptimal shimming. Poor fat suppression (*arrows*) is evident in a 76 year old woman, presenting for breast MRI to evaluate extent of disease, in the cleavage on the T1-weighted first post contrast series obtained at 3 T (**a**). Incomplete fat suppression is noted in the mastectomy bed (*arrow*) in a 57-year-old woman presenting for high risk screening on the T1-weighted first post contrast series obtained at 1.5 T (**b**). In both cases, unique anatomic considerations (pendulous breasts in (**a**), asymmetry due to mastectomy in (**b**)) contributed to pronounced B_0 inhomogeneity. Patient adaptive shimming techniques can help decrease these effects

primarily related to inadequate shimming causing B_0 inhomogeneity or to incorrectly selected water center frequency (Fig. 1.6). At higher magnetic field strength (e.g. 3 T), B_1 inhomogeneity (discussed more below) can also lead to inhomogeneous fat suppression. Fat suppression also can be more challenging in women with fatty breasts (due to high fat signal relative to water) or pendulous breasts (due to shimming difficulties for bilateral imaging). Review by the MRI technologist of the location of water and fat peaks and adjustment, if necessary, of the water center frequency automatically selected by the system software may improve frequency-selective fat saturation. Alternate shimming approaches, through manual adjustment of the shim volume or use of advanced higher order shimming techniques, may improve magnetic field homogeneity and resulting uniformity of fat suppression.

1.8.4 Metallic/Susceptibility Artifacts

Metallic objects, including biopsy marker clips, chemotherapy ports, jewelry, etc. can cause disturbances in the main magnetic field, resulting in metallic/susceptibility artifacts in images (Fig. 1.7). Such artifacts can be helpful (e.g. for confirming biopsy clip placement) or a hindrance if they are large and may obscure cancer [30]. The degree of magnetic field distortion is determined by the size, shape, and composition of the metallic object [31]. Metallic artifacts typically appear as signal voids, sometimes also accompanied by signal flares in some types of sequences (e.g. spin echo). Metallic biopsy markers are available in non-ferromagnetic

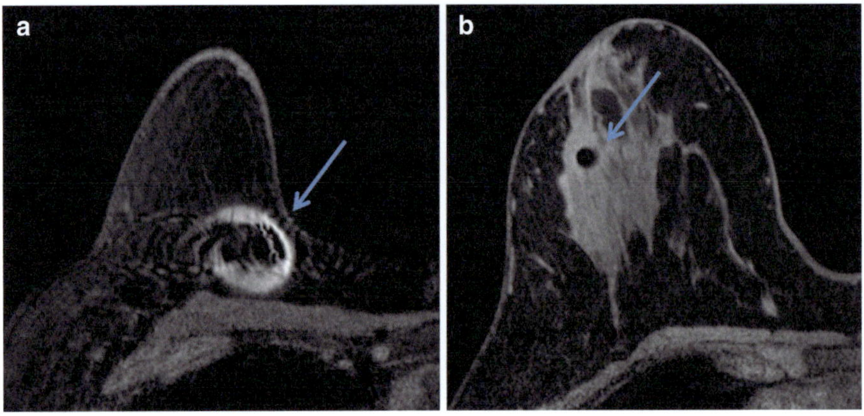

Fig. 1.7 Magnetic susceptibility artifacts. Signal void and surrounding incomplete fat suppression (*arrow*) due to magnetic susceptibility related to the presence of a port catheter in the superior right breast on first post-contrast T1-weighted DCE image with fat suppression in a 64-year old woman during mid-therapy monitoring (**a**). Signal void in the subareolar right breast (*arrow*) due to magnetic susceptibility related to the presence of a titanium metallic biopsy marker clip from a prior needle biopsy on first post-contrast T1-weighted DCE image with fat suppression in a 43-year old woman presenting for breast MRI to evaluate extent of disease (**b**)

titanium, which cause less distortion than markers made of stainless steel. Use of titanium markers may be preferable for 3 T imaging, as magnet susceptibility is greater at higher field strengths. Susceptibility artifacts can be further reduced in size by using fast spin echo rather than gradient echo sequences, reducing TE, and increasing readout gradient strength (increasing bandwidth).

1.8.5 Aliasing/Phase Wrap Artifacts

Tissue outside of the prescribed field-of-view can alias and overlay on the opposite side of the image. This phenomenon is observed in the phase-encoding direction as MR manufacturers have implemented techniques to automatically suppress image wrap in the frequency encoding directions. Because the phase-encoding gradient is typically applied in the left—right direction to minimize the effects of cardiac motion, axial images can suffer wrap artifacts of the patient's arms (Fig. 1.8) if they are positioned at the patient's sides, or wrap artifacts from the non-imaged contralateral breast in the case of unilateral acquisitions [7]. 3D acquisitions utilize two phase-encoding directions and therefore also exhibit phase wrap in the slice-select direction. Means to mitigate phase wrap include appropriate selection of phase-encoding direction, widening the imaging FOV to include all tissue in the phase-encoding direction, applying saturation bands to suppress the signal from outside the FOV, or phase oversampling (also known as 'no phase wrap') techniques.

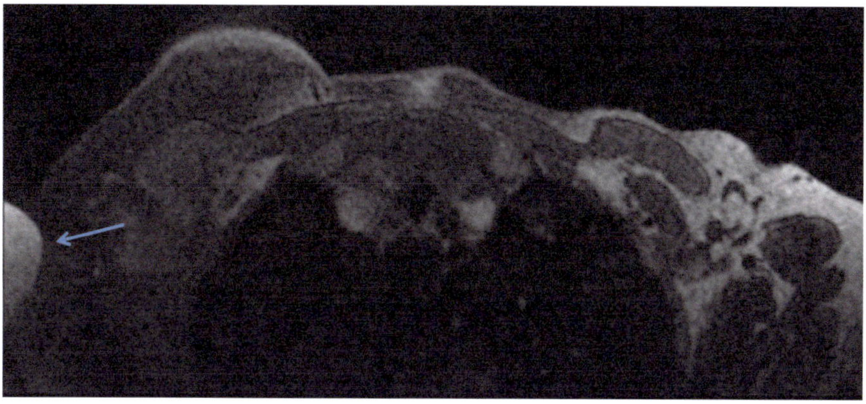

Fig. 1.8 Phase wrap artifact in a 57-year old woman presenting for high-risk screening MRI. Selected image from a T1-weighted fast gradient recalled echo sequence obtained at 1.5 T demonstrates phase wrap artifact of the left arm (which was positioned along the patient's torso for comfort in this woman status post left mastectomy with lymphedema) in the region of the right axilla (*arrow*). Note also incomplete fat suppression in the left axilla due to B_0 inhomogeneity

Other general MRI artifacts that may affect breast MR examinations include chemical shift artifacts resulting from differences in the resonant frequencies of hydrogen in fat and water, which causes spatial misregistration between the "fat image" and the "water image" in the frequency-encoding direction and manifests as bright or dark bands at fat-tissue interfaces. RF noise artifacts can also occur due to interference from external RF sources, potentially resulting from inadequate shielding of the scan room during image acquisition.

1.9 3 T Breast MR Considerations

Imaging at higher magnetic field strength holds potential advantages, primarily related to increased spatial and temporal resolution. As a result, clinical use of MRI scanners with field strength greater than 1.5 T has increased substantially in recent years. While clinical scanning has been reported in up to 7 T magnetic field strengths [32, 33], 3 T is much more readily available [34] and thus merits further discussion.

Scanning at 3 T provides a near doubling of the SNR when compared with 1.5 T, and this increased SNR can be used to obtain higher spatial resolution images at comparable imaging times or to shorten imaging times. Breast MR examinations can also benefit from improved fat suppression because of the greater spectral separation of fat and water at 3 T. Studies have reported significant improvement in accuracy at 3 T compared with 1.5 T in the same patients for differential diagnosis of enhancing breast lesions [35] and for assessing extent of disease in ductal carcinoma in situ [36]. However, specific refinement of breast imaging protocols is required to address the technical and safety challenges of imaging at higher field strength. Such challenges include increased RF energy deposition, increased spatial inhomogeneities of the main magnetic field (B_0) and applied radiofrequency field (B_1), and increased susceptibility effects [34].

1.9.1 Specific Absorption Rate (SAR)

SAR is a measure of radiofrequency (RF) energy deposition that causes tissue heating. When compared to 1.5 T, SAR for breast MRI increases approximately four fold at 3 T when imaging parameters are held constant. Parallel imaging is a primary means to reduce MR imaging times and resulting RF power deposition. Use of reduced flip angles also directly reduces SAR, but with resulting effects on contrast. Additional strategies to mitigate SAR effects require tradeoffs in image acquisition rates, resolution, and slice coverage. Multi-source parallel RF transmission techniques (e.g. dual-source [37, 38]) may also help to reduce SAR by enabling greater control of the distribution of magnetic and electric fields produced in tissue, as well as shortening RF pulse durations.

1.9.2 B_0 Inhomogeneity

Variations of the main magnetic field can cause magnetic susceptibility effects and incomplete fat suppression (Fig. 1.6), particularly at the interfaces between soft tissue (breast) and air. Uniform B_0 throughout the entire field of view is especially important for T1-weighted gradient echo imaging with fat saturation. B_0 inhomogeneities are more problematic at 3 T than 1.5 T due to increased magnetic susceptibility at higher magnetic field strengths [39]. Higher order image-based shimming methods can substantially improve B_0 uniformity for breast imaging.

1.9.3 B_1 Inhomogeneity

Variations in the applied magnetic field are also more pronounced at 3 T vs. 1.5 T due to the higher RF transmit frequency causing standing wave and/or dielectric effects. B_1 inhomogeneities cause the applied flip angle and signal measured to be nonuniform across the field of view, resulting in shading and variations in tissue contrast depending on location [40]. B_1 inhomogeneities can be particularly problematic in breast imaging due to the large field of view required for bilateral imaging and the off-center positioning of the breasts within the transmitting whole-body RF birdcage coil [41]. Use of 3D imaging and increased flip angles can minimize such effects and newer dual source parallel RF excitation techniques substantially improve B_1 homogeneity for breast imaging [42].

1.10 Advanced MRI Techniques

Emerging advanced functional MRI sequences such as diffusion-weighted imaging (DWI) and MR spectroscopy (MRS) can provide potentially useful in vivo measurements of tissue microstructure and metabolism to complement the anatomic and vascular information provided by conventional breast MRI examinations [43]. These techniques are under investigation to improve disease detection and characterization, but have not yet been widely incorporated into clinical breast MRI protocols and interpretations. There are specific challenges and considerations to successfully implementing such advanced sequences. Generally, higher field strength and high performance gradients are advantageous to maximize signal strength and data quality for advanced MRI techniques. In particular, excellent shimming and fat suppression are essential to reduce artifacts in both DWI and MRS. These advanced approaches are described in more detail in a later chapter on multiparametric imaging.

1.11 Summary

Breast MRI is a widely utilized imaging tool for a variety of clinical indications. There are multiple ways to achieve high quality breast MR images, and each approach must be tailored to the specific equipment available. When performed consistently using a DCE technique that balances spatial and temporal resolution, achieves homogeneous fat suppression, and minimizes artifacts, breast MRI offers unparalleled anatomic detail combined with useful physiologic information. The resulting high quality MR images, paired with interpretations by experienced radiologists, provide the most sensitive imaging test for detection and characterization of breast cancer.

References

1. Damadian R. Tumor detection by nuclear magnetic resonance. Science (New York, NY). 1971;171(3976):1151–3. PubMed PMID: 5544870. Epub 1971/03/19. eng
2. Bovee WM, Getreuer KW, Smidt J, Lindeman J. Nuclear magnetic resonance and detection of human breast tumor. J Natl Cancer Inst. 1978;61(1):53–5. PubMed PMID: 276638. Epub 1978/07/01. eng
3. Kaiser WA, Zeitler E. MR imaging of the breast: fast imaging sequences with and without Gd-DTPA. Preliminary observations. Radiology. 1989;170(3 Pt 1):681–6. PubMed PMID: 2916021. Epub 1989/03/01. eng
4. D'Orsi CJ, Sickles EA, Mendelson EB, Morris EA, et al. ACR BI-RADS® Atlas, breast imaging reporting and data system. Reston, VA, American College of Radiology; 2013.
5. Nnewihe AN, Grafendorfer T, Daniel BL, Calderon P, Alley MT, Robb F, et al. Custom-fitted 16-channel bilateral breast coil for bidirectional parallel imaging. Magn Reson Med. 2011;66(1):281–9. PubMed PMID: 21287593. Pubmed Central PMCID: 3128917. Epub 2011/02/03. eng

6. Ladd ME. High-field-strength magnetic resonance: potential and limits. Top Magn Reson Imaging. 2007;18(2):139–52. PubMed PMID: 17621228
7. Rausch DR, Hendrick RE. How to optimize clinical breast MR imaging practices and techniques on Your 1.5-T system. Radiographics. 2006;26(5):1469–84. PubMed PMID: 16973776. Epub 2006/09/16. eng
8. Hendrick RE, Haacke EM. Basic physics of MR contrast agents and maximization of image contrast. J Magn Reson Imaging. 1993;3(1):137–48. PubMed PMID: 8428081. Epub 1993/01/01. eng
9. The American College of Radiology Breast Magnetic Resonance Imaging (MRI) Accreditation Program Requirements [updated 07/31/2015; cited 2015 12/14/2015] Available from: http://www.acr.org/~/media/ACR/Documents/Accreditation/BreastMRI/Requirements.pdf.
10. Hendrick RE. Breast MRI: fundamentals and technical aspects. Springer Science + Business Media, New York, LLC.; 2008.
11. Kuhl CK. Current status of breast MR imaging. Part 2. Clinical applications. Radiology. 2007;244(3):672–91. PubMed PMID: 17709824
12. Wang LC, DeMartini WB, Partridge SC, Peacock S, Lehman CD. MRI-detected suspicious breast lesions: predictive values of kinetic features measured by computer-aided evaluation. AJR Am J Roentgenol. 2009;193(3):826–31. PubMed PMID: 19696298. Epub 2009/08/22. eng
13. Middleton MS. MR evaluation of breast implants. Radiol Clin North Am. 2014;52(3):591–608. PubMed PMID: 24792659
14. Kuhl CK, Schild HH, Morakkabati N. Dynamic bilateral contrast-enhanced MR imaging of the breast: trade-off between spatial and temporal resolution. Radiology. 2005;236(3):789–800. PubMed PMID: 16118161
15. Gutierrez RL, Strigel RM, Partridge SC, DeMartini WB, Eby PR, Stone KM, et al. Dynamic breast MRI: does lower temporal resolution negatively affect clinical kinetic analysis? AJR Am J Roentgenol. 2012;199(3):703–8. PubMed PMID: 22915415
16. Friedman PD, Swaminathan SV, Smith R. SENSE imaging of the breast. AJR Am J Roentgenol. 2005;184(2):448–51. PubMed PMID: 15671362
17. Griswold MA, Jakob PM, Heidemann RM, Nittka M, Jellus V, Wang J, et al. Generalized autocalibrating partially parallel acquisitions (GRAPPA). Magn Reson Med. 2002;47(6):1202–10. PubMed PMID: 12111967
18. Griswold MA, Jakob PM, Nittka M, Goldfarb JW, Haase A. Partially parallel imaging with localized sensitivities (PILS). Magn Reson Med. 2000;44(4):602–9. PubMed PMID: 11025516
19. Pruessmann KP, Weiger M, Scheidegger MB, Boesiger P. SENSE: sensitivity encoding for fast MRI. Magn Reson Med. 1999;42(5):952–62. PubMed PMID: 10542355
20. Herrmann KH, Baltzer PA, Dietzel M, Krumbein I, Geppert C, Kaiser WA, et al. Resolving arterial phase and temporal enhancement characteristics in DCE MRM at high spatial resolution with TWIST acquisition. J Magn Reson Imaging. 2011;34(4):973–82. PubMed PMID: 21769981
21. Le Y, Kipfer H, Majidi S, Holz S, Dale B, Geppert C, et al. Application of time-resolved angiography with stochastic trajectories (TWIST)-Dixon in dynamic contrast-enhanced (DCE) breast MRI. J Magn Reson Imaging. 2013;38(5):1033–42. PubMed PMID: 24038452
22. Saranathan M, Rettmann DW, Hargreaves BA, Clarke SE, Vasanawala SS. DIfferential Subsampling with Cartesian Ordering (DISCO): a high spatio-temporal resolution Dixon imaging sequence for multiphasic contrast enhanced abdominal imaging. J Magn Reson Imaging. 2012;35(6):1484–92. PubMed PMID: 22334505. Pubmed Central PMCID: 3354015
23. Saranathan M, Rettmann DW, BA H, JA L, BL D. Variable spatiotemporal resolution three-dimensional dixon sequence for rapid dynamic contrast-enhanced breast MRI. J Magn Reson Imaging. 2013;40(6):1392–9. PubMed PMID: 24227703
24. Tudorica LA, Oh KY, Roy N, Kettler MD, Chen Y, Hemmingson SL, et al. A feasible high spatiotemporal resolution breast DCE-MRI protocol for clinical settings. Magn Reson

Imaging. 2012;30(9):1257–67. PubMed PMID: 22770687. Pubmed Central PMCID: 3466402

25. Pinker K, Grabner G, Bogner W, Gruber S, Szomolanyi P, Trattnig S, et al. A combined high temporal and high spatial resolution 3 Tesla MR imaging protocol for the assessment of breast lesions: initial results. Invest Radiol. 2009;44(9):553–8. PubMed PMID: 19652611
26. American College of Radiology Practice Parameter for the Performance of Contrast-Enhanced MRI of the Breast [updated 10/01/2014, cited 12/14/2015]. Available from: http://www.acr.org/~/media/2a0eb28eb59041e2825179afb72ef624.pdf.
27. Dixon WT. Simple proton spectroscopic imaging. Radiology 1984;153(1):189–194. PubMed PMID: 6089263.
28. Reeder SB, Pineda AR, Wen Z, Shimakawa A, Yu H, Brittain JH, et al. Iterative decomposition of water and fat with echo asymmetry and least-squares estimation (IDEAL): application with fast spin-echo imaging. Magn Reson Med. 2005;54(3):636–44. PubMed PMID: 16092103
29. Glover GH, Schneider E. Three-point Dixon technique for true water/fat decomposition with B0 inhomogeneity correction. Magn Reson Med. 1991;18(2):371–83. PubMed PMID: 2046518
30. Yitta S, Joe BN, Wisner DJ, Price ER, Hylton NM. Recognizing artifacts and optimizing breast MRI at 1.5 and 3 T. AJR Am J Roentgenol. 2013;200(6):W673–82. PubMed PMID: 23701101
31. Harvey JA, Hendrick RE, Coll JM, Nicholson BT, Burkholder BT, Cohen MA. Breast MR imaging artifacts: how to recognize and fix them. Radiographics. 2007;27(Suppl 1):S131–45. PubMed PMID: 18180223
32. van der Velden TA, Schmitz AM, Gilhuijs KG, Veldhuis WB, Luijten PR, Boer VO, et al. Fat suppression techniques for obtaining high resolution dynamic contrast enhanced bilateral breast MR images at 7 tesla. Magn Reson Imaging. 2016;34(4):462–8. doi:10.1016/j.mri.2015.12.012. Epub 2015/12/ 17.
33. Schmitz AM, Veldhuis WB, Menke-Pluijmers MB, van der Kemp WJ, van der Velden TA, Kock MC, et al. Multiparametric MRI with dynamic contrast enhancement, diffusion-weighted imaging, and 31-phosphorus spectroscopy at 7 T for characterization of breast cancer. Invest Radiol. 2015;50(11):766–71. PubMed PMID: 26135017
34. Rahbar H, Partridge SC, DeMartini WB, Thursten B, Lehman CD. Clinical and technical considerations for high quality breast MRI at 3 Tesla. J Magn Reson Imaging. 2013;37(4):778–90. PubMed PMID: 23526757
35. Kuhl CK, Jost P, Morakkabati N, Zivanovic O, Schild HH, Gieseke J. Contrast-enhanced MR imaging of the breast at 3.0 and 1.5 T in the same patients: initial experience. Radiology. 2006;239(3):666–76. PubMed PMID: 16549623
36. Rahbar H, DeMartini WB, Lee AY, Partridge SC, Peacock S, Lehman CD. Accuracy of 3 T versus 1.5 T breast MRI for pre-operative assessment of extent of disease in newly diagnosed DCIS. Eur J Radiol. 2015;84(4):611–6. PubMed PMID: 25604909. Pubmed Central PMCID: 4348176
37. Nelles M, Konig RS, Gieseke J, Guerand-van Battum MM, Kukuk GM, Schild HH, et al. Dual-source parallel RF transmission for clinical MR imaging of the spine at 3.0 T: intraindividual comparison with conventional single-source transmission. Radiology. 2010;257(3):743–53. PubMed PMID: 20858848. Epub 2010/09/23. eng
38. Willinek WA, Gieseke J, Kukuk GM, Nelles M, Konig R, Morakkabati-Spitz N, et al. Dual-source parallel radiofrequency excitation body MR imaging compared with standard MR imaging at 3.0 T: initial clinical experience. Radiology. 2010;256(3):966–75. PubMed PMID: 20720078. Epub 2010/08/20. eng
39. Rakow-Penner R, Hargreaves B, Glover GH, Daniel B. Breast MRI at 3 T. Appl Radiol. 2009;March:6–13.
40. Kuhl CK, Kooijman H, Gieseke J, Schild HH. Effect of B1 inhomogeneity on breast MR imaging at 3.0 T. Radiology. 2007;244(3):929–30. PubMed PMID: 17709843
41. Azlan CA, Di Giovanni P, Ahearn TS, Semple SI, Gilbert FJ, Redpath TW. B1 transmission-field inhomogeneity and enhancement ratio errors in dynamic contrast-enhanced MRI (DCE-MRI) of the breast at 3 T. J Magn Reson Imaging. 2010;31(1):234–9. PubMed PMID: 20027594. Epub 2009/12/23. eng

42. Rahbar H, Partridge SC, Demartini WB, Gutierrez RL, Parsian S, Lehman CD. Improved B(1) homogeneity of 3 tesla breast MRI using dual-source parallel radiofrequency excitation. J Magn Reson Imaging. 2012;35(5):1222–6. PubMed PMID: 22282269. Epub 2012/01/28. Eng
43. Rahbar H, Partridge SC. Multiparametric MR imaging of breast cancer. Magn Reson Imaging Clin N Am. 2016;24(1):223–38. PubMed PMID: 26613883. Pubmed Central PMCID: 4672390

Chapter 2
Breast MRI: Standard Terminologies and Reporting

Dipti Gupta, Lilian Wang, and Sarah Friedewald

Abstract Breast MRI is a highly sensitive imaging modality valuable for screening women at high risk for developing breast cancer and for diagnostic imaging, including evaluation of extent of disease in women with a known breast malignancy. The ACR Breast Imaging Reporting and Data System (BI-RADS®) developed a common language to describe MRI findings in a clear and concise manner, which led to the breast MRI lexicon. The language used in the lexicon not only allows standardized reporting and triggers appropriate management recommendations, but also facilitates communication between the radiologist and ordering physician.

Keywords MRI • BI-RADS • Lexicon • Standard reporting • Background parenchymal enhancement • Focus • Mass • Non-mass enhancement • Kinetic curve • Assessment categories

2.1 Introduction

Breast MRI is the most sensitive imaging modality for detection of breast cancer, with sensitivity cited as ranging from 77 to 100 % [1]. Because of this high sensitivity, screening breast MRI is recommended as an adjunct to mammography for high risk women. These include women with BRCA mutations and their untested first degree relatives as well as women with a 20 % or greater lifetime risk of breast cancer. Women who have received radiation therapy to the chest between ages 10 and 30 are also considered high risk because of the

D. Gupta, MD (✉)
Department of Radiology, Feinberg School of Medicine, Northwestern University, Chicago, IL, USA
e-mail: dipti.gupta3@gmail.com

L. Wang, MD
Department of Radiology, Prentice Women's Hospital, Northwestern Medicine, Chicago, IL, USA

S. Friedewald, MD
Department of Radiology, Northwestern Memorial Hospital, Chicago, IL, USA

S.L. Heller, L. Moy (eds.), *Breast Oncology: Techniques, Indications, and Interpretation*, DOI 10.1007/978-3-319-42563-4_2

radiosensitivity of developing breast tissue resulting in significant incidence of breast cancer in this population. Finally, other conditions such as Li Fraumeni and Cowden syndrome predispose patients to breast cancer and therefore have been included in the high risk category of patients that would benefit from surveillance with breast MRI [2].

Diagnostic applications of breast MRI include delineating extent of disease in women with recently diagnosed breast cancer and assessing response to neoadjuvant chemotherapy. In certain clinical scenarios with equivocal mammographic and sonographic findings, MRI can help with definitive problem solving. Patients with a negative mammogram and ultrasound (US) and known breast cancer metastasis to axillary lymph nodes also benefit from breast MRI due to its high sensitivity in detection of primary breast cancer.

2.2 MRI Lexicon in BI-RADS® (2013)

The American College of Radiology (ACR) Breast Imaging Reporting and Data System (BI-RADS®) MRI subcommittee developed a lexicon to describe MRI findings in a manner that is standardized, clear and concise (Table 2.1) [3]. Similar to the ACR BIRADS for mammography and ultrasound, use of the standardized terminology reduces confusion in interpretation and reporting, triggers appropriate management recommendations, and guides principles of an audit.

The standardized language used in the lexicon facilitates communication between the radiologist and ordering physician regarding morphologic and kinetic features of the pertinent findings, and promoting collaborative management.

2.2.1 Amount of Fibroglandular Tissue (FGT)

The amount of FGT correlates with breast density on mammography and is divided into quartiles. The proportion of fat and fibroglandular tissue varies widely and may be dependent on the patient's age, hormonal influences and individual characteristics. While there are substantial individual variations, generally there is a greater proportion of fat in older women and more FGT in younger women.

The amount of FGT is assessed on T1W imaging with or without fat suppression and is divided into *almost entirely fatty, scattered fibroglandular tissue, heterogeneous fibroglandular tissue* and *extreme fibroglandular tissue* (Fig. 2.1). In contrast to mammography, the amount of FGT does not limit the sensitivity of breast MRI.

Table 2.1 American College of Radiology BI-RADS® MRI Lexicon

Amount of fibroglandular tissue (FGT) Almost entirely fat Scattered fibroglandular tissue Heterogeneous fibroglandular tissue Extreme fibroglandular tissue	**Background Parenchymal Enhancement** Level Minimal Mild Moderate Marked Symmetric or Asymmetric
Focus **Masses** *Shape* Oval Round Irregular *Margin* Circumscribed Not circumscribed Irregular Spiculated *Internal enhancement patterns* Homogeneous Heterogeneous Rim enhancement Dark internal septations **Non-mass enhancement (NME)** *Distribution* Focal Linear Segmental Regional Multiple regions Diffuse *Internal enhancement pattern* Homogeneous Heterogeneous Clumped Clustered ring	**Non-enhancing findings** Ductal pre-contrast high signal on T1 W Cyst Post-operative collections (hematoma/seroma) Post-therapy skin and trabecular thickening Non-enhancing mass Architectural distortion Signal void from foreign bodies, clips, etc **Associated features** Nipple retraction Nipple invasion Skin retraction Skin thickening Skin invasion a. Direct invasion b. Inflammatory cancer Axillary adenopathy Pectoralis muscle invasion Chest wall invasion Architectural distortion **Kinetic Curve Assessment** Initial phase Slow Medium Fast Delayed phase Persistent Plateau Washout

From American College of Radiology: ACR BI-RADS®—MRI, In *ACR Breast Imaging and Reporting and Data System, breast imaging atlas*, Reston, VA, 2013, American College of Radiology, Table 1. Implant section is not included in this table and is covered in Chap. 6

2.2.2 *Background Parenchymal Enhancement (BPE)*

BPE is the normal enhancement of fibroglandular tissue and should be assessed on the first set of post-contrast images, which are obtained 90 seconds after contrast administration. BPE does not necessarily correlate with the amount of fibroglandular

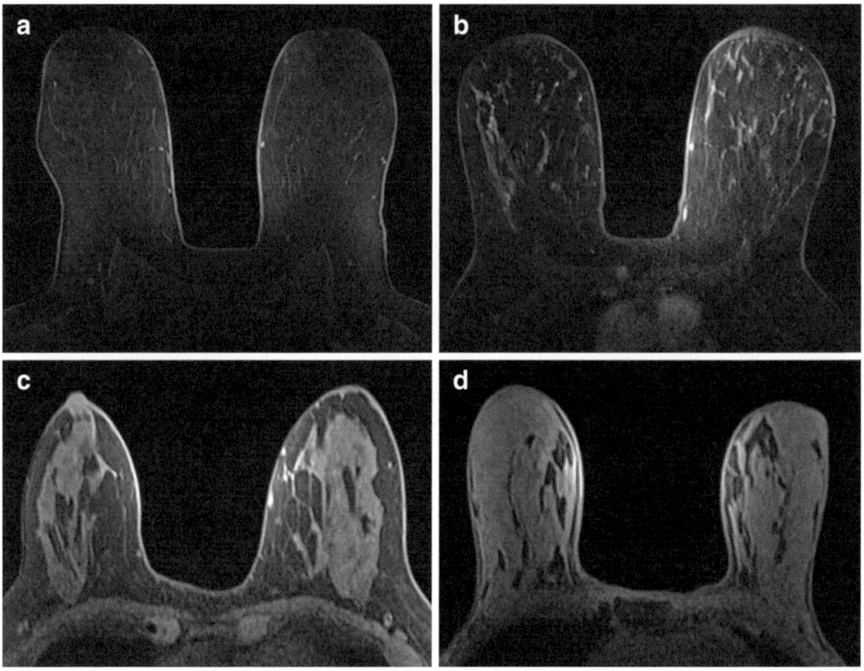

Fig. 2.1 Amount of fibroglandular tissue. Axial T1 pre-contrast images demonstrate entirely fatty (**a**), scattered (**b**), heterogeneous (**c**) and extreme (**d**) fibroglandular tissue

tissue. For example, women with heterogeneously or extremely dense breast tissue counterintuitively may have minimal BPE (Fig. 2.2) and those with scattered fibroglandular tissue may have marked BPE.

Due to the masking effects of BPE, there is the potential for decreased lesion conspicuity. Studies have shown that breast cancers can be detected regardless of BPE. However, the reduced specificity of breast MRI from BPE may lead to increased recommendations for follow-up or biopsy [4].

In general, BPE is more prominent during the luteal phase of the menstrual cycle in pre-menopausal women. As BPE is least prominent during week 2 of the menstrual cycle, screening breast MRI exams should be scheduled during this time whenever possible [5]. During weeks 1 and 4, the enhancement is more avid, and screening breast MRI exams should be avoided. When MRI is performed to assess extent of disease in women with known breast cancer, imaging should be performed regardless of the timing of the menstrual cycle, to avoid delay in care.

The **level** of BPE is divided into *minimal* (<25 % of FGT enhancement), *mild* (25–50 % of FGT enhancement), *moderate* (>50–75 % of FGT enhancement) and *marked* (>75 % of FGT enhancement) Fig. 2.3.

In addition to the level of BPE, it is also important to observe whether BPE is **symmetric or asymmetric**. Bilateral *symmetric* BPE appears as mirror image

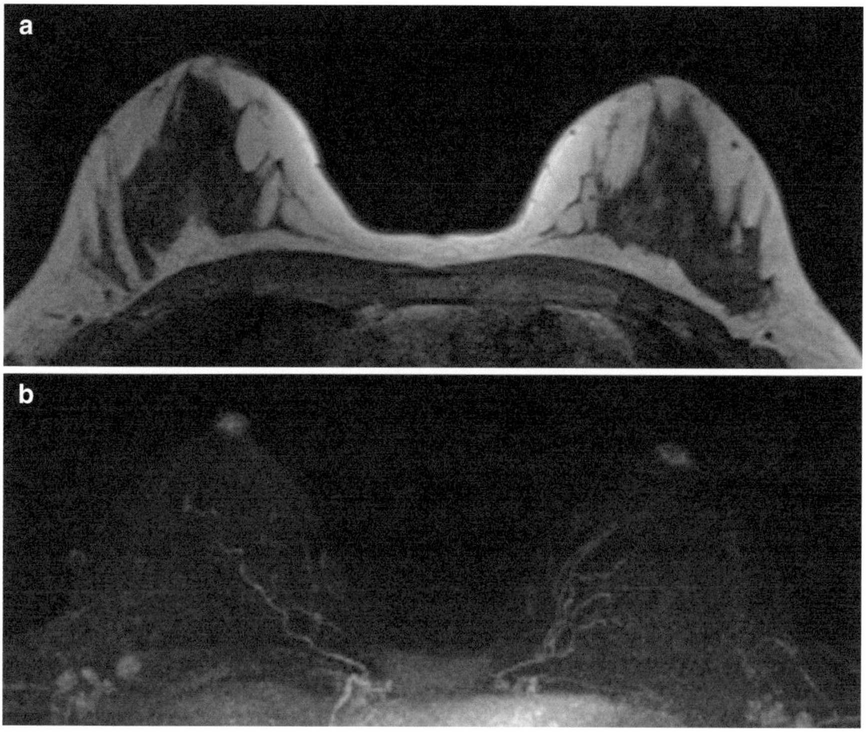

Fig. 2.2 The amount of FGT does not necessarily correlate with the degree of BPE. 54-year-old woman with heterogeneous FGT (**a**) has minimal BPE (**b**)

enhancement which is physiologic and likely related to the vascular supply of the breast. Preferential enhancement typically occurs in a peripheral and posterior distribution, creating a "picture frame appearance." This pattern of enhancement is suggestive of benign BPE.

Asymmetric BPE, on the other hand, may be due to benign or malignant causes. Asymmetry denotes more enhancement in one breast relative to the other, and may be physiologic in a patient who has received radiation therapy, post breast conservation. The radiated breast has less BPE than the non-radiated breast, possibly due to localized decrease in vascularity from radiation therapy. In the absence of radiation, asymmetric BPE is suspicious for extensive disease and should be biopsied (Fig. 2.4).

2.2.3 *Focus*

A focus is defined as a punctuate dot of enhancement which is smaller than 5 mm and too small for its shape and margin to be accurately characterized (Fig. 2.5). A focus has no corresponding finding on the pre-contrast scan and is unlikely to have

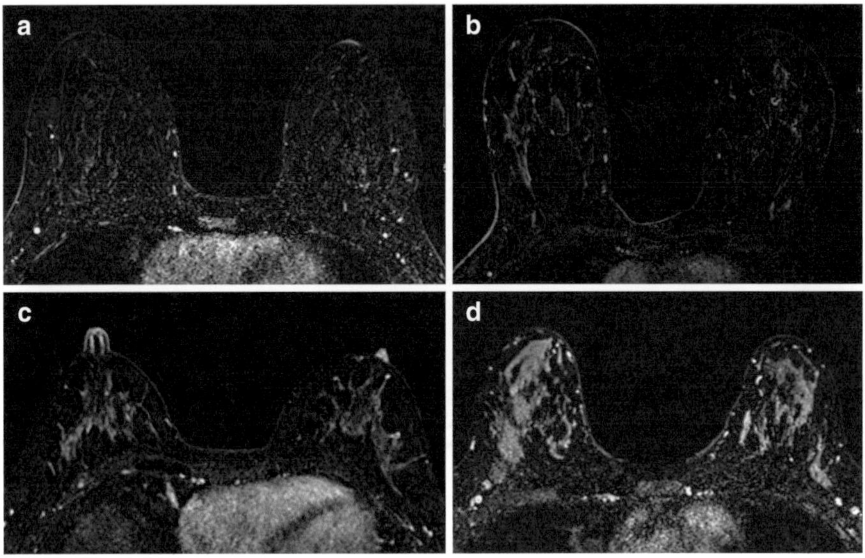

Fig. 2.3 Level of BPE. Axial T1 post-contrast subtracted images with minimal (**a**), mild (**b**), moderate (**c**) and marked (**d**) amount of background parenchymal enhancement

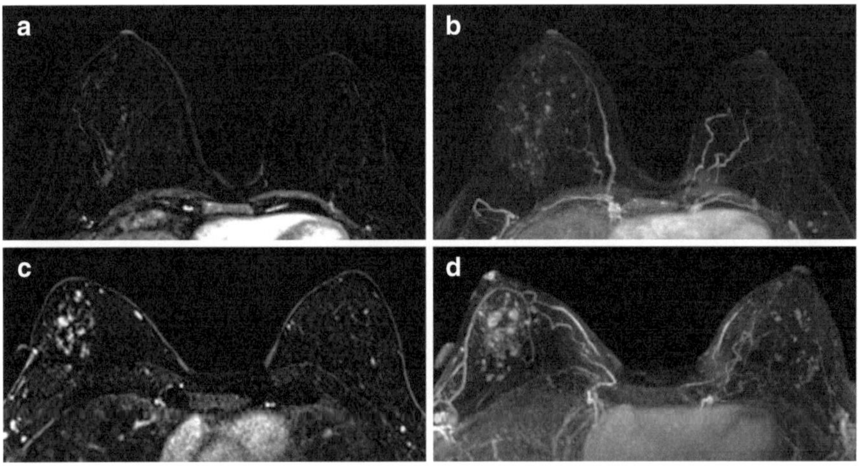

Fig. 2.4 Asymmetric BPE. Axial T1 post contrast subtracted (**a**) and axial MIP (**b**) images demonstrate asymmetric, increased background parenchymal enhancement within the right breast in this patient with history of left lumpectomy and radiation therapy. Axial T1 post contrast subtracted (**c**) and axial MIP (**d**) images in another patient demonstrate asymmetric increased enhancement within the right breast compared to the left in this patient with extensive right breast DCIS

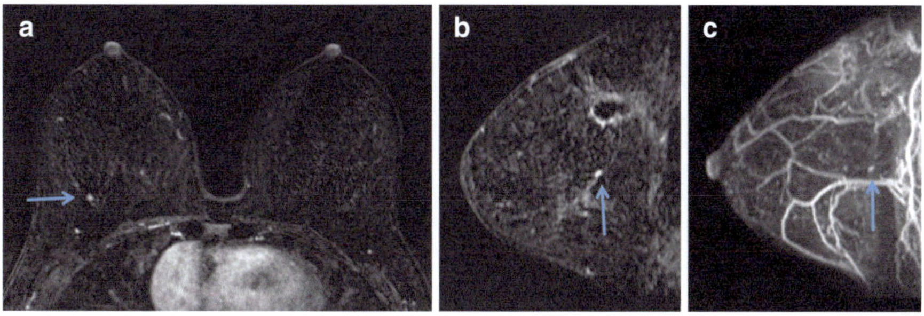

Fig. 2.5 Focus. Solitary punctate dot of enhancement inferior to site of recent surgical excision for DCIS in the upper central right breast on axial post contrast subtracted (**a**), sagittal (**b**) and sagittal MIP (**c**) images (*arrows*). MRI biopsy yielded DCIS involving a radial scar and intraductal papilloma

a correlate on ultrasound. A focus may be benign or malignant and should be evaluated in the clinical context. Tiny foci of enhancement widely separated by normal breast parenchyma represent BPE and should be assessed as benign. Other features that support benignity include high T2 signal, persistent enhancement kinetics, and stability from prior exams. Features of a focus that are more suspicious include low signal on T2 weighted images, washout kinetics, increased size and interval development compared to prior exams.

2.2.4 *Masses*

As in mammography and ultrasound, a mass is three dimensional and occupies space. It has a convex outward contour and is usually larger than or equal to 5 mm. Analysis of the **shape, margin and internal enhancement** can help differentiate benign masses like fibroadenomas from invasive breast cancer. The mass should be assessed on pre- and post-contrast images as well as on T2 weighted imaging.

Masses may be *oval, round,* or *irregular* in **shape** (Fig. 2.6). The descriptor *oval* is used for a mass that is elliptical and includes gentle lobulation with up to three undulations (Fig. 2.7). A *round* mass is one that is spherical, ball shaped, circular or globular (Fig. 2.8). By definition, a mass that is neither round nor oval is *irregular* (Fig. 2.9).

Margin is the edge or border of the lesion and is an important predictor of the likelihood of malignancy of a mass. Margins are *circumscribed* or *not circumscribed.* A *circumscribed* margin is one that is well defined or sharp, with an abrupt transition between the lesion and the surrounding tissue (Fig. 2.10). Unlike mammography, for MRI, the entire margin of a mass must be well defined in order to be characterized as having a *circumscribed* margin. If any portion of the mass is not

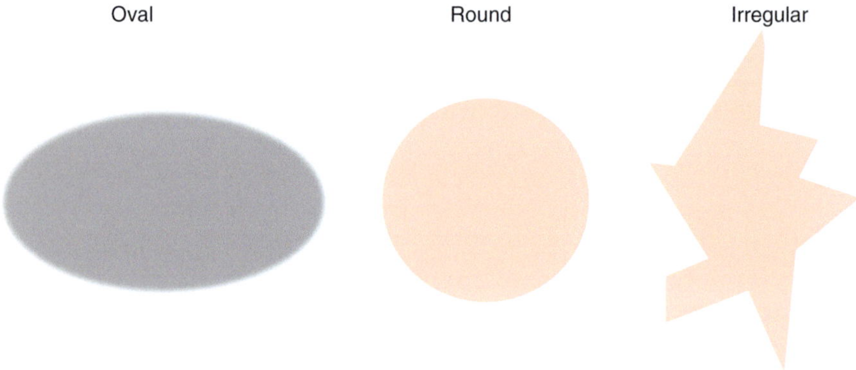

Fig. 2.6 Schematic of shape

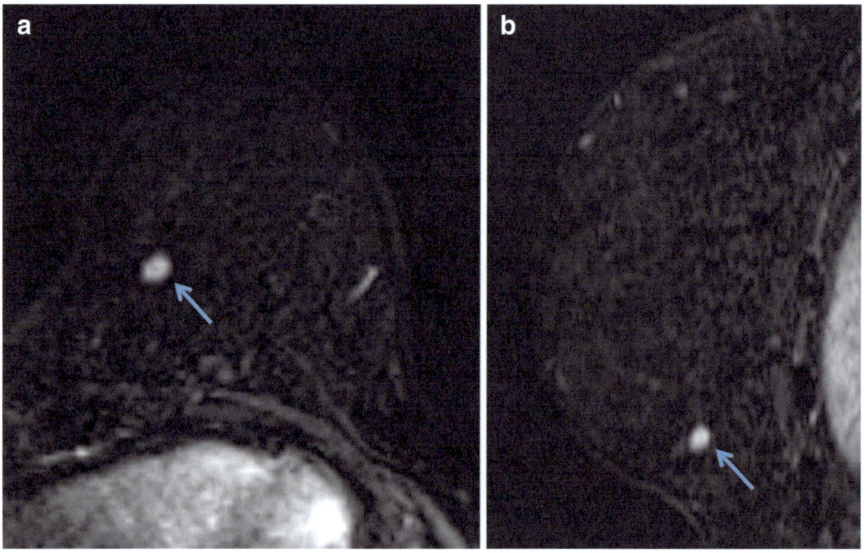

Fig. 2.7 Mass shape – oval. Post contrast axial (**a**) and sagittal (**b**) images demonstrate a 0.8 cm oval enhancing mass in the left lower inner breast (*arrows*). MR biopsy revealed breast tissue with chronic inflammation, histiocytic reaction, and fat necrosis

well defined, the mass is assessed as being *not circumscribed.* Margin and shape analysis should be performed on the first post contrast sequence to avoid lesion washout or progressive enhancement of the background parenchyma. Nunes et al. reported that 97–100 % of masses with circumscribed margin were benign [6, 7].

The *not circumscribed* descriptor includes *irregular* (Fig. 2.11) and *spiculated* categories (Fig. 2.12). An *irregular* margin has edges that may be uneven or jagged and is suspicious. A *spiculated* margin has sharp lines radiating from the mass and often

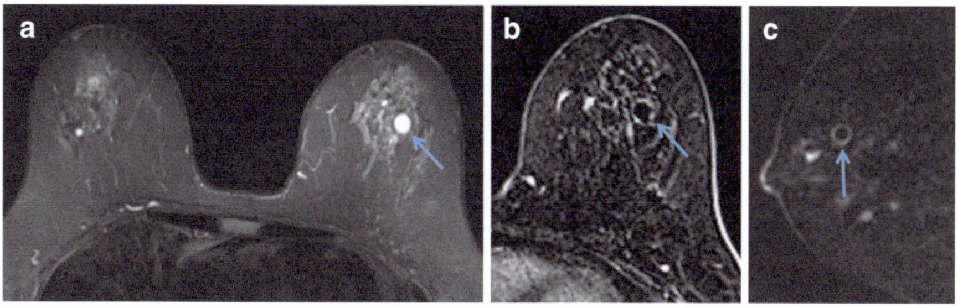

Fig. 2.8 Mass shape – round. Round mass with circumscribed margins in the upper central left breast has high T2 signal (**a**) and uniform rim enhancement on the axial (**b**) and sagittal (**c**) post contrast images (*arrows*), consistent with a benign inflamed cyst

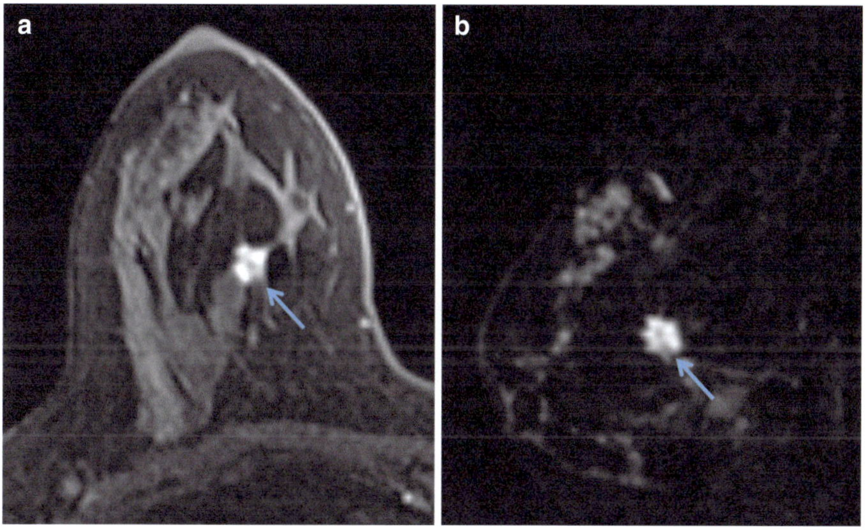

Fig. 2.9 Mass shape – irregular. MRI performed for extent of disease in a 42 year old female with a biopsy proven invasive ductal carcinoma in the right breast. Axial (**a**) and sagittal (**b**) post contrast images show an irregular 7 mm enhancing mass (*arrows*) which corresponds with the known cancer

indicates malignancy. Masses with *irregular* and *spiculated* margins have a high positive predictive value (PPV) for malignancy, ranging from 80 to 100 % [6, 8].

Internal enhancement describes the enhancement pattern within an enhancing mass. *Homogeneous* enhancement is confluent and uniform whereas *heterogeneous* enhancement is non-uniform with variable signal intensity. While *heterogeneous* enhancement is more characteristic of malignancy (Fig. 2.13) and homogeneous enhancement is more often seen with benign masses (Fig. 2.14), there is considerable overlap. Small cancers may have homogeneous enhancement.

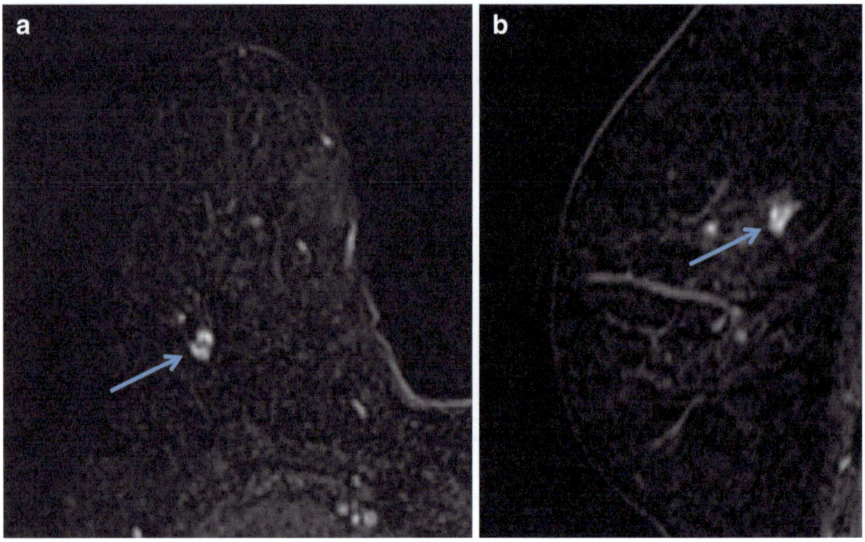

Fig. 2.10 Margin – circumscribed. Oval enhancing mass with circumscribed margins and non-enhancing internal septations in the right upper outer breast on post contrast axial (**a**) and sagittal (**b**) images (*arrows*) is consistent with a fibroadenoma

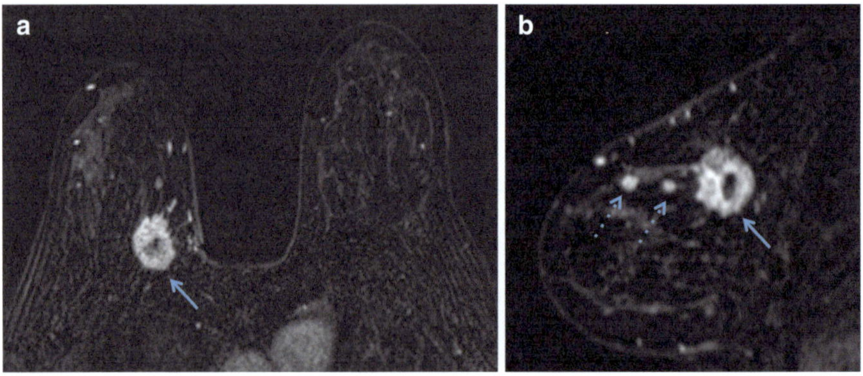

Fig. 2.11 Mass margin: not circumscribed – Irregular margin. Extent of disease MRI shows an irregular enhancing mass in the right upper inner breast consistent with biopsy proven malignancy on axial post-contrast image (**a**) (*solid arrow*). There are 2 smaller satellite masses (*dashed arrows*) extending anterior to the dominant mass (*solid arrow*) on the sagittal view (**b**)

Special enhancement patterns include *rim enhancement* and *dark internal septations*. When enhancement is more pronounced at the periphery of the mass, it is referred to as *rim enhancement* (Fig. 2.15). Rim enhancement can be seen with inflamed cysts, which have central T2 hyperintensity, and with fat necrosis, which demonstrates internal T1 hyperintensity on non-fat suppressed images. A study by Goto et al. found that while the prevalence of malignancy with rim enhancement is low at about 25 %, the finding has a specificity of 93 % for carcinoma [9].

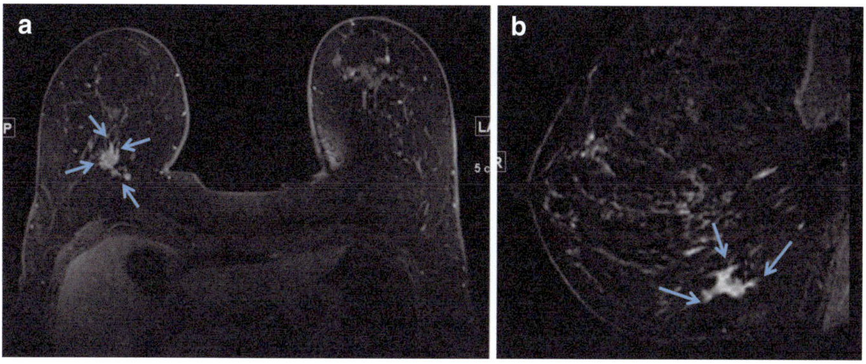

Fig. 2.12 Mass margin: not circumscribed – spiculated margin. A 2.5 cm irregular mass in the right lower central breast has lines radiating from it forming a spiculated margin as seen on axial (**a**) and sagittal (**b**) post-contrast images (*arrows*). Biopsy showed invasive ductal carcinoma, grades 2 and 3

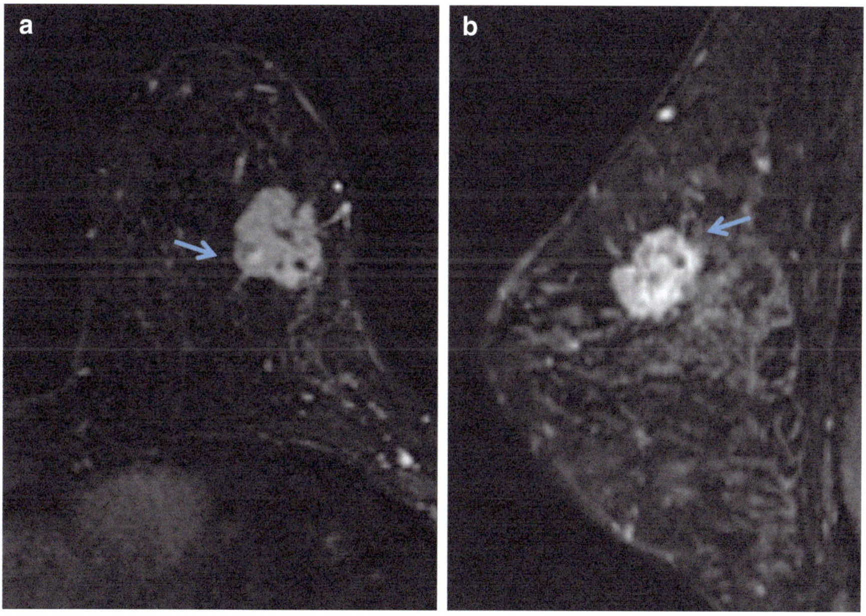

Fig. 2.13 Masses: internal enhancement – heterogeneous. Extent of disease MRI in a 29 year old with invasive ductal carcinoma shows an irregular heterogeneously enhancing mass in the left upper outer quadrant, consistent with the known malignancy on axial (**a**) and sagittal (**b**) post-contrast images (*arrows*)

Non-enhancing *dark internal septations* are most often seen with fibroadenomas, when associated with an oval, circumscribed, high T2 signal mass with persistent enhancement kinetics (Fig. 2.16). While *dark internal septations* support the diagnosis of a fibroadenoma, they are not pathognomonic for benignity and should not dissuade the radiologist from biopsy of a mass with suspicious morphology or kinetics.

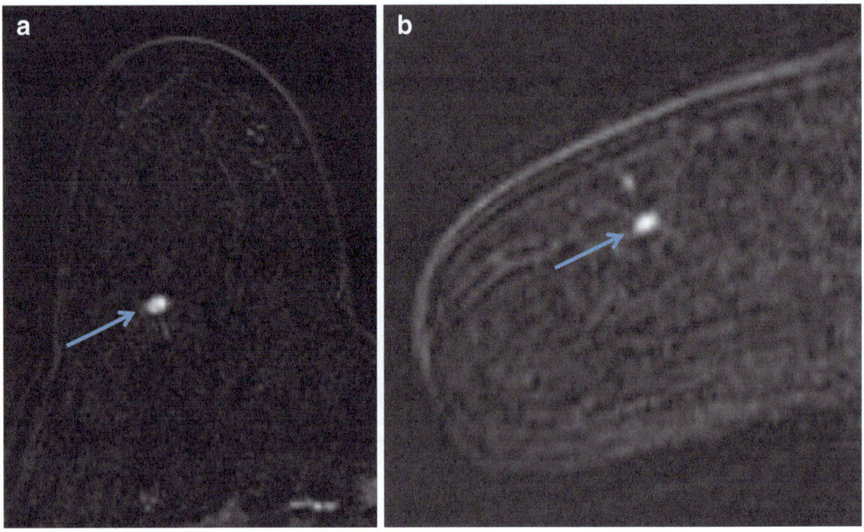

Fig. 2.14 Masses: internal enhancement – homogeneous. Oval, circumscribed, homogeneously enhancing mass detected on axial (**a**) and sagittal (**b**) screening breast MRI images (*arrows*) was biopsied with benign histology

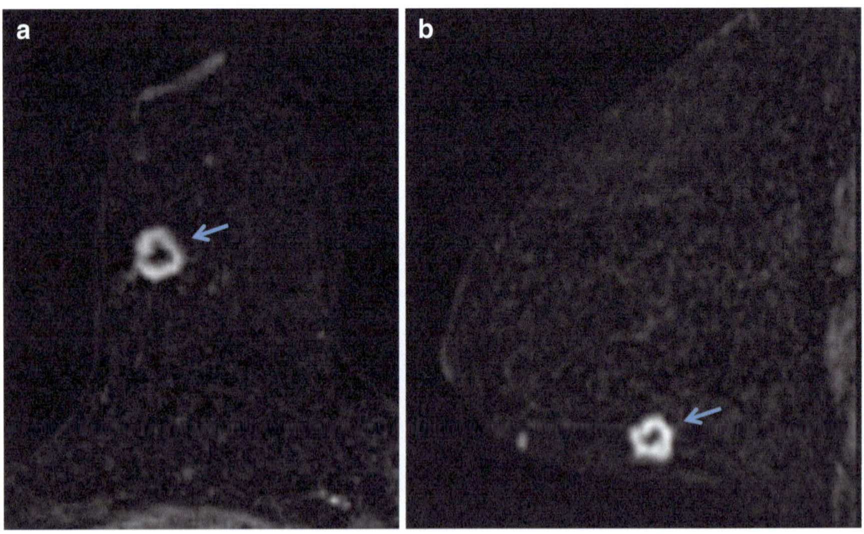

Fig. 2.15 Masses: rim enhancement. Fifty-six year old with a known invasive ductal carcinoma with tubular features presents as a mass with irregular rim enhancement on axial (**a**) and sagittal (**b**) post-contrast images (*arrows*). Contrast this with the thin, uniform, rim enhancement of an inflamed cyst as seen on Fig. 2.8

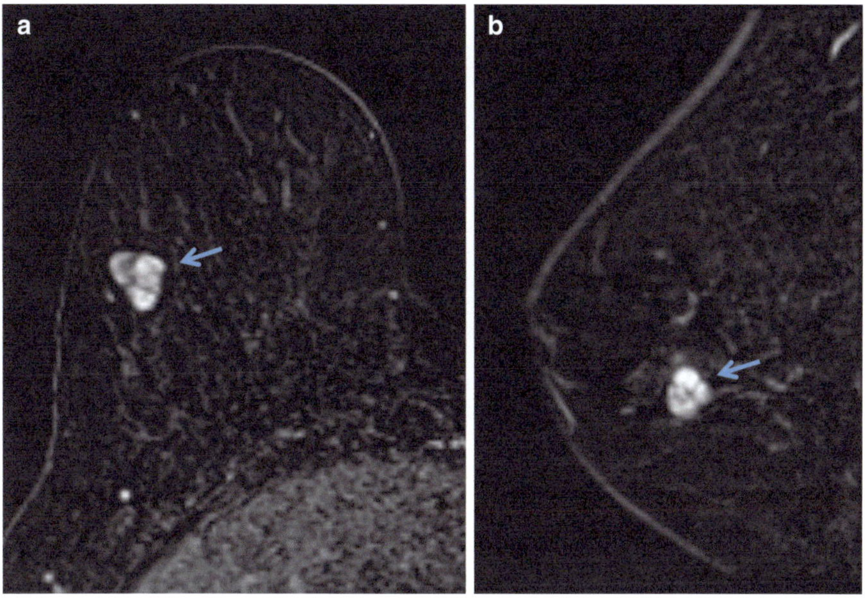

Fig. 2.16 Masses: dark internal septations. Oval enhancing mass in the right lower outer breast with dark internal septations consistent with a biopsy proven fibroadenoma as seen on axial (**a**) and sagittal (**b**) post-contrast images (*arrows*)

2.2.5 Non-mass Enhancement (NME)

NME is used to describe an area that is neither a mass nor a focus and may extend over small or large regions. NME appears discrete from the normal surrounding background parenchymal enhancement. Within the area of abnormal NME, there may be regions of normal fibroglandular tissue or fat interspersed within the abnormally enhancing components.

Distribution of NME can be described as *focal, linear, segmental, regional, multiple regions or diffuse*. A *focal* area of NME describes a confined area in the breast, which involves less than a quadrant and is within a single duct system (Fig. 2.17). *Linear* NME is enhancement along a single duct which appears as a line (Fig. 2.18) that may or may not be straight, and may have branches. This pattern of enhancement is suspicious for malignancy, with a PPV ranging from 26 to 58.5 % [10, 11]. *Segmental* NME is triangular or cone shaped, with the apex of the cone at the nipple (Fig. 2.19). *Segmental* enhancement indicates involvement of a duct or ducts and their branches, and is suspicious for extensive or multifocal malignancy, with a PPV ranging from 67 to 100% [12]. Linear and segmental enhancement is the most frequent manifestation of DCIS on MRI [13].

Regional enhancement involves a larger area than a single duct system (Fig. 2.20). This distribution may be geographic and spans at least one quadrant. *Multiple regions of non-mass enhancement* encompasses at least 2 broad areas separated by

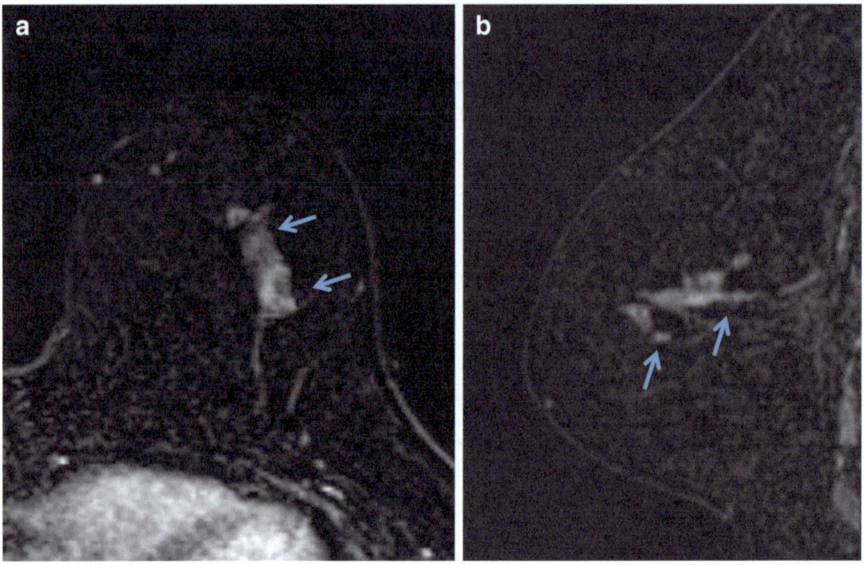

Fig. 2.17 NME: focal. Sixty year old with biopsy proven DCIS in the left upper outer breast underwent MRI for extent of disease. The known DCIS presents as an area of focal, clumped NME on axial (**a**) and sagittal (**b**) images (*arrows*)

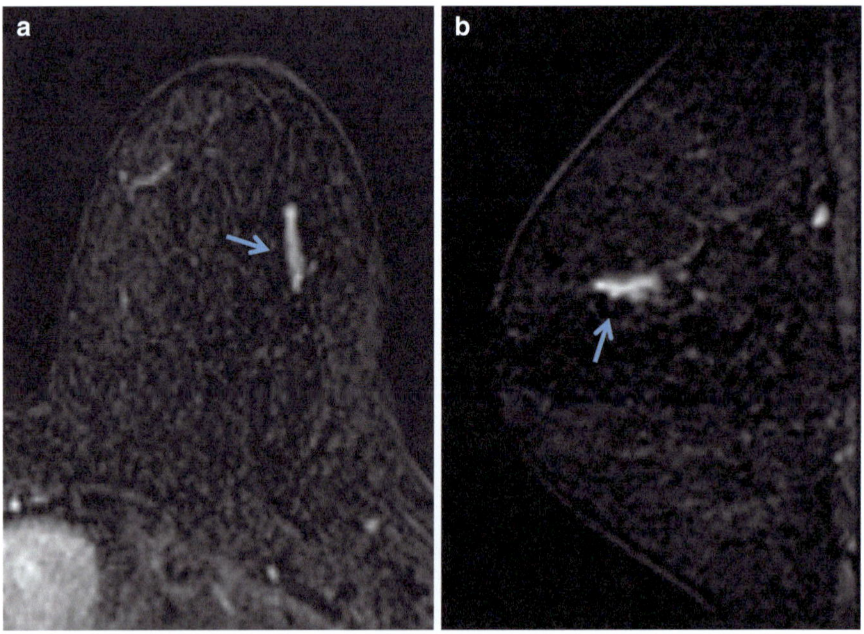

Fig. 2.18 NME: linear. Forty-six year old underwent high risk screening MRI which showed a 1.8 cm area of homogeneous, linear NME in the left upper outer breast on axial (**a**) and sagittal (**b**) images (*arrows*). MR biopsy was significant for DCIS, cribriform, solid, papillary, and micropapillary types, nuclear grade 2, with microcalcifications, necrosis, and lobular extension

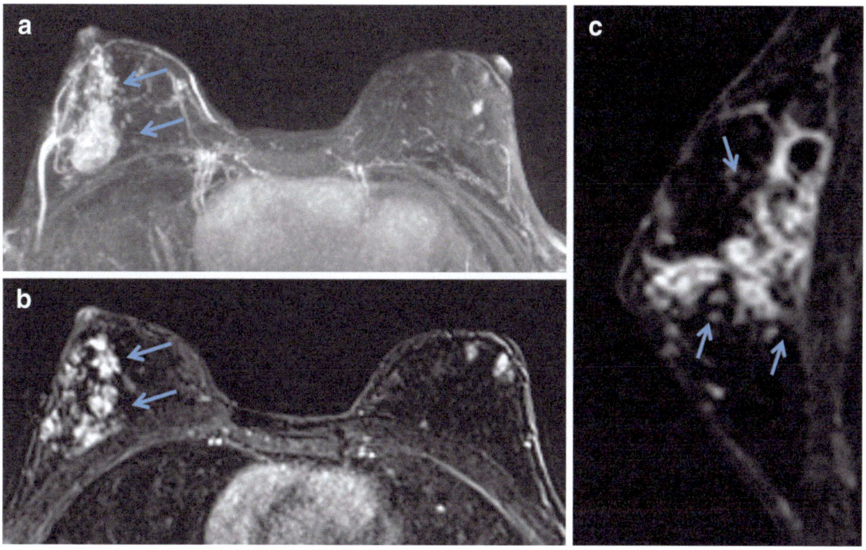

Fig. 2.19 NME – segmental. Markedly abnormal heterogeneous NME in a segmental distribution involving the right upper outer breast is consistent with biopsy proven invasive ductal carcinoma. The abnormal enhancement is striking on the MIP images (**a**) in addition to the axial (**b**) and sagittal (**c**) images (*arrows*)

normal tissue, and does not conform to a ductal distribution (Fig. 2.21). As this involves many areas of geographic enhancement, it has a patchy appearance. *Diffuse* NME describes similar appearing, widely scattered and evenly distributed enhancement throughout the breast tissue (Fig. 2.22). *Regional, multiple regions and diffuse* NME are more characteristic of benign processes such as proliferative changes; however, multicentric carcinoma may have this appearance.

NME can be further described using **internal enhancement patterns** which includes *homogeneous, heterogeneous, clumped or clustered ring enhancement.* As with masses, *homogeneous* enhancement is uniform and confluent (Fig. 2.18), while *heterogeneous* enhancement is non-uniform and random (Fig. 2.19). *Clumped* enhancement appears as an aggregation of foci with a cobblestone appearance and is suspicious for malignancy (Fig. 2.23). *Clumped* NME may appear as a cluster of grapes when it is focal or may have a beaded appearance when in a linear distribution. *Clustered ring* enhancement is also suspicious for malignancy and describes enhancement of the periductal stroma appearing as rings of enhancement clustered around the ducts (Fig. 2.24).

2.2.6 Associated Features

Associated features include *nipple retraction, nipple invasion, skin thickening, skin retraction, skin invasion, pectoralis muscle invasion, chest wall invasion, architectural distortion, axillary lymphadenopathy and architectural distortion.* Associated

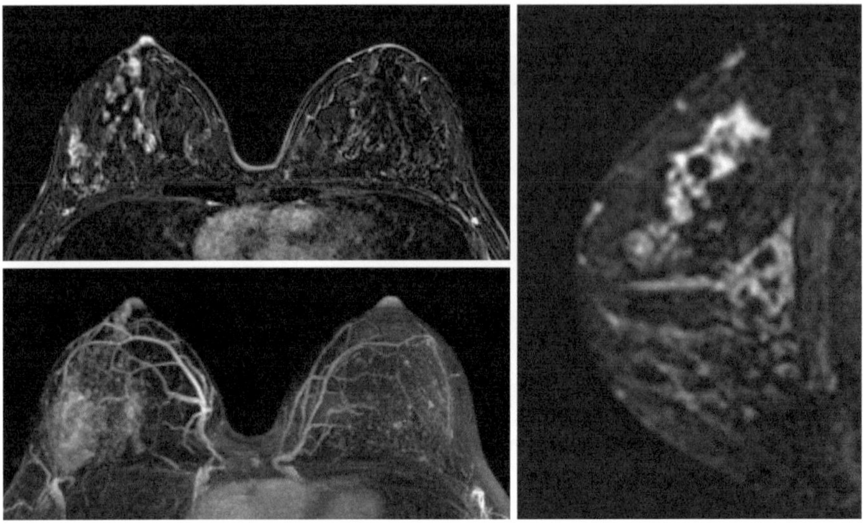

Fig. 2.20 NME – regional. Forty year old with regional enhancement throughout the right outer breast on the axial (**a**), axial MIP (**b**) and sagittal (**c**) post contrast images, consistent with biopsy proven DCIS. Suspicious calcifications showed a similar distribution on mammography

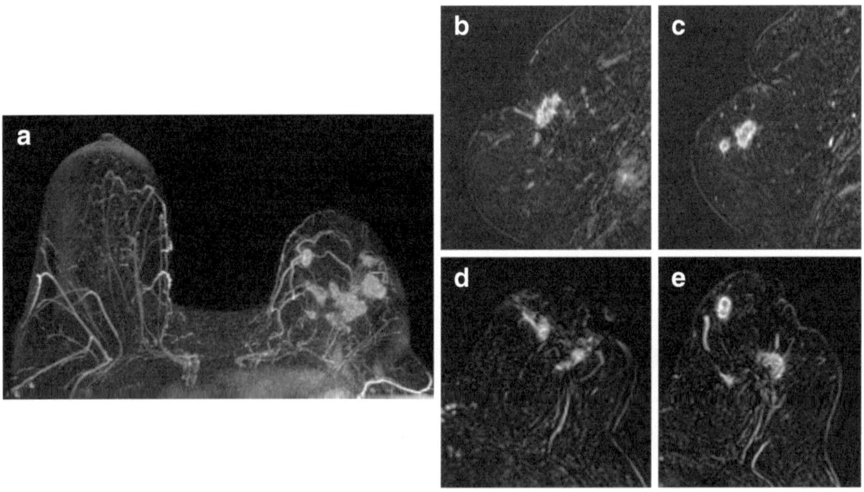

Fig. 2.21 NME – multiple regions. Seventy-four year old with history of left lumpectomy for invasive lobular carcinoma 10 years ago had multiple prior biopsies showing fat necrosis. MRI shows multiple regions of NME on the axial MIP (**a**), sagittal post contrast (**b**, **c**) and axial post contrast (**d**, **e**) images. Second look ultrasound and biopsy was performed, also showing fat necrosis

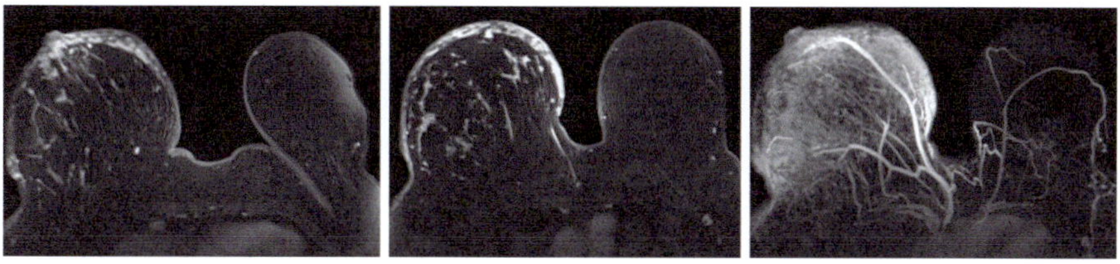

Fig. 2.22 NME – diffuse. Fifty-five year old with history of invasive ductal carcinoma, grade 3 on skin punch biopsy shows diffuse right breast and skin enhancement on the axial post contrast (**a**, **b**) and MIP (**c**) images

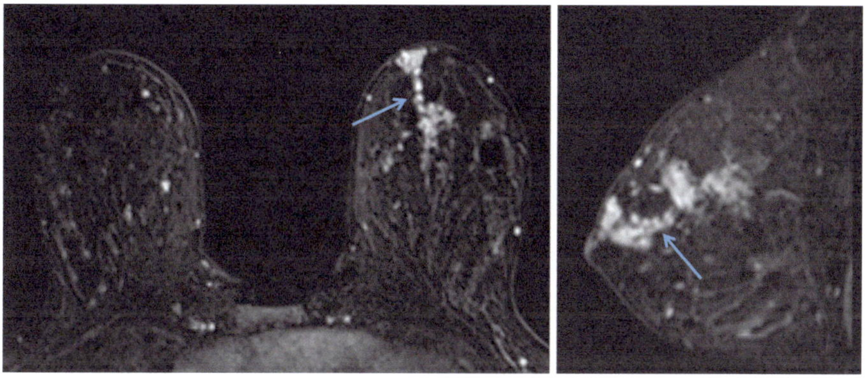

Fig. 2.23 NME – internal enhancement: clumped. Linear, clumped nonmass enhancement extending to the nipple from a known malignancy in the upper central left breast as seen on axial (**a**) and sagittal (**b**) post contrast images (*arrows*). MR biopsy of the anterior extent revealed grade 3 DCIS

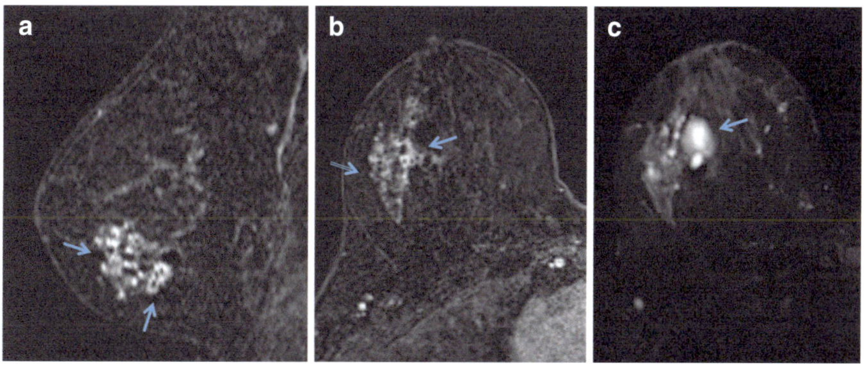

Fig. 2.24 NME – internal enhancement: clustered ring. Clustered ring enhancement in the lower outer right breast on sagittal (**a**) and axial (**b**) post contrast images, with associated increased signal on T2 weighted images (**c**) (*arrows*). This enhancement pattern can be seen with DCIS. MR biopsy in this case yielded fibrocystic changes and duct ectasia

features are often seen with suspicious enhancing masses or NME, but may stand alone as the only finding if no other abnormality is present. These features elevate the degree of suspicion when seen with other findings and may alter surgical management as well as staging.

2.2.7 *Kinetic Curve Assessment*

Dynamic contrast-enhanced MRI (DCE-MRI) allows lesion characterization using both its morphology as well as contrast enhancement over time. Dynamic measurements of signal intensity are made following contrast administration and plotted over time to generate enhancement kinetic curves.

Initial phase enhancement reflects enhancement within the first 2 min or until the peak enhancement is achieved (Fig. 2.25). Initial enhancement is classified as *slow, medium* and *fast* based on changes in signal intensity from the pre- and first post contrast sequences (<50 %, 50–100 %, and >100 %, respectively).

Delayed phase enhancement occurs after the first 2 min or after the curve starts to change, and describes the shape of the curve. *Persistent* curves show increasing signal intensity throughout the delayed phase (≥10 % increase from peak initial enhancement), *plateau* curves remain constant after peak enhancement (±10 % of initial enhancement) and *washout* curves show decreasing signal intensity over time (≤10 % of peak initial enhancement).

As cancers have dense, highly permeable vasculature and rapid blood flow, malignant lesions generally have washout kinetics while benign lesions tend to have persistent delayed phase kinetics. It is important to note, however, that there is considerable overlap between kinetic curves of benign and malignant lesions. Kinetic analysis is only one aspect of lesion characterization. Persistent enhancement

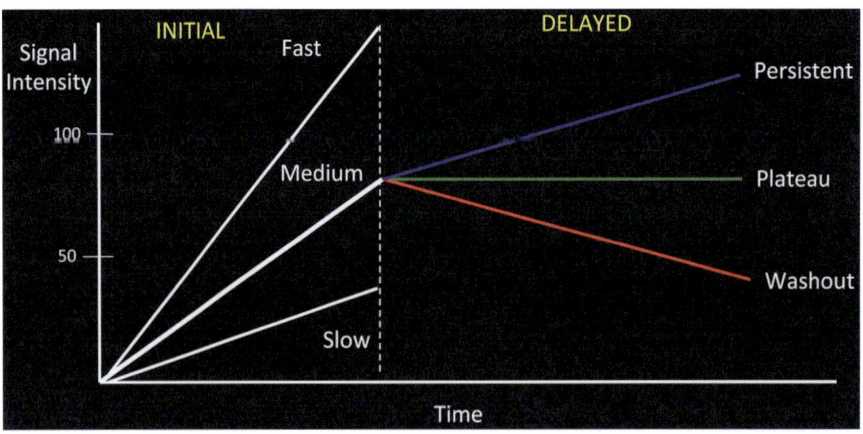

Fig. 2.25 Kinetic curve assessment

kinetics are not reassuring in the setting of suspicious morphology, which should prompt biopsy for further evaluation.

Conclusion Based on the analysis of both the morphologic and kinetic features of breast lesions as described in the MRI lexicon, appropriate BI-RADS® assessment category is assigned which in turn triggers appropriate management.

2.3 Reporting System

The assessment categories used for breast MRI are based on the BI-RADS® categories developed for mammography. The MRI report should be assigned an ACR BI-RADS® final assessment code indicating the level of suspicion for cancer and follow-up management recommendations (Table 2.2).

2.3.1 Category 0: Incomplete – Need Additional Imaging Evaluation

This category may be used for a technically unacceptable exam or when more information is needed from mammography or ultrasound to render a final assessment. An assessment of *incomplete* may be useful when the finding on MRI is suspicious but may represent a benign finding such as a lymph node or fat necrosis, which

Table 2.2 ACR BI-RADS® assessment categories

BIRADS category	Definition	Likelihood of malignancy	Management recommendation
0	Incomplete	N/A	Recommend additional imaging: Mammogram or Targeted US
1	Negative	Essentially 0 %	Routine breast MRI screening if cumulative lifetime ≥20 %
2	Benign	Essentially 0 %	Routine breast MRI screening if cumulative lifetime ≥20 %
3	Probably benign	> 0 % but ≤2 %	Short-interval (6-month) follow-up
4	Suspicious	> 2 % to <95 %	Tissue diagnosis
5	Highly suggestive of malignancy	≥ 95 %	Tissue diagnosis
6	Known biopsy-proven malignancy	N/A	Surgical excision when clinically appropriate

From ACR BI-RADS®-Breast MRI, In *ACR BI-RADS® Atlas, Breast Imaging Reporting and Data System*. Reston, VA, 2013, American College of Radiology, Table 5 could be confirmed on mammography or US, and used to avert a biopsy. *Incomplete* assessment should be used very rarely, as there is usually enough information on the MRI exam to provide the appropriate management recommendation.

2.3.2 Category 1: Negative

This is used for a normal exam, where no abnormal enhancement is present and routine follow up is recommended. Normal description of breast composition and degree of BPE should be included.

2.3.3 Category 2: Benign

This is also a normal assessment and routine follow up is recommended. The only difference from an assessment of *negative* is that the radiologist describes specific benign findings such as lymph nodes, implants, cysts, fibroadenomas or biopsy clips. If benign findings are reported, the assessment category is *benign* and if these benign findings are not included in the report (even if they are present), the assessment category is *negative.*

2.3.4 Category 3: Probably Benign

This category is used for lesions with a ≤2 % chance of malignancy. Imaging surveillance of these lesions is recommended to avoid the risks and costs of tissue sampling. BPE should not be recommended for follow up, unless there is a question of whether the enhancement is related to the hormonal status of the patient or if the patient is scanned in the suboptimal phase of her menstrual cycle. If the morphology, kinetics and T2 signal of a focus or mass are reassuring, then in certain clinical settings, short interval follow up imaging may be appropriate. There is insufficient evidence to support follow up of areas of NME at this time. The use of *probably benign* assessment on MRI is based on limited data and is discussed in more detail in Chap. 14.

2.3.5 Category 4: Suspicious

This category is used for the majority of findings that lead to a biopsy recommendation. The probability of malignancy when a lesion is assessed as *suspicious* is between 2 and 95 %. Masses that are assessed as *suspicious* on MRI, warrant a targeted breast ultrasound, and if a correlate is identified, ultrasound guided core biopsy can be performed.

2.3.6 Category 5: Highly Suggestive of Malignancy

Lesions assessed as *highly suggestive of malignancy* have a ≥95 % probability of malignancy. If the biopsy of a category 5 lesion is benign, the biopsy results are considered discordant and surgical excision is recommended. As with mammography and US, appropriate combination of suspicious findings is needed for a category 5 assessment.

2.3.7 Category 6: Known Biopsy-Proven Malignancy

This category is reserved for cases in which the only pertinent MRI finding is the previously biopsied cancer, and no other MRI abnormalities needing additional evaluation are present. When there are findings other than the known cancer which need tissue sampling, the overall assessment should be category 4 or 5. The final assessment should be most actionable category as it needs more prompt intervention.

References

1. Saslow D et al. American Cancer Society guidelines for breast screening with MRI as an adjunct to mammography. CA Cancer J Clin. 2007;57(2):75–89.
2. Mainiero MB et al. ACR appropriateness criteria breast cancer screening. J Am Coll Radiol. 2013;10(1):11–4.
3. Morris EA, Comstock CE, Lee CH, et al. ACR BI-RADS® Magnetic Resonance Imaging. In: ACR BI-RADS® Atlas, Breast Imaging Reporting and Data System. Reston: American College of Radiology; 2013.
4. Hambly NM et al. Background parenchymal enhancement on baseline screening breast MRI: impact on biopsy rate and short-interval follow-up. AJR Am J Roentgenol. 2011;196(1):218–24.
5. Giess CS et al. Background parenchymal enhancement at breast MR imaging: normal patterns, diagnostic challenges, and potential for false-positive and false-negative interpretation. Radiographics. 2014;34(1):234–47.
6. Nunes LW, Schnall MD, Orel SG. Update of breast MR imaging architectural interpretation model. Radiology. 2001;219(2):484–94.
7. Nunes LW et al. Breast MR imaging: interpretation model. Radiology. 1997;202(3):833–41.
8. Tozaki M, Igarashi T, Fukuda K. Positive and negative predictive values of BI-RADS-MRI descriptors for focal breast masses. Magn Reson Med Sci. 2006;5(1):7–15.
9. Goto M et al. Diagnosis of breast tumors by contrast-enhanced MR imaging: comparison between the diagnostic performance of dynamic enhancement patterns and morphologic features. J Magn Reson Imaging. 2007;25(1):104–12.

10. Liberman L et al. Ductal enhancement on MR imaging of the breast. AJR Am J Roentgenol. 2003;181(2):519–25.
11. Schnall MD et al. Diagnostic architectural and dynamic features at breast MR imaging: multicenter study. Radiology. 2006;238(1):42–53.
12. Agrawal G et al. Significance of breast lesion descriptors in the ACR BI-RADS MRI lexicon. Cancer. 2009;115(7):1363–80.
13. Morakkabati-Spitz N et al. Diagnostic usefulness of segmental and linear enhancement in dynamic breast MRI. Eur Radiol. 2005;15(9):2010–7.

Part II
Indications

Chapter 3
MRI and Screening

Sabrina Rajan and Barbara J.G. Dall

Abstract Identifying women at higher risk is a combination of assessment of family history, genetic testing and review of clinical history. The management of women at increased risk of breast cancer presents a challenge and includes chemoprevention, risk-reducing surgery and intensified imaging surveillance. Recommendations for imaging surveillance are based on the individual's risk dividing the population into low, moderate, high and very high risk. MRI has a significantly higher sensitivity in comparison to mammography and ultrasound, and this is not affected by age, mutation status or breast density. Additional cancers detected by MRI alone are smaller and less likely to involve lymph nodes than cancers detected by conventional imaging. The majority of invasive cancers demonstrate typical malignant morphology and enhancement kinetics. However, in a small proportion of high-risk women, cancers may present as a morphologically benign mass with smooth borders and this emphasises the importance of considering a wider range of diagnostic features that could represent malignant disease in this group. A consistent and high quality MRI examination is required, complying with recommendations of a robust quality assurance programme with prospective collection and audit of data. In the future, personalised screening based on accurate risk assessment and gene testing in specialised family history clinics will facilitate the development of a tailored screening programme.

Keywords Breast MRI • Screening • Family history

S. Rajan, BMed Sci(Hons), BMBS, MRCP, FRCR (✉)
MRI Department, Leeds Teaching Hospitals NHS Trust, St. James's University Hospital, Leeds, West Yorkshire, UK
e-mail: sabrinarajan@nhs.net

B.J.G. Dall, MB ChB, FRCR, FRCP
Department of Radiology, Leeds Teaching Hospitals NHS Trust, St. James's University Hospital, Leeds, West Yorkshire, UK

S.L. Heller, L. Moy (eds.), *Breast Oncology: Techniques, Indications, and Interpretation*, DOI 10.1007/978-3-319-42563-4_3

3.1 Risk Assessment

MRI is an established screening test in women who have a higher than population risk of developing breast cancer. Identifying women at higher risk is a combination of three factors; family history assessment, genetic testing and review of clinical history. Important factors within the family history are young age at onset of disease, bilateral disease, multiple cases on one side of the family, male relatives with breast cancer, other related early onset cancers including ovary, prostate and sarcoma.

The highest risk of breast cancer is among women with an inherited predisposition to breast cancer due to genetic mutations of BRCA1 or BRCA2. Birth prevalence of BRCA1 is 0.07–0.09 % and BRCA2 is 0.14–2.22 % and mutations in these genes account for 5–10 % of all breast cancers [1]. Among these women, the cumulative lifetime risk of breast cancer is 50–85 % [2, 3]. The peak decade for occurrence of breast cancer in these women is 40–50 years [4]. Other genes with a high risk of breast cancer are TP53 (Li-Fraumeni syndrome) and PTEN (Cowden and Bannayan-Riley-Ruvalcaba syndromes); these are much less common but most cases of breast cancer occur between 30 to 40 years and these individuals are at increased risk of multiple cancers. Genetic testing should ideally start with an affected individual which is essentially mutation searching. It can then be offered to adult members of families with a known gene. If a gene has been identified in a family and a family member tests negative, his or her breast cancer risk drops to population risk. However in a high-risk family without a known gene, failure to find a mutation does not reduce an individual's risk [5].

Careful review of the clinical history including a personal history of breast cancer, breast atypia or ovarian cancer must be noted. The greatest risk to women presenting with a breast cancer is recurrence of that breast cancer. They are however also at increased risk of a second breast cancer, as are women presenting with premalignant conditions such as atypical ductal hyperplasia and lobular neoplasia. Supra-diaphragmatic irradiation conveys a risk similar to BRCA1/2 mutation carriers; the risk varies with the estimated dose to the breast, age at treatment, and modifying factors such as dose to ovaries and chemotherapy, which are protective. A number of epidemiological factors convey a modest increased risk and these act multiplicatively. These include parity, age at menopause, hormone use (oral contraceptive and hormone replacement therapy), alcohol consumption, obesity and breast density. These epidemiological factors become increasingly relevant in women who have a family history or a personal history of breast cancer.

3.2 Management Options

The management of women at increased risk of breast cancer presents a challenge. Women who are mutation carriers have cancer risk management options that include chemoprevention and risk-reducing mastectomy and salpingo-oophorectomy.

Prophylactic bilateral mastectomies for such women reduce mortality by more than 90 % [6, 7]. Despite this, the majority of women still opt for intensified imaging surveillance [8]. The effectiveness of a screening test can be demonstrated by showing that it reduces patient mortality, as opposed to simply increasing lead-time. This may be inferred from evidence that the screening test detects additional cases of disease with a reduction in rates of interval cancers and incidence of disease in subsequent screening rounds [9].

A second consideration is the imaging modality utilised for screening, taking into consideration that the relative cancer risk in women with predisposing mutations is particularly high at younger ages. Mammography is an effective screening method in the normal population particularly in those over 50 with an overall sensitivity of about 86 % [10]. However, with the early onset of disease in the high-risk population, there is a need to screen at a younger age where the higher proportion of glandular breast tissue can result in high density mammograms which have a reduced sensitivity for malignancy [11, 12]. Although ultrasound is readily available and relatively inexpensive, it has no evidence-based role as a primary screening test although, in the United States, ultrasound may be considered in high-risk women who are unable to tolerate MRI [13]. Contrast-enhanced breast MRI does not use ionising radiation, which is particularly relevant in this younger age group with active glandular breast tissue that is more radiosensitive. In addition, MRI maintains a high sensitivity for cancer detection even in breast with a dense parenchymal pattern [14].

3.3 Efficacy of MRI Screening

The greatest challenge in reviewing the evidence on the effectiveness of MRI screening is the lack of randomised trials. Riedl et al. recently reported on a prospective non-randomised comparison study that offered BRCA mutation carriers and women with a lifetime risk of breast cancer >20 % annual screening with mammography, ultrasound and MRI [15]. Of the 559 women screened, 40 cancers (invasive n = 26, DCIS n = 14) were identified. The sensitivity of MRI (90 %) was significantly higher than that of mammography (38 %) and ultrasound (38 %). Of the 40 cancers, 45 % were detected by MRI alone, 5 % by mammography alone and no cancers were detected by ultrasound alone. The two cases detected by mammography alone were areas of microcalcification representing ductal carcinoma in situ (DCIS) with microinvasion and DCIS with <10 mm invasive component. Importantly, age, mutation status and breast density had no influence on the sensitivity of MRI. Similarly, in the Italian multicentre screening study, Sardanelli prospectively compared clinical breast examination, mammography, ultrasound and MRI in the surveillance of asymptomatic women at high risk of inherited breast cancer [16]. MRI had a significantly higher sensitivity at 91 % in comparison to mammography and ultrasound, with 31 % of all cancers detected by MRI only.

The EVA trial which was a prospective multicentre observational cohort study based in Germany screened 687 asymptomatic women with a lifetime risk ≥20 % [17]. The sensitivity of MRI (93 %) was significantly higher than mammography (33 %) or ultrasound (37 %). Cancer yield by MRI alone was significantly higher and this was not significantly improved by adding mammography and did not change by adding ultrasound. In this study, MRI was not only superior to mammography for diagnosing invasive breast cancer, but also for DCIS with more than half of the cases of DCIS diagnosed by MRI only. Whilst there is concern that the increased detection of DCIS may lead to overdiagnosis, all cases of DCIS identified on MRI were biologically relevant intermediate or high nuclear grade. The is because the detection of cancer on MRI is determined by angiogenic activity that underpins tissue alterations implicated in cancer proliferation, therefore serving as a biomarker for cancer vitality. The only mammographically detected case of DCIS that was occult on MRI had a low nuclear grade.

The UK Magnetic Resonance Imaging in Breast Cancer Screening (MARIBS) trial compared MRI with mammography in a prospective multicentre cohort study including 649 women with a strong family history of breast cancer or a high probability of carrying mutations in BRCA1, BRCA2 or TP53 [18]. MRI was almost twice as sensitive as mammography in this high-risk group and combining both techniques gave an overall sensitivity of 94 % and specificity of 77 %. Despite a high proportion of grade 3 cancers, 52 % were less than 15 mm in size and 81 % of women with invasive cancer were node negative. Similarly, Kuhl et al. reported that in patients with a lifetime risk of breast cancer of at least 20 %, additional cancers detected by MRI alone, were statistically significantly smaller and less likely to involve lymph nodes than cancers detected by mammography and ultrasound [19]. Warner et al. reported on a Canadian prospective observational study that followed 1,275 women with BRCA1 or BRCA2 mutations, of which 445 women underwent annual MRI screening and 830 women in the comparison group were screened with protocols that did not include MRI [20]. This study demonstrated a stage shift with a significant reduction in the incidence of advanced-stage breast cancer (stages II–IV) in BRCA1 and BRCA2 carriers who were in the MRI screening group.

Although there is an association between tumour size and lymph node involvement for most tumour types, this pattern is not invariable. In North America, data from 276 BRCA1-related breast cancers demonstrated that there was no consistent relationship between tumour size and lymph node status [21]. Such cancers grow faster than non-hereditary breast cancer with the propensity to metastasise to distant sites through the bloodstream, independent of local lymphatic spread and this contributes to the poorer prognosis associated with BRCA1-related breast cancers. A national population-based study of Israeli women reported that tumour size had minimal impact on survival among women with BRCA1-related breast cancer [22]. If the size-survival relationship is attenuated, then it is unclear how much can be gained from detecting a cancer when it is small. These findings have important implications for evaluating the effectiveness of early diagnosis in BRCA1-related breast cancers.

In a Norwegian study, Hagen et al. assessed the sensitivity of MRI in comparison to conventional screening in the diagnosis of BRCA-associated breast cancer [23]. In 491 BRCA mutation carriers (BRCA1 n = 445, BRCA2 n = 46) screened, there were 25 cancers detected, with a MRI sensitivity of 86 % and mammography sensitivity of 50 %. Of note, 20 % of the cancers presented as interval cancers between scheduled screening investigations, with a mean time of 8.4 months since the last examination. This higher rate of interval cancers may reflect the underlying aggressive tumour biology with a shorter doubling time in BRCA1 mutation carriers, which represented 90 % of the study population. Further analysis of the UK MARIBS study [18], the Canadian study [24] and the Dutch MRI study [25, 26] subsequently highlighted subtle differences between BRCA1 and BRCA2-associated breast cancer [27]. In total, 1,275 BRCA1/2 mutation carriers participated in the studies, with a total of 124 cancers detected. BRCA2 mutation carriers were diagnosed with relatively more DCIS and T1a/b tumours and fewer interval cancers in comparison to BRCA1 mutation carriers. The predicted duration of the preclinical detectable phase was longer for BRCA2 than for BRCA1, which means that BRCA2 cancers grow more slowly and therefore have a higher probability of being screen-detected. The differences in the natural history of BRCA1 and BRCA2 mutation carriers suggest the optimal screening regimen may differ in both groups.

At present, there is no convincing evidence that annual breast MRI surveillance reduces breast-cancer specific mortality, especially in women who are BRCA mutation carriers. The Dutch MRI screening study is a non-randomised multicentre prospective cohort study that included 2,157 women with a cumulative lifetime risk of breast cancer of ≥15 %, who were screened every 6 months with a clinical breast examination and annually with mammography and MRI [26]. Within the group, there were 599 carriers of a pathogenic gene mutation in BRCA1 (n = 422), BRCA2 (n = 172) and PTEN/TP53 (n = 5). In the BRCA1/2 mutation carriers who developed invasive cancer, the cumulative distant-metastasis free survival was 84 % and overall survival was 93 % at 6 years. In comparison, in the non-mutation carriers who developed cancer, the cumulative distant-metastasis free survival and overall survival was 100 %.

In Norway, as part of a national initiative, women with a BRCA1 mutation were offered annual screening with breast MRI in addition to mammography [28]. The 5-year breast cancer-specific survival for BRCA1 women with cancer was 75 % and the 10-year survival was 69 %. In addition, the 5-year survival for BRCA1 women with stage 1 breast cancer was 82 % compared to 98 % in the population based on the Norwegian Cancer Registry. In an updated analysis that compared the survival in BRCA1 breast cancer cases detected through annual screening with mammography and MRI with cases detected through annual screening with mammography only, although tumours did appear to be downstaged in the MRI series, the expected survival benefit was not observed [29].

3.4 Imaging Recommendations

The recommendations below are based on UK National Institute for Health and Care Excellence (NICE) Familial Breast Cancer Guidance [30] with reference to imaging recommendations from the Society of Breast Imaging, American College of Radiology (ACR) [13] and American Cancer Society (ACS) [31]. The European Society of Breast Imaging also has its own recommendations that will not be addressed in detail in this chapter [32]. The UK NICE guidance is a comprehensive document on how to assess an individual's risk, dividing the population into low, moderate, high and very high risk and how to manage that risk. Individuals at low risk are considered to be equivalent to population risk and do not require any specialist surveillance. They should be reassured, educated about breast awareness and encouraged to undergo routine screening surveillance. Individuals at moderate risk and above do benefit from referral to specialist family history clinics. These clinics provide expert advice using risk assessment models and have access to gene testing if considered appropriate.

LOW risk: Breast cancer risk between age 40 and 50 years is <3 %, lifetime risk <17 %

- MRI: NOT recommended for lifetime risk <15 % (UK or ACR) because low incidence means harm of false positives outweighs benefits of true positives.
- Mammography: 3 yearly from 50 years (UK); opportunity to begin annual screening between ages 40 and 44 (ACS) and annually from 40 years (ACR).

MODERATE risk: Breast cancer risk between age 40 and 50 years is 3–8 %, lifetime risk 17–30 %

- MRI: NOT recommended in UK. In the US, MRI may be considered in women with between 15 and 20 % lifetime risk for breast cancer on the basis of personal history of breast or ovarian cancer or biopsy proven lobular neoplasia or atypical ductal hyperplasia (ACR). For US guidelines for women with >20 % lifetime risk of breast cancer, please see HIGH risk section below.
- Mammography: recommended annually 40–60 years and then 3 yearly (UK); annually from 40 years (ACR). For US guidelines for women with >20 % lifetime risk of breast cancer, please see HIGH risk section below.

HIGH risk: Breast cancer risk between age 40 and 50 years is >8 %, lifetime risk >30 %, untested but 20–30 % chance of faulty gene

- MRI: NOT recommended in UK unless there is a personal history of breast cancer where it would be advised annually until 50 years. Annual MRI recommended by ACR for women ≥20 % lifetime risk on the basis of family history starting at 30 but not before age 25, or 10 years before the age of the youngest affected relative, whichever is later.
- Mammography: consider annually 30–40 years, recommended annually 40–60 years and then 3 yearly (UK). Annual mammogram recommended by ACR for women ≥20 % lifetime risk on the basis of family history starting at 30

but not before age 25, or 10 years before the age of the youngest affected relative, whichever is later.

VERY HIGH risk: Lifetime risk 50–85 %, gene positive, untested but >30 % chance of faulty gene (note that guidelines in the US do not make a distinction between HIGH risk and VERY HIGH risk groups)

- TP53: MRI 20–69 years, mammography not recommended at any age.
- >30 % equivalent risk of TP53: as for TP53 but reassess at 60 years, if no personal history of breast cancer then risk of gene is reduced and can be screened as normal population.
- BRCA1/2: MRI and mammography annually 30–49 years; mammography only 50–69 years unless dense breast tissue when MRI should continue (UK). In the US, annual mammogram and annual MRI starting by age 30 but not before age 25 (ACR).
- >30 % equivalent risk of BRCA1/2: as for BRCA1/2 but reassess at 60 years; if no personal history of breast cancer then risk of gene is reduced and can be screened as normal population (UK). In the US, annual mammogram and annual MRI starting by age 30 but not before age 25 (ACR).
- Supra-diaphragmatic irradiation: the risk is delayed and therefore surveillance should not start until a minimum of 8 years following treatment. UK recommends annual MRI from 30 years and annual mammography from 40 years. ACR recommends annual MRI; mammography is not recommended before 25 years.

3.4.1 *Higher Risk Screening in Pregnancy*

The incidence of breast cancer during pregnancy is estimated to be 1.3–2.4/10,000 live births, which equates to 2–3 % of total breast cancers. MRI may be useful in the first trimester, but there are safety concerns around its effects on the foetus, due to the heating effect, noise and potential toxicity of the gadolinium-based contrast agent. Later in pregnancy, the capacity of MRI scans to detect small tumours will fall due to intense background enhancement. The collective expert opinion from MRI specialists in the UK is that MRI screening during pregnancy and lactation is not recommended but can be resumed 6 weeks after cessation of breast feeding [33].

3.5 MRI Technique

A consistent and high quality MRI examination is required. In the UK, very high risk screening has been incorporated into the National Health Service Breast Screening Programme (NHSBSP) and complies with the recommendations of the Quality Assurance programme [34]. This ensures that all examinations are performed and reported to the same high standard and there is prospective collection and audit of data. In the US and in continental Europe, there are similarly stringent requirements for MRI quality control, reporting and documentation [32, 35].

3.5.1 Equipment and Protocols

MRI scanners have high-level maintenance contracts that apply manufacturer's thresholds. In addition, weekly quality control tests of signal to noise ratio and suppression effectiveness should be carried out. Training of staff, adherence to protocol and recording of data are all monitored. A 1.5 T MRI machine is required with a dedicated breast coil to ensure patient movement is minimised and there is uniform signal homogeneity across the coils. The scanning parameters should be set up to image both breasts. High spatial resolution is required to assess lesion morphology i.e. a slice thickness of ≤2 mm and in plane resolution of <1 mm. To assess lesion kinetics, high temporal resolution is required with a scan time of ≤60 s and the scan should be repeated out to 7 min following the administration of a gadolinium-based contrast agent (pump injection of at least 0.1 mmol/kg is recommended with a 3 cc/sec flow rate and a 20 ml bolus of saline). Standard sequences should be set up and should include the following:

- T2-weighted fast spin echo
- T1-weighted spoiled gradient echo
- T1-weighted spoiled gradient echo with fat suppression post-contrast

Attention to the timing of the breast MRI study with respect to the menstrual cycle is important. There is a higher prevalence of contrast-enhancing lesions during week 1 and 4 of the menstrual cycle [36]. Therefore, the examination should be carried out in the first half of the menstrual cycle, ideally day 6–16 (in the US, day 7–14), when the background physiological enhancement is less marked [34, 37]. This helps to improve specificity with a reduction in the number of unnecessary recommendations for biopsy of benign lesions and improve sensitivity by minimising the likelihood of a subtle lesion being obscured by marked background physiological glandular enhancement.

Data storage is necessary to store the basic examination in a way that ensures that it can be reprocessed if required in the future. A reporting workstation is required that allows post-processing of images with creation of dynamic enhancement curves, interrogation of subtracted images and maximum intensity projections.

3.5.2 Reporting and Image Interpretation

Reporters embarking on MRI screening should be experienced and the UK NHSBSP and the US ACR requires that each reader should report a minimum of 100 breast MRI examinations per year with double reporting as the gold standard in the UK [34, 38]. The MRI is reported in conjunction with the screening mammogram and review of the previous MRI examinations. The images should be reported in line with the updated BI-RADS system and conclude with an MRI score of 1–5 to indicate the level of concern (1 indicating normal and 5 indicating malignant) [39] and in the US in accordance with BI-RADS assessment (ACR) [35].

Schrading and Kuhl have reviewed the MRI features of invasive cancer and DCIS in women at familial risk and reported the imaging phenotypes of cancers differ among risk categories [40]. The most frequent finding in women with invasive cancers was an enhancing mass that exhibited typical malignant features in terms of morphology (ill-defined margins, irregular or spiculate shape), enhancement pattern (heterogeneous or rim-enhancement) and the enhancement kinetics (rapid uptake followed by a plateau or washout of contrast). However, the study also reported that 23 % of invasive cancers appeared as a benign enhancing mass with smooth borders, a round or oval configuration, homogenous internal enhancement but suspicious enhancement kinetics. Of these cases, 80 % occurred in women at high risk and documented BRCA1 mutation carriers.

It is increasingly recognised that the imaging features of tumours arising in BRCA1 mutation carriers differs from the characteristics of sporadic tumours. Differing tumour biology in BRCA1 carriers with a high grade and high mitotic activity is associated with rapid growth and reflected in prominent pushing margins around the tumours [41]. The imaging features of such aggressive lesions have a more rounded configuration with sharp, smooth margins, which are morphological characteristics that are more commonly attributed to benign lesions [42]. In contrast, low grade tumours are more likely to incite a desmoplastic reaction within the surrounding tissue, giving rise to the classical appearance of a malignant mass with spiculated margins [43]. However, MRI provides additional functional information with the enhancement pattern and kinetics that allows the level of suspicion to be raised despite the reassuring benign morphology.

In addition, Schrading and Kuhl reported that non-mass like enhancement was the dominant imaging feature of 20 % of invasive cancers and 92 % of DCIS cases. These lesions do not exhibit a correlate on T1 or T2 weighted MRI sequences, do not cause distortion of the normal fibroglandular architecture and do not exhibit space-occupying effects. It is conceivable that this represents another reason for the lower sensitivity of unenhanced imaging modalities such as mammography and ultrasound in the detection of familial breast cancer. This emphasises the importance of considering a wider range of diagnostic features that could represent malignant disease in this high-risk group (Figs. 3.1 and 3.2).

The MRI report should include a management plan. This should indicate if a MR-directed ultrasound +/– biopsy is required and whether an MRI biopsy would be feasible if the ultrasound is normal. The lesions that do raise concern are a new mass lesion ≥5 mm or new isolated area of enhancement ≥10 mm in breasts which otherwise demonstrate minimal enhancement [39]. Careful directed ultrasound will

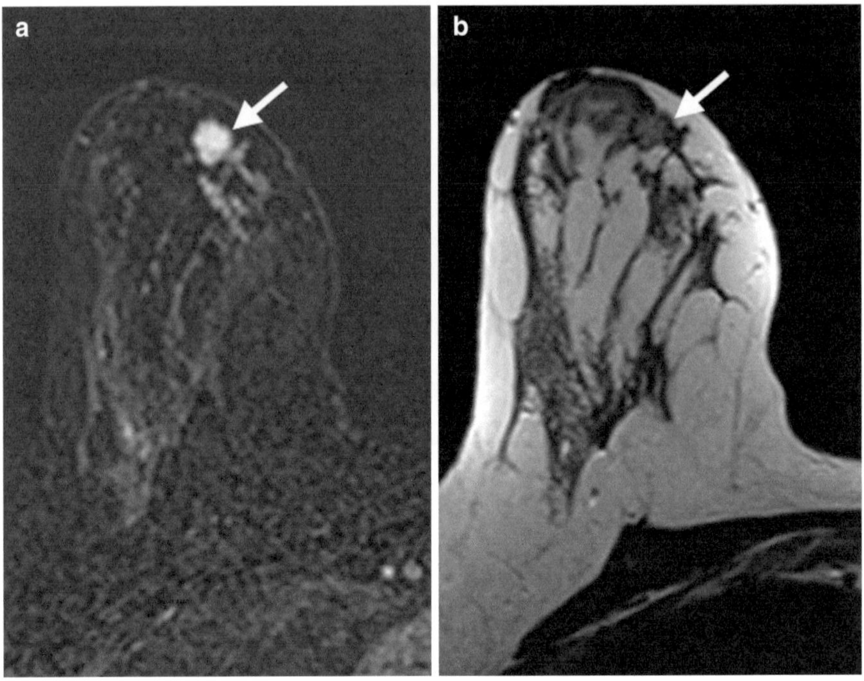

Fig. 3.1 High risk family history patient with normal mammograms. A suspicious 10 mm well-circumscribed rounded enhancing mass in the right upper inner quadrant on post-contrast subtraction images (*white arrow*) (**a**) with a morphological correlate on T2 (*white arrow*) (**b**). Histology confirms grade 2 invasive ductal carcinoma

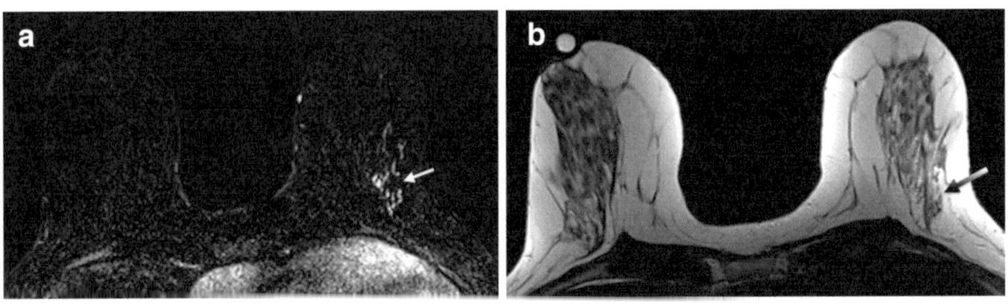

Fig. 3.2 BRCA1 positive patient with normal mammograms. An indeterminate area of segmental stippled enhancement in the lateral aspect of the left breast on post-contrast subtraction images (*white arrow*) (**a**) with no morphological correlate on T2 (*gray arrow*) (**b**). Histology confirms high-grade DCIS

identify about 60 % of these lesions, particularly if there is a mass. Lesions not seen on ultrasound should have an MRI biopsy with clip placement. Facilities that perform MRI should be able to perform MRI biopsy or have an established pattern of referral to a site that can perform these procedures.

3.6 Limitations of MRI Screening

MRI is more expensive and less readily available in comparison to mammography and ultrasound. It also requires the use of an intravenous gadolinium-based contrast agent that may not be suitable for patients with renal disease. MRI may not be feasible for certain women such as those with pacemakers, aneurysm clips or claustrophobia [44]. It is important that patients are appropriately counselled and aware of the methods and frequency of screening investigations, benefits and risks including the possibility of false-positive and false-negative studies with the development of interval cancers.

The increased sensitivity of screening with MRI should be considered with evidence suggesting a 3–5 fold higher risk of patient recall for investigation of false-positive results [45]. Biopsies that do not yield malignancy are considered false-positive results and a disadvantage of MRI screening as this generates unnecessary patient anxiety and has its associated costs in time and money. In the UK MARIBS study, the recall rate was 3.9 % for mammography and 10.7 % for MRI with an overall recall rate of 12.7 % combining both techniques. Overall, there were 8.5 recalls and 0.21 benign surgical biopsies per cancer detected. Therefore, although the absolute recall rate is high, taking into account the high annual risk of cancer in this group at high familial risk, the recall and intervention rate per cancer detected are similar to that found in screening the normal population [46].

In the United States, a multicentre study prospectively evaluated the biopsy rates, positive predictive value and cancer yield of screening mammography, ultrasound and MRI in asymptomatic women who were identified as genetically at high risk including BRCA1/2 carriers or women with at least a 20 % probability of carrying the gene [47]. Findings on MRI prompted biopsy in 8.2 %, while mammography and ultrasound prompted biopsy in 2.3 % of patients. The positive predictive value of biopsies performed as a result of MRI was 43 % with a diagnostic yield of 3.5 % in comparison to 1.2 % for mammography and 0.6 % for ultrasound. This study demonstrated that although screening MRI had a higher biopsy rate, it did help to detect more cancers than either mammography or ultrasound. This suggests that MRI is potentially cost-effective for screening younger women at very high risk of breast cancer, but less cost-effective for screening populations with a wider risk or wider age distribution.

False-negative results can occur when the MRI is reported as normal and fails to diagnose a cancer that is already present. This may be due to a suboptimal study causing difficulties in interpretation due to inadequate contrast agent administration, poor fat suppression or movement artefact. Lesion size and location can also affect accuracy of interpretation with difficulties arising when the abnormality is small (<5 mm) or if the lesion is located close to the boundary of the field of view [48]. In some cases, the lesion may be missed or misinterpreted by the reader [49].

3.7 Conclusion

Standardised high quality MRI examinations achieving a high sensitivity, in addition to available evidence of the efficacy of MRI screening, have allowed expert opinion to support MRI as a screening test in higher risk women who have been appropriately assessed in a specialist clinic. It is different from mammographic screening where the stronger evidence allows it to be applied to a whole population. Women who are choosing between risk-reducing mastectomy and screening should be counselled that although the sensitivity of MRI in combination with mammography is excellent, it will always be less than 100 %. In addition, some very small tumours will already be incurable at the time of detection. Women who opt for screening should be willing to accept the risk of a false negative result as well as the extra investigations generated by a false positive examination. Ideally in the future, personalised screening based on accurate risk assessment and the increased availability and speed of gene testing in specialised family history clinics will facilitate the development of a tailored screening programme. This may require more intensive screening strategies in some younger women, although the cost benefit of this in terms of increased surveillance, recalls for further work-up and economics would have to be considered.

References

1. Prevalence and penetrance of BRCA1 and BRCA2 mutations in a population-based series of breast cancer cases. Anglian Breast Cancer Study Group. Br J Cancer. 2000;83(10):1301–8.
2. Narod SA, Foulkes WD. BRCA1 and BRCA2: 1994 and beyond. Nat Rev Cancer. 2004;4(9):665–76.
3. Ford D, Easton DF, Stratton M, Narod S, Goldgar D, Devilee P, et al. Genetic heterogeneity and penetrance analysis of the BRCA1 and BRCA2 genes in breast cancer families. The Breast Cancer Linkage Consortium. Am J Hum Genet. 1998;62(3):676–89.
4. Evans DG, Shenton A, Woodward E, Lalloo F, Howell A, Maher ER. Penetrance estimates for BRCA1 and BRCA2 based on genetic testing in a clinical cancer genetics service setting: risks of breast/ovarian cancer quoted should reflect the cancer burden in the family. BMC Cancer. 2008;8:155.
5. Saslow D, Boetes C, Burke W, Harms S, Leach MO, Lehman CD, et al. American Cancer Society guidelines for breast screening with MRI as an adjunct to mammography. CA Cancer J Clin. 2007;57(2):75–89.
6. Hartmann LC, Schaid DJ, Woods JE, Crotty TP, Myers JL, Arnold PG, et al. Efficacy of bilateral prophylactic mastectomy in women with a family history of breast cancer. N Engl J Med. 1999;340(2):77–84.
7. Rebbeck TR, Friebel T, Lynch HT, Neuhausen SL, van't Veer L, JE G, et al. Bilateral prophylactic mastectomy reduces breast cancer risk in BRCA1 and BRCA2 mutation carriers: the PROSE Study Group. J Clin Oncol. 2004;22(6):1055–62.
8. van Dijk S, van Roosmalen MS, Otten W, Stalmeier PF. Decision making regarding prophylactic mastectomy: stability of preferences and the impact of anticipated feelings of regret. J Clin Oncol. 2008;26(14):2358–63.
9. Irwig L, Houssami N, Armstrong B, Glasziou P. Evaluating new screening tests for breast cancer. BMJ. 2006;332(7543):678–9.

10. Banks E, Reeves G, Beral V, Bull D, Crossley B, Simmonds M, et al. Influence of personal characteristics of individual women on sensitivity and specificity of mammography in the Million Women Study: cohort study. BMJ. 2004;329(7464):477.
11. Kolb TM, Lichy J, Newhouse JH. Comparison of the performance of screening mammography, physical examination, and breast US and evaluation of factors that influence them: an analysis of 27,825 patient evaluations. Radiology. 2002;225(1):165–75.
12. Mandelson MT, Oestreicher N, Porter PL, White D, Finder CA, Taplin SH, et al. Breast density as a predictor of mammographic detection: comparison of interval- and screen-detected cancers. J Natl Cancer Inst. 2000;92(13):1081–7.
13. Lee CH, Dershaw DD, Kopans D, Evans P, Monsees B, Monticciolo D, et al. Breast cancer screening with imaging: recommendations from the Society of Breast Imaging and the ACR on the use of mammography, breast MRI, breast ultrasound, and other technologies for the detection of clinically occult breast cancer. J Am Coll Radiol. 2010;7(1):18–27.
14. Sardanelli F, Giuseppetti GM, Panizza P, Bazzocchi M, Fausto A, Simonetti G, et al. Sensitivity of MRI versus mammography for detecting foci of multifocal, multicentric breast cancer in Fatty and dense breasts using the whole-breast pathologic examination as a gold standard. Am J Roentgenol. 2004;183(4):1149–57.
15. Riedl CC, Luft N, Bernhart C, Weber M, Bernathova M, Tea MK, et al. Triple-modality screening trial for familial breast cancer underlines the importance of magnetic resonance imaging and questions the role of mammography and ultrasound regardless of patient mutation status, age, and breast density. J Clin Oncol. 2015;33(10):1128–35.
16. Sardanelli F, Podo F, Santoro F, Manoukian S, Bergonzi S, Trecate G, et al. Multicenter surveillance of women at high genetic breast cancer risk using mammography, ultrasonography, and contrast-enhanced magnetic resonance imaging (the high breast cancer risk italian 1 study): final results. Invest Radiol. 2011;46(2):94–105.
17. Kuhl C, Weigel S, Schrading S, Arand B, Bieling H, Konig R, et al. Prospective multicenter cohort study to refine management recommendations for women at elevated familial risk of breast cancer: the EVA trial. J Clin Oncol. 2010;28(9):1450–7.
18. Leach MO, Boggis CR, Dixon AK, Easton DF, Eeles RA, Evans DG, et al. Screening with magnetic resonance imaging and mammography of a UK population at high familial risk of breast cancer: a prospective multicentre cohort study (MARIBS). Lancet. 2005;365(9473):1769–78.
19. Kuhl CK, Schrading S, Leutner CC, Morakkabati-Spitz N, Wardelmann E, Fimmers R, et al. Mammography, breast ultrasound, and magnetic resonance imaging for surveillance of women at high familial risk for breast cancer. J Clin Oncol. 2005;23(33):8469–76.
20. Warner E, Hill K, Causer P, Plewes D, Jong R, Yaffe M, et al. Prospective study of breast cancer incidence in women with a BRCA1 or BRCA2 mutation under surveillance with and without magnetic resonance imaging. J Clin Oncol. 2011;29(13):1664–9.
21. Foulkes WD, Metcalfe K, Hanna W, Lynch HT, Ghadirian P, Tung N, et al. Disruption of the expected positive correlation between breast tumor size and lymph node status in BRCA1-related breast carcinoma. Cancer. 2003;98(8):1569–77.
22. Rennert G, Bisland-Naggan S, Barnett-Griness O, Bar-Joseph N, Zhang S, Rennert HS, et al. Clinical outcomes of breast cancer in carriers of BRCA1 and BRCA2 mutations. N Engl J Med. 2007;357(2):115–23.
23. Hagen AI, Kvistad KA, Maehle L, Holmen MM, Aase H, Styr B, et al. Sensitivity of MRI versus conventional screening in the diagnosis of BRCA-associated breast cancer in a national prospective series. Breast. 2007;16(4):367–74.
24. Warner E, Plewes DB, Hill KA, Causer PA, Zubovits JT, Jong RA, et al. Surveillance of BRCA1 and BRCA2 mutation carriers with magnetic resonance imaging, ultrasound, mammography, and clinical breast examination. JAMA. 2004;292(11):1317–25.
25. Kriege M, Brekelmans CT, Boetes C, Besnard PE, Zonderland HM, Obdeijn IM, et al. Efficacy of MRI and mammography for breast-cancer screening in women with a familial or genetic predisposition. N Engl J Med. 2004;351(5):427–37.
26. Rijnsburger AJ, Obdeijn IM, Kaas R, Tilanus-Linthorst MM, Boetes C, Loo CE, et al. BRCA1-associated breast cancers present differently from BRCA2-associated and familial cases: long-term follow-up of the Dutch MRISC Screening Study. J Clin Oncol. 2010;28(36):5265–73.

27. Heijnsdijk EA, Warner E, Gilbert FJ, Tilanus-Linthorst MM, Evans G, Causer PA, et al. Differences in natural history between breast cancers in BRCA1 and BRCA2 mutation carriers and effects of MRI screening-MRISC, MARIBS, and Canadian studies combined. Cancer Epidemiol Biomarkers Prev. 2012;21(9):1458–68.
28. Moller P, Stormorken A, Jonsrud C, Holmen MM, Hagen AI, Clark N, et al. Survival of patients with BRCA1-associated breast cancer diagnosed in an MRI-based surveillance program. Breast Cancer Res Treat. 2013;139(1):155–61.
29. Tharmaratnam K, Hagen AI, Moller P. MRI screening of women with hereditary predisposition to breast cancer: diagnostic performance and survival analysis. Breast Cancer Res Treat. 2014;148(3):687–8.
30. Familial breast cancer: classification and care of people at risk of familial breast cancer and management of breast cancer and related risks in people with a family history of breast cancer. Clinical guideline developed for NICE by the National Collaborating Centre for Cancer 2013.
31. Oeffinger KC, Fontham ET, Etzioni R, Herzig A, Michaelson JS, Shih YC, et al. Breast cancer screening for women at average risk: 2015 guideline update from the American Cancer Society. JAMA. 2015;314(15):1599–614.
32. Mann RM, Balleyguier C, Baltzer PA, Bick U, Colin C, Cornford E, et al. Breast MRI: EUSOBI recommendations for women's information. Eur Radiol. 2015;25(12):3669–78.
33. Screening for breast cancer in high-risk women during pregnancy and lactation. NHS Cancer Screening Programmes 2012. Available from www.cancerscreening.nhs.uk.
34. Technical guidelines for magnetic resonance imaging for the surveillance of women at higher risk of developing breast cancer. NHSBSP Publication No 68. NHS Cancer Screening Programmes 2012. Available from www.cancerscreening.nhs.uk.
35. ACR Practice Parameter for the Performance of Contrast-enhanced Magnetic Resonance Imaging (MRI) of the Breast. 2014. Available at http://www.acr.org/~/media/ACR/Documents/PGTS/guidelines/MRI_Breast.pdf.
36. Kuhl CK, Bieling HB, Gieseke J, Kreft BP, Sommer T, Lutterbey G, et al. Healthy premenopausal breast parenchyma in dynamic contrast-enhanced MR imaging of the breast: normal contrast medium enhancement and cyclical-phase dependency. Radiology. 1997;203(1):137–44.
37. Giess CS, Raza S, Birdwell RL. Patterns of nonmasslike enhancement at screening breast MR imaging of high-risk premenopausal women. Radiographics. 2013;33(5):1343–60.
38. ACR Practice Parameter for Performing and Interpreting Magnetic Resonance Imaging. 2014. Available at http://www.acr.org/~/media/EB54F56780AC4C6994B77078AA1D6612.pdf.
39. Dall BJ, Vinnicombe S, Gilbert FJ. Reporting and management of breast lesions detected using MRI. Clin Radiol. 2011;66(12):1120–8.
40. Schrading S, Kuhl CK. Mammographic, US, and MR imaging phenotypes of familial breast cancer. Radiology. 2008;246(1):58–70.
41. Tilanus-Linthorst M, Verhoog L, Obdeijn IM, Bartels K, Menke-Pluymers M, Eggermont A, et al. A BRCA1/2 mutation, high breast density and prominent pushing margins of a tumor independently contribute to a frequent false-negative mammography. Int J Cancer. 2002;102(1):91–5.
42. Veltman J, Mann R, Kok T, Obdeijn IM, Hoogerbrugge N, Blickman JG, et al. Breast tumor characteristics of BRCA1 and BRCA2 gene mutation carriers on MRI. Eur Radiol. 2008;18(5):931–8.
43. Lamb PM, Perry NM, Vinnicombe SJ, Wells CA. Correlation between ultrasound characteristics, mammographic findings and histological grade in patients with invasive ductal carcinoma of the breast. Clin Radiol. 2000;55(1):40–4.
44. Kanal E, Borgstede JP, Barkovich AJ, Bell C, Bradley WG, Felmlee JP, et al. American College of Radiology white paper on MR safety. Am J Roentgenol. 2002;178(6):1335–47.
45. Lord SJ, Lei W, Craft P, Cawson JN, Morris I, Walleser S, et al. A systematic review of the effectiveness of magnetic resonance imaging (MRI) as an addition to mammography and ultrasound in screening young women at high risk of breast cancer. Eur J Cancer. 2007;43(13):1905–17.

46. Leach MO. Breast cancer screening in women at high risk using MRI. NMR Biomed. 2009;22(1):17–27.
47. Lehman CD, Isaacs C, Schnall MD, Pisano ED, Ascher SM, Weatherall PT, et al. Cancer yield of mammography, MR, and US in high-risk women: prospective multi-institution breast cancer screening study. Radiology. 2007;244(2):381–8.
48. Teifke A, Hlawatsch A, Beier T, Werner Vomweg T, Schadmand S, Schmidt M, et al. Undetected malignancies of the breast: dynamic contrast-enhanced MR imaging at 1.0 T. Radiology. 2002;224(3):881–8.
49. Obdeijn IM, Loo CE, Rijnsburger AJ, Wasser MN, Bergers E, Kok T, et al. Assessment of false-negative cases of breast MR imaging in women with a familial or genetic predisposition. Breast Cancer Res Treat. 2010;119(2):399–407.

Chapter 4
MRI and Preoperative Staging in Women Newly Diagnosed with Breast Cancer

Su-Ju Lee and Mary C. Mahoney

Abstract Breast magnetic resonance imaging (MRI) is well established as the most sensitive and accurate imaging modality for local-regional staging of breast cancer. It is superior to clinical examination, mammography and ultrasound, alone or combined, in delineation of size and extent of tumor, additional sites of disease, pectoralis muscle and chest wall invasion, nipple and skin involvement, as well as lymph node metastasis. However, the use of MRI for staging of newly diagnosed breast cancer has been a subject of intense debate, because the expected clinical benefits of improved staging by MRI have been called into question. The clinical outcome literature on the benefits of preoperative MRI shows conflicting results regarding re-excision rates and local recurrence rates, and the data do not support a benefit on long-term survival. There are also concerns that preoperative MRI causes delayed definitive therapy and increased mastectomy rates. This chapter details the advantages of MRI staging of newly diagnosed breast cancer, discusses the benefit of MRI staging for a subset of patients and certain clinical scenarios, and reviews the current literature with respect to the pros and cons of MRI staging.

Keywords Breast MRI • Breast cancer staging • MRI staging • Benefits of preoperative breast MRI • Size and extent of disease • Multifocal/multicentric disease • Contralateral disease • Regional lymph node staging • Surgical planning • Re-excision rate • Mastectomy rate • Utility in clinical scenarios

S.J. Lee, MD (✉) • M.C. Mahoney, MD, FACR
Department of Radiology, University of Cincinnati Medical Center,
234 Goodman Street, Mail Location 0772, Cincinnati, OH 45219-2316, USA
e-mail: su-ju.lee@uc.edu; Mary.Mahoney@uc.edu

S.L. Heller, L. Moy (eds.), *Breast Oncology: Techniques, Indications, and Interpretation*, DOI 10.1007/978-3-319-42563-4_4

Abbreviations

ADC	Apparent diffusion coefficient
AJCC	American Joint Committee on Cancer
ALND	Axillary lymph node dissection
BCT	Breast conservation therapy
BPE	Background parenchymal enhancement
DCIS	Ductal carcinoma in situ
EIC	Extensive intraductal component
ER	Estrogen receptor
Her2	Human epidermal growth factor receptor 2
IBC	Inflammatory breast cancer
ILC	Invasive lobular cancer
IM	Internal mammary
MIP	Maximal-intensity projection
MLO	Mediolateral oblique
MRI	Magnetic resonance imaging
NAC	Nipple-areolar complex
NME	Nonmass enhancement
NSM	Nipple sparing mastectomy
PBI	Partial breast irradiation
PR	Progesterone receptor
SLNB	Sentinel lymph noe biopsy

4.1 Introduction

The TNM system developed by American Joint Committee on Cancer (AJCC) is routinely used for determination of prognosis and treatment options for breast cancer (see Tables 4.1, 4.2, 4.3, and 4.4) [1]. The TNM system categorizes the stage of disease based on data from the primary tumor (T), regional lymph nodes (N), and distant metastases (M). Prior to the advent of breast magnetic resonance imaging (MRI), clinical staging and treatment planning for newly diagnosed breast cancer were based on clinical examination, mammography, and ultrasound. This is then replaced by pathologic staging after resection of the primary tumor and lymph node sampling. Breast cancer biologic markers, including estrogen receptor (ER), progesterone receptor (PR), and human epidermal growth factor receptor 2 (HER2) also play a role in treatment planning.

Breast MRI is the most sensitive and accurate imaging modality for local-regional staging of breast cancer [2–7]. It is superior to clinical examination,

Table 4.1 The American Joint Committee on Cancer staging system: breast primary tumor (T)

TX	Primary tumor cannot be assessed
T0	No evidence of primary tumor
Tis	Carcinoma in situ
Tis (DCIS)	Ductal carcinoma in situ
Tis (LCIS)	Lobular carcinoma in situ
Tis (Paget's)	Paget's disease of the nipple not associated with invasive carcinoma or carcinoma in situ (DCIS and/or LCIS) in the underlying breast parenchyma
T1	Tumor ≤20 mm in greatest dimension
T1mi	Tumor ≤1 mm in greatest dimension
T1a	Tumor >1 mm but ≤5 mm in greatest dimension
T1b	Tumor >5 mm but ≤10 mm in greatest dimension
T1c	Tumor >10 mm but ≤20 mm in greatest dimension
T2	Tumor >20 mm but ≤50 mm in greatest dimension
T3	Tumor >50 mm in greatest dimension
T4	Tumor of any size with direct extension to the chest wall and/or to the skin (ulceration or skin nodules) Note: Invasion of the dermis alone does not qualify as T4
T4a	Extension to the chest wall, not including only pectoralis muscle adherence/invasion
T4b	Ulceration and/or ipsilateral satellite nodules and/or edema (including peau d'orange) of the skin, which do not meet the criteria for inflammatory carcinoma
T4c	Both T4a and T4b
T4d	Inflammatory carcinoma

Source: Edge et al. [1] (Used with the permission of the American Joint Committee on Cancer (AJCC), Chicago, Illinois)

mammography and ultrasound, alone or combined, in delineation of the size and extent of tumor, additional sites of disease, pectoralis muscle and chest wall invasion, nipple and skin involvement, as well as lymph node metastasis. The ability of MRI to assess the size and extent of the index tumor and to identify additional, otherwise occult disease of the index and contralateral breasts has added sensitivity and complexity to clinical staging and surgical planning.

4.2 Size and Extent of Index Tumor

All published studies show that breast MRI is the most accurate imaging tool for evaluation of the size and extent of breast tumor [2–7]. Lesion size as determined by MRI correlates best with the pathologic size assessment among all imaging modalities (Fig. 4.1), although overestimation and underestimation do occur. MRI may

Table 4.2 The American Joint Committee on Cancer staging system: breast regional lymph nodes (N)

Clinical	
NX	Regional lymph nodes cannot be assessed (e.g. previously removed)
N0	No regional lymph node metastases
N1	Metastases to movable ipsilateral level I, II axillary lymph node(s)
N2	Metastases in ipsilateral level I, II axillary lymph nodes that are clinically fixed or matted; or in clinically detected[a] ipsilateral internal mammary nodes in the absence of clinically evident axillary lymph node metastases
N2a	Metastases in ipsilateral level I, II axillary lymph nodes fixed to one another (matted) or to other structures
N2b	Metastases only in clinically detected[a] ipsilateral internal mammary nodes and in the absence of clinically evident level I, II axillary lymph node metastases
N3	Metastases in ipsilateral infraclavicular (level III axillary) lymph node(s) with or without level I, II axillary lymph node involvement; Or in clinically detected[a] ipsilateral internal mammary lymph node(s) with clinically evident level I, II axillary lymph node metastases; Or metastases in ipsilateral supraclavicular lymph node(s) with or without axillary or internal mammary lymph node involvement
N3a	Metastases in ipsilateral infraclavicular lymph node(s)
N3b	Metastases in ipsilateral internal mammary lymph node(s) and axillary lymph node(s)
N3c	Metastases in ipsilateral supraclavicular lymph node(s)

Source: Edge et al. [1] (Used with the permission of the American Joint Committee on Cancer (AJCC), Chicago, Illinois)

[a]*Clinically detected* is defined as detected by imaging studies (excluding lymphoscintigraphy) or by clinical examination and having characteristics highly suspicious for malignancy or a presumed pathologic macrometastasis based on fine needle aspiration biopsy with cytologic examination

Table 4.3 The American Joint Committee on Cancer staging system: breast distant metastases (M)

Mo	No clinical or radiographic evidence of distant metastases
cM0(i+)	No clinical or radiographic evidence of distant metastases, but deposits of molecularly or microscopically detected tumor cells in circulating blood, bone marrow, or other nonregional nodal tissue that are no larger than 0.2 mm in a patient without symptoms or signs of metastases
M1	Distant detectable metastases as determined by classic clinical and radiographic means and/or histologically proven larger than 0.2 mm

Source: Edge et al. [1] (Used with the permission of the American Joint Committee on Cancer (AJCC), Chicago, Illinois)

overestimate tumor size (by greater than 5 mm) in up to 35 % of cases and underestimate size in 13 % of cases [5, 6]. The causes of over- or under-estimation have yet to be defined. Some studies suggest that MRI tumor size correlates better with pathologic measurement with high-grade invasive tumor and high-grade ductal carcinoma in-situ (DCIS), and tends to underestimate size in low-grade tumors [8, 9]. However, a recent report showed high-grade tumor and DCIS to be the strongest negative factors resulting in overestimation of tumor size on MRI [10]. There is a greater tendency for tumor size overestimation when tumors are larger than 2 cm in

Table 4.4 The American Joint Committee on Cancer staging system: breast anatomic stage/prognostic groups

Stage	Tumor	Node	Metastasis
0	Tis	N0	M0
IA	T1[a]	N0	M0
IB	T0 T1[a]	N1mi N1mi	M0 M0
IIA	T0 T1[a] T2	N1[b] N1[b] N0	M0 M0 M0
IIB	T2 T3	N1 N0	M0 M0
IIIA	T0 T1[a] T2 T3 T3	N2 N2 N2 N1 N2	M0 M0 M0 M0 M0
IIIB	T4 T4 T4	N0 N1 N2	M0 M0 M0
IIIC	Any T	N3	M0
IV	Any T	Any N	M1

Source: Edge et al. [1] (Used with the permission of the American Joint Committee on Cancer (AJCC), Chicago, Illinois)

[a]T1 includes T1mi

[b]T0 and T1 tumors with nodal micrometastases only are excluded from Stage IIA and are classified as Stage IB disease

size [6, 10]. The MRI sequence on which the tumors are measured may also be a factor. A recent report suggests that index tumor size is best measured on T2 weighted images, whereas the whole extent of disease is best estimated on early-subtracted dynamic contrast enhanced T1 weighted images [11].

MRI is more accurate than mammography or ultrasound for detection of an intraductal component of an invasive cancer (Figs 4.2 and 4.3). However, it may overestimate this finding in 11–28 % and underestimate it in 17–28 % of cases [12–14]. Overestimation may be due to enhancement of normal glandular tissue, other coexisting benign entities, or lymphovascular invasion [15]. Since extensive intraductal component (EIC) is a contributing factor for positive surgical margins at breast conserving surgery, preoperative delineation of the extent of EIC is essential.

Contrary to early reports, MRI has been shown to be more sensitive in detection of DCIS than mammography and ultrasound (Fig. 4.4). This is largely attributable to a greater emphasis on high spatial resolution over high temporal resolution in MRI technique [16]. Reported MRI sensitivity for DCIS in the more recent literature is 79–97 %, compared with only 52–56 % by mammography. The sensitivity reaches 98 % in high-grade or comedo type DCIS [16, 17]. Several recent studies investigated the utility of MRI in the detection of invasive component in DCIS diag-

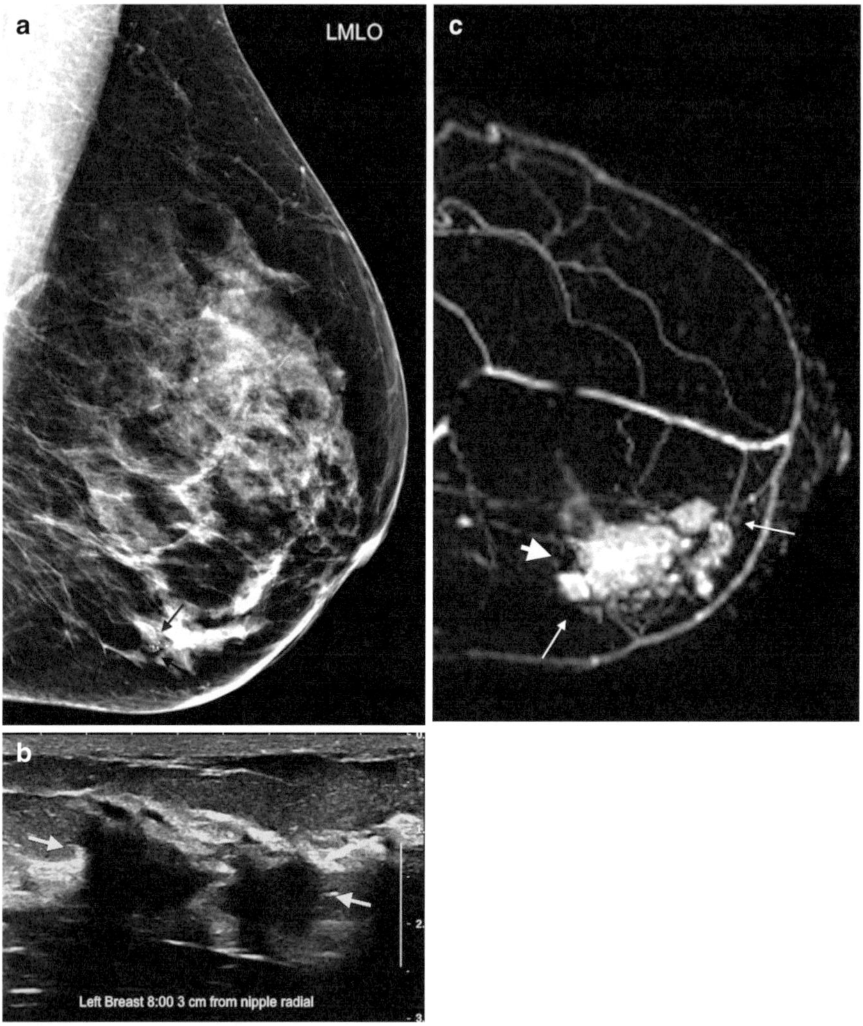

Fig. 4.1 Clinical stage IIA, T2N0M0 tumor in a 52-year-old with a palpable mass in the left breast and discordant tumor size between breast examination, mammography, and ultrasound. (**a**) Left mediolateral oblique view (MLO) mammogram reveals a small group of microcalcifications (*black arrow*). Biopsy revealed invasive lobular carcinoma. (**b**) Ultrasound of the left breast at the biopsy site shows two adjacent irregular hypoechoic masses, measuring 2.7 × 1.5 cm in aggregate. (**c**) Sagittal post contrast T1-weighted maximal-intensity projection (MIP) MR image reveals an irregular enhancing mass, 3.7 × 2.5 × 2.0 cm in size (between *arrows*). *Arrowhead* denotes focal susceptibility artifact caused by a tissue marker at the site of microcalcifications. Histopathology confirmed the large tumor size

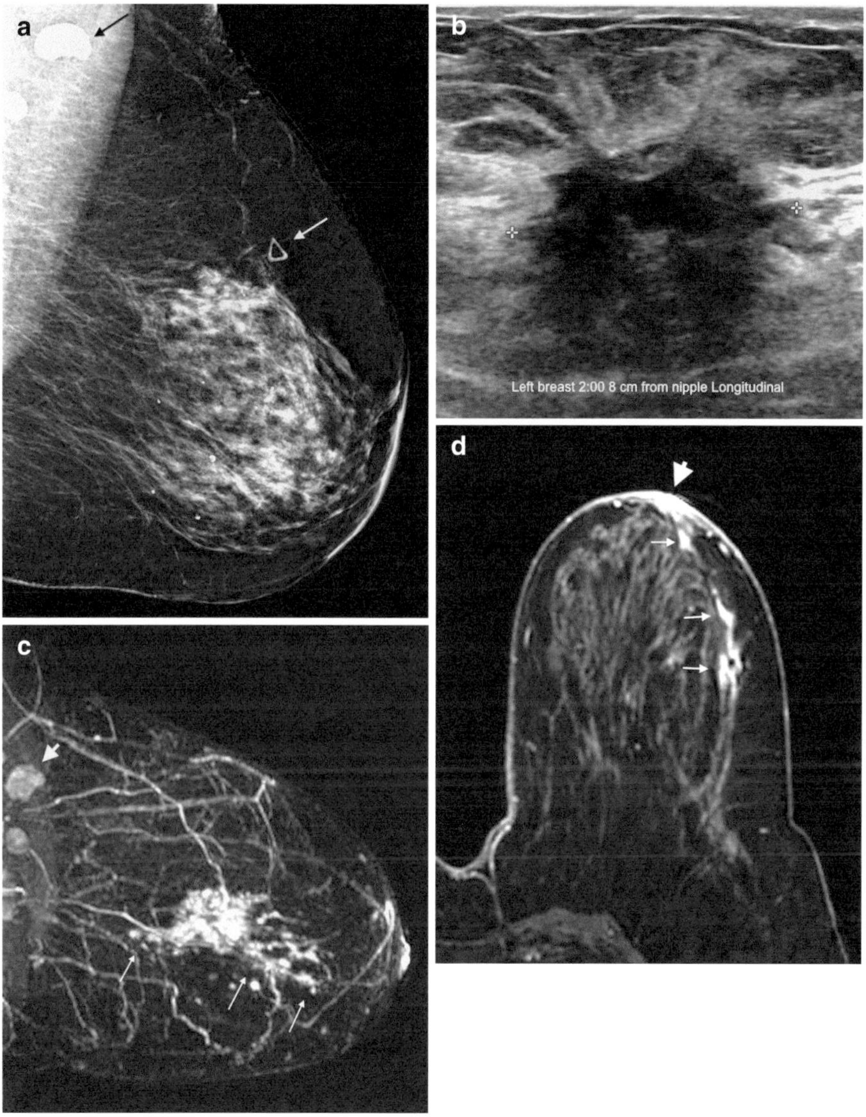

Fig. 4.2 Clinical stage IIIA, T3N1M0 tumor in a 72-year-old with extensive intraductal component (EIC) and unsuspected nipple involvement. (**a**) Left MLO view mammogram shows heterogeneously dense breast tissue with a triangular marker (*white arrow*) indicating a palpable mass. The mass is not visible on mammography. An abnormal high-density axillary lymph node is visible (*black arrow*). (**b**) Ultrasound of the palpable mass reveals a 2.7 cm irregular mass. Ultrasound guided biopsy confirmed invasive ductal carcinoma. Fine needle aspiration of the suspicious lymph node was positive for metastasis. (**c**) Sagittal post contrast T1 MIP MR image demonstrates an irregular enhancing mass corresponding to the known invasive cancer, with nonmass enhancement (*long arrows*) extending from the mass both anteriorly and posteriorly, consistent with EIC. The maximal anteroposterior extent of the tumor is 12 cm. Note the metastatic node with loss of fatty hilum (*arrowhead*). (**d**) Axial post contrast fat-saturated T1 MR image reveals nonmass enhancement in a ductal distribution (*short arrows*) extending to the nipple, with enhancement of the nipple-areolar complex (NAC) (*arrowhead*) consistent with tumor invasion

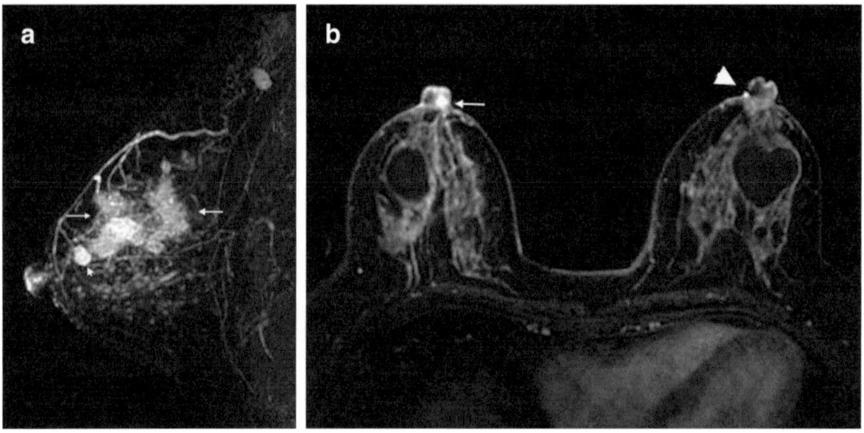

Fig. 4.3 Clinical stage IIIA, T3N1M0 tumor in a 42-year-old woman with multicentric right breast cancer, EIC, and nipple involvement. (**a**) Sagittal post contrast subtraction T1 MIP MR image of the right breast shows a small known invasive tumor (*arrowhead*) and extensive nonmass enhancement consistent with EIC, involving the upper outer and upper inner quadrants (between *arrows*). There is a metastatic lymph node in the axilla. (**b**) Bilateral axial post contrast fat-saturated T1 MR image demonstrates nodular enhancement in the right nipple (*arrow*), compared to non-enhancement of the left nipple. The focal signal abnormality in the left nipple (*arrowhead*) is an artifact

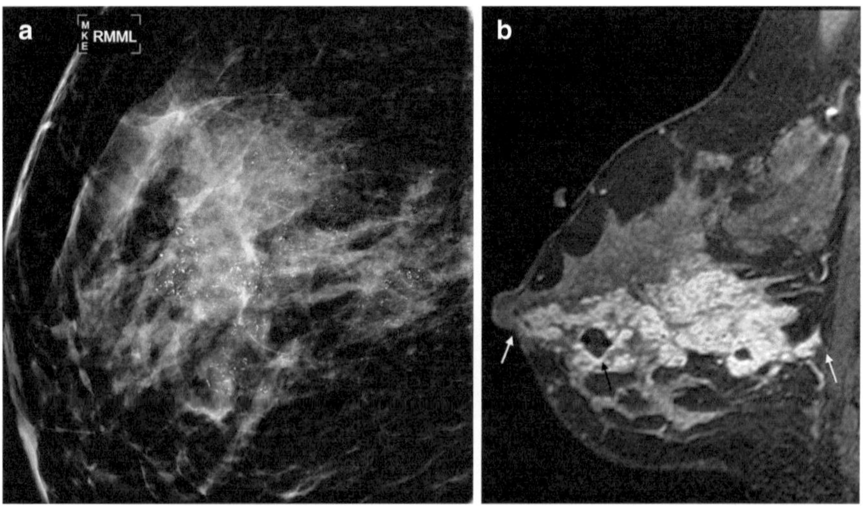

Fig. 4.4 Clinical stage 0, TisN0M0 tumor in a 39-year-old woman with extensive DCIS. (**a**) Spot magnification mediolateral view mammogram of the right breast demonstrates dense breast tissue with extensive pleomorphic microcalcifications that did not extend to the nipple. Biopsy confirmed high grade DCIS. (**b**) Sagittal post contrast fat-saturated T1 MR image shows extensive clumped nonmass enhancement. The tumor extends to within 2 mm of the nipple anteriorly and 3 mm of the pectoral muscle posteriorly (*white arrows*). A small hematoma from biopsy is present (*black arrow*). The patient is not an appropriate candidate for nipple-sparing mastectomy because the close proximity of tumor to the nipple suggests occult nipple invasion

nosed on needle biopsies. The presence of a mass, rapid initial enhancement, washout kinetics, larger lesion size, higher lesion to background signal intensity ratios, higher number of tissue cores involved by tumor nests, and lower apparent diffusion coefficient (ADC) values have been linked to the presence of occult invasion [18–20].

4.3 Additional Sites of Disease

Multifocal disease is defined as two or more tumor foci in the same quadrant of the breast (Fig. 4.5). Multicentric disease is a condition with two or more tumor foci in different quadrants of the breast (Fig. 4.6). Although TNM staging system does not

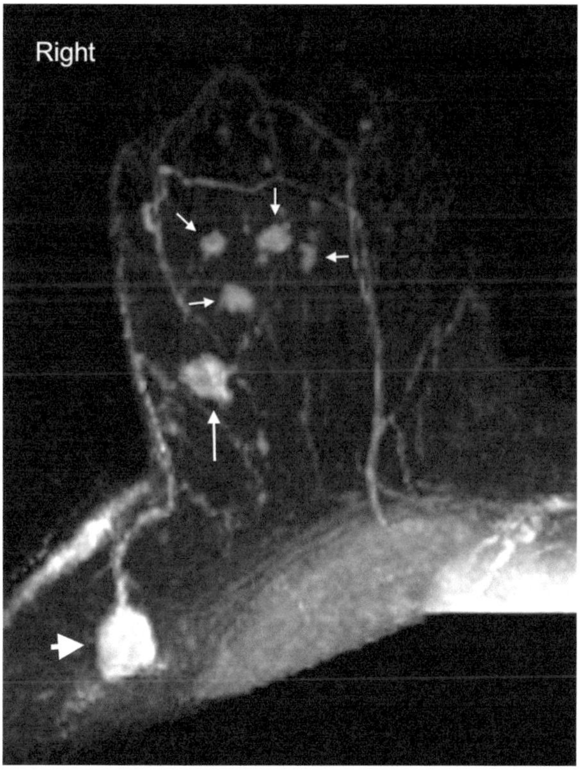

Fig. 4.5 Clinical stage IIA, T1N1M0 tumor in a 52-year-old woman with multifocal carcinoma. Axial post contrast subtraction T1 MIP MR image of the right breast demonstrates multiple enhancing masses in the central and lateral aspects of right upper breast. The largest, 1.2 cm mass is a known invasive carcinoma (*long arrow*). Four additional tumors (*short arrows*) are seen anterior to it. An enlarged level I right axillary lymph node with loss of reniform shape and fatty hilum (*arrowhead*) was positive for metastatic disease on fine needle aspiration

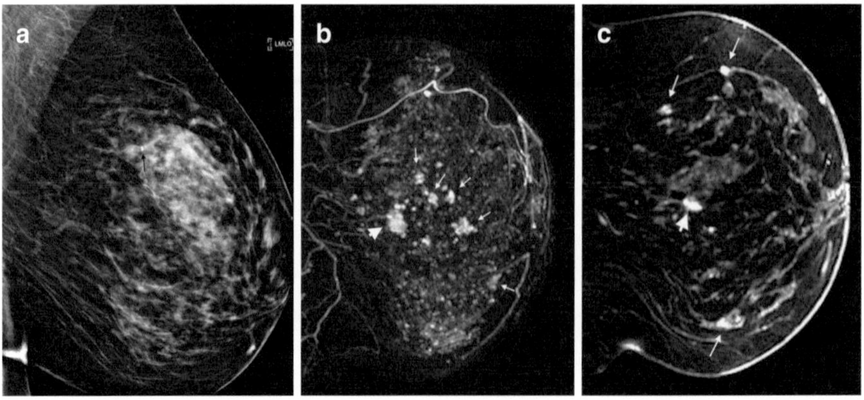

Fig. 4.6 Clinical stage IIA, T1N0M0 tumor in a 48-year-old woman with multicentric tumors. An architectural distortion on her screening mammogram led to the ultrasound biopsy of a 1.2 cm mass, which revealed invasive lobular carcinoma. (**a**) Left MLO view mammogram shows heterogeneously dense breast with a biopsy marker at the site of the index tumor (*black arrow*). No other suspicious abnormality is visible. (**b**) Sagittal post contrast T1 MIP MR image demonstrates the lobulated index mass (*arrowhead*) and multiple additional small irregular enhancing masses (*small arrows*). (**c**) Sagittal post contrast fat-saturated T1 MR image shows part of the known index tumor (*arrowhead*). Multiple tumors in different quadrants (*long arrows*) are better appreciated. Biopsies of two additional masses confirmed multicentric invasive lobular cancers

take these into consideration, the detection of additional sites of disease greatly impacts surgical management. While multifocal disease may be amenable to breast conservation, multicentric disease is usually treated with mastectomy. MRI is superior to conventional imaging for identifying additional cancer foci in the same breast as the index tumor, and in the opposite breast [21–26]. The preoperative identification of these additional tumor foci may alter surgical and radiation therapy. In a recent meta-analysis of 50 studies, Plana and associates found that preoperative MRI detected additional, otherwise occult, cancers in the ipsilateral breast in 20 % of cases, with a summary positive predictive value (PPV) of 67 % and accuracy of 93 %. The PPV increased to 75 % when MR scanner ≥1.5 T was used [23]. These results are similar to the findings of an earlier meta-analysis of 19 studies, showing detection of additional disease in 16 % of cases with a summary PPV of 66 % and accuracy of 86 % [24]. In this and another meta-analysis, MRI found additional cancer in the contralateral breast in 4.1–5.5 % of patients (Fig. 4.7) at the time of diagnosis [23, 25]. This is similar to the 3.1 % rate reported by the ACRIN 6667 multicenter prospective trial [26].

Many studies have examined the surgical impact of finding additional sites of disease. Plana's meta-analysis of 26 studies found an appropriate change in surgical management in 12.8 % of patients with confirmed additional malignancy, with 8.3 % of patients converted from breast conservation therapy (BCT) to mastectomy and 4.5 % receiving more extensive excision [23]. However, false positive cases resulted in inappropriate alteration in surgical treatment in 6.3 % of cases, including

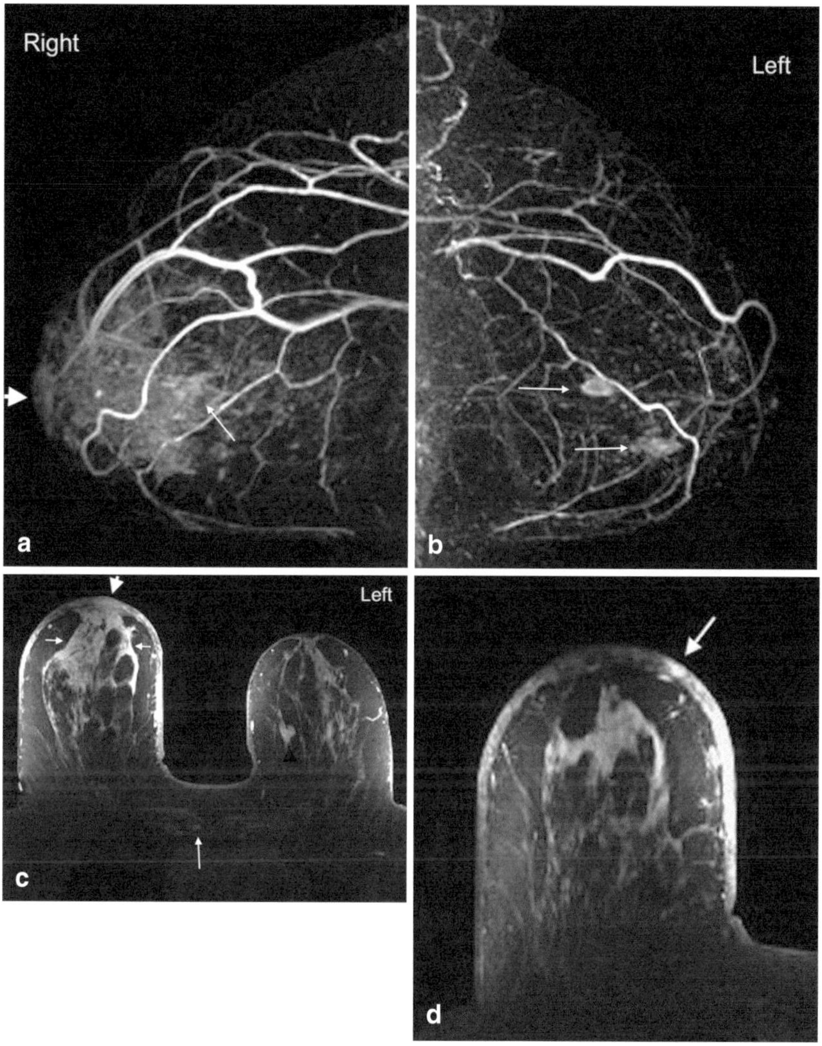

Fig. 4.7 Clinical stage IV, T4dN1M1 tumor in a 63-year-old woman with diffuse erythema of the right breast. Skin punch biopsy confirmed inflammatory breast cancer (IBC). Staging MRI showed contralateral left breast cancers and positive right axillary level I, II nodes. (**a**) Sagittal T1 MIP MR image of the right breast reveals extensive nonmass enhancement (between *arrow* and *arrowhead*) and enhancement of the nipple consistent with invasion (*arrowhead*). A partially obscured irregular mass is seen more posteriorly (*long arrow*). (**b**) Sagittal T1 MIP MR image of the left breast shows two masses with heterogeneous enhancement. Biopsy confirmed both to be invasive ductal carcinoma. (**c**) Bilateral axial post contrast fat-saturated T1 MR image demonstrates asymmetric enlargement of the right breast with diffuse thickening and heterogeneous enhancement of the skin. Nipple invasion (*white arrowhead*) and extensive subareolar nonmass enhancement (between *short arrows*) are obvious. An enhancing mass is seen in the left breast (*black arrowhead*). An enhancing focus in the right sternum (*long white arrow*) was positive on PET/CT scan, consistent with distant metastasis. (**d**) Axial post contrast fat-saturated T1 MR image of the right breast demonstrates enhancing nodule in the skin (*arrow*) caused by dermal lymphatic embolus (the "punched out" lesion). Diffuse thickening and heterogeneous enhancement of the skin are evident

1.7 % undergoing mastectomy and 4.6 % receiving more extensive excision [23]. These results parallel the findings of another meta-analysis, which showed a 1.1 % conversion rate to mastectomy and a 5.5 % rate of more extensive surgery due to false positive MRI [24]. The false positive cases illustrate the importance of histologic confirmation of suspicious MRI findings before performing more extensive surgery.

Occasionally, additional tumor may be present, but not detected by MRI. These false negative cases may be caused by non-enhancing tumor or obscuration by moderate to marked background parenchymal enhancement (BPE) of normal tissue [2, 27, 28]. BPE is mediated by hormonal activity, and is not correlated with mammographic density [28]. Attempts should be made to schedule breast MRI during the second week of the menstrual cycle or discontinuing exogenous hormone therapy for several months before MRI to reduce BPE. However, to avoid delay in therapy, this is not possible in patients newly diagnosed with breast cancer.

4.4 Pectoral Muscle and Chest Wall Involvement

Knowledge of pectoral or chest wall invasion by breast cancer prior to surgery is important, because of its impact on tumor staging, surgical planning and overall therapeutic approach. Chest wall invasion is defined as tumor infiltration of ribs, intercostal muscles and/or serratus anterior muscle [29]. Breast tumor with chest wall invasion is considered locally advanced disease with a tumor classification of T4a and a minimum TNM stage of IIIB with a 5-year survival rate of 23 % [30, 31]. Breast tumor with chest wall invasion may require neoadjuvant chemotherapy, with or without chest wall radiation, followed by more extensive surgery including chest wall resection [30, 31]. A tumor that invades only the pectoral muscle may require partial excision of the muscle if the invasion is superficial, or radical mastectomy with resection of the entire muscle if full thickness of the muscle is involved (Fig. 4.8) [30].

Evaluation of the pectoral muscle and chest wall underlying a posteriorly located breast tumor is usually limited on physical examination, mammography and ultrasound [30–32]. Far posterior tumors are difficult to include in the field of view on mammography. On sonography, the strong acoustic shadowing by breast cancer often obscures the underlying pectoral muscle. By contrast, the pectoral muscle and chest wall are well demonstrated on MRI (Fig. 4.9) [32]. Previous studies showed that contrast enhancement of the pectoral muscle or chest wall structures, either infiltrative or mass-like (Figs. 4.8 and 4.10a), are the only reliable MRI finding to predict invasion [32, 33]. Proximity of the tumor or violations of the fat plane alone are not sufficient evidence of muscle invasion (Fig. 4.11a) [32, 33]. Pectoral muscle enhancement caused by recent biopsy of nearby primary tumor is a known cause of false positive interpretation [33].

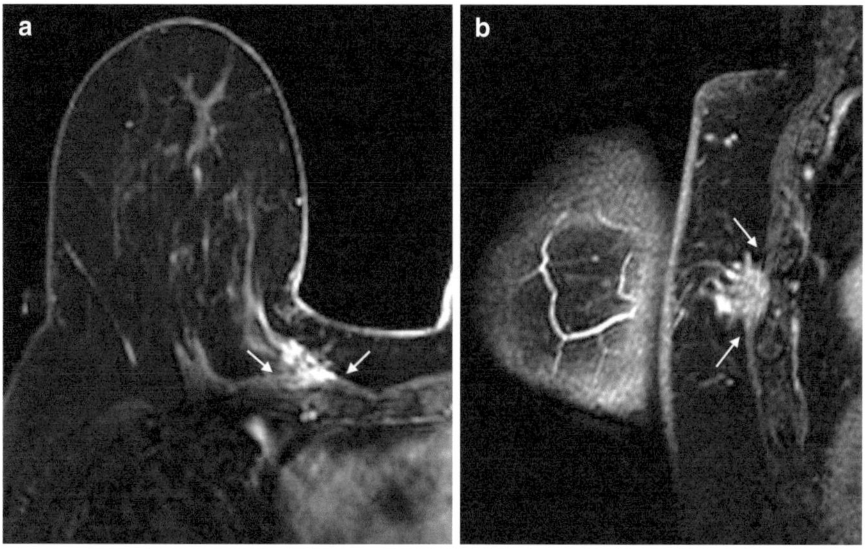

Fig. 4.8 Clinical stage IIA, T2N0M0 tumor in a 70-year-old woman with invasive ductal carcinoma of the right breast. (**a**) Axial post contrast fat-saturated T1 MR image demonstrates a posteriorly located tumor in the right breast with full thickness involvement of the pectoral muscle (between *arrows*). The tumor has a maximum dimension of 2.2 cm. (**b**) Sagittal post contrast fat-saturated T1 MR image shows the irregular mass invading the pectoral muscle (between *arrows*) without affecting the underlying intercostal muscles

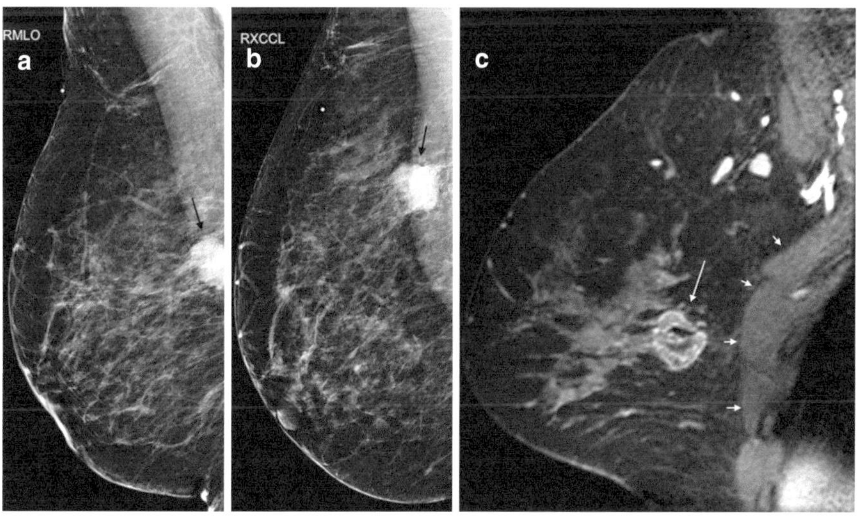

Fig. 4.9 Clinical stage IIA, T2N0M0 tumor in a 44-year-old woman with a posteriorly located invasive ductal carcinoma of the right breast. (**a**) Right MLO view mammogram demonstrates a 2.5 cm mass (*black arrow*) in the posterior breast, incompletely imaged and inseparable from pectoral muscle. A BB on the breast skin denotes a palpable mass. (**b**) On the laterally exaggerated CC view, the tumor again overlaps with the pectoral muscle. (**c**) Sagittal post contrast fat-saturated T1 MR image shows the mass (*long arrow*) not in close proximity or invading the pectoral muscle (*four small arrows*)

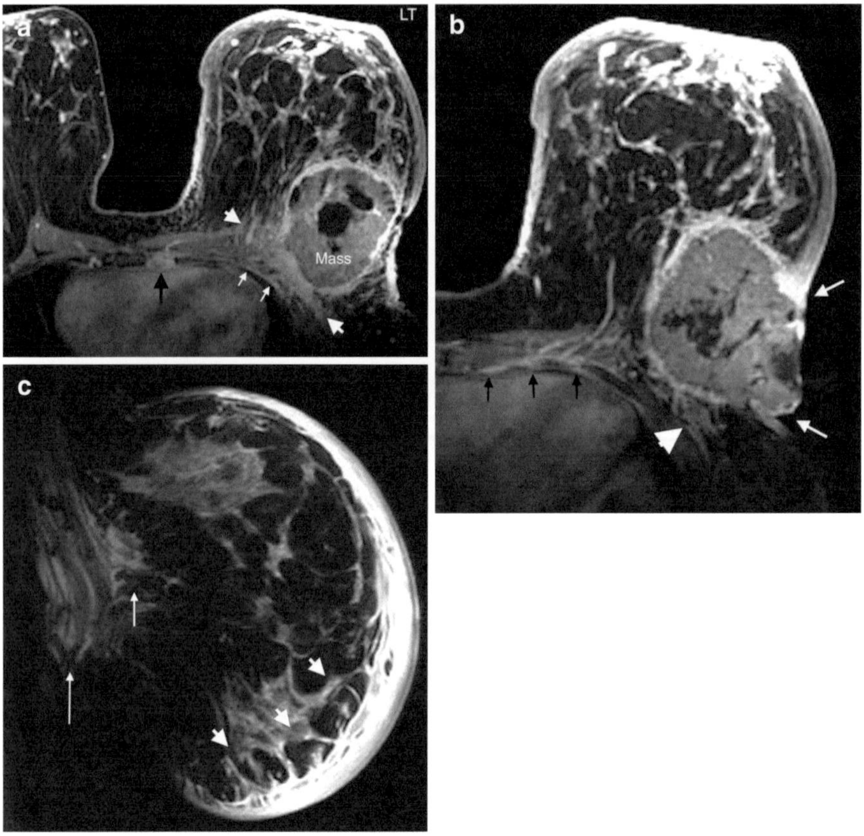

Fig. 4.10 Clinical stage IIIC, T4dN3Mx tumor in a 41-year-old woman with triple-negative invasive ductal carcinoma, and clinical evidence of inflammatory carcinoma of the left breast. (**a**) Axial post contrast fat-saturated T1 MR image demonstrates a 10 cm left breast mass with enhancement of the pectoral muscle, indicating invasion (between *arrowheads*). Enhancement of intercostal muscles and pleura (*small white arrows*) indicates chest wall invasion. An enlarged left internal mammary lymph node (*black arrow*) and palpable left axillary nodes constitute N3 nodal status. Diffuse thickening and enhancements of the skin and Cooper ligaments are consistent with inflammatory carcinoma. (**b**) Axial post contrast fat-saturated T1 MR image shows the locally advanced tumor invading the skin with ulceration (between *small white arrows*), the pectoral muscle (*arrowhead*) and the intercostal muscle (*black arrows*). (**c**) Sagittal fat-saturated T2 image demonstrates diffuse cutaneous and subcutaneous edema (*arrowheads*), prepectoral edema (*short arrow*), and intramuscular edema (*long arrow*). These are differential features in favor of IBC

4.5 Skin and Nipple Involvement

According to AJCC TNM system for clinical staging of breast cancer, ulceration and/or satellite nodules and/or edema (including peau d'orange) of the skin which do not meet the criteria for inflammatory carcinoma, are classified as T4b tumor, resulting in at least stage IIIB disease (Tables 4.1 and 4.4). Invasion of the dermis

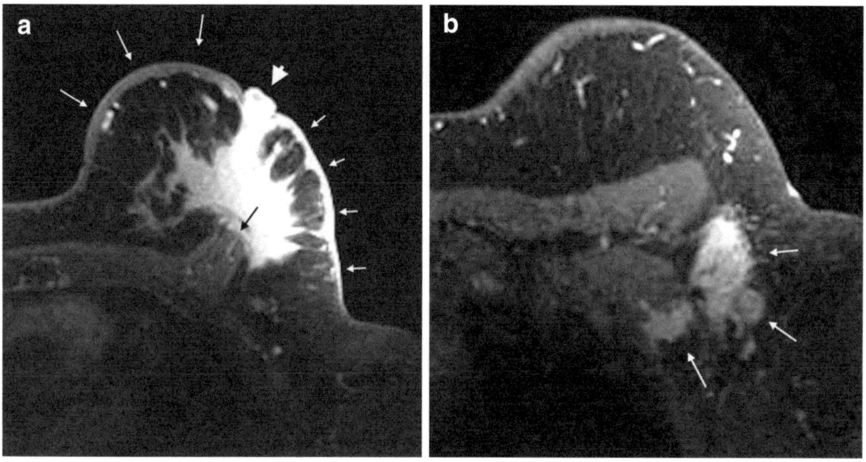

Fig. 4.11 Clinical stage IIIA, T3N2M0 tumor in a 54-year-old woman with a left breast mass and left nipple retraction. (**a**) Axial post contrast fat-saturated T1 MR image of the left breast reveals a large (7.1 cm) spiculated enhancing mass abutting the pectoral muscle (*black arrow*). Obliteration of the muscle fascia and tenting of the muscle are present, but there is no muscle enhancement to indicate invasion. Enhancement and retraction of the nipple (*arrowhead*) indicates nipple invasion. Diffuse thickening and enhancement of the skin in the lateral aspect of the breast (*four short arrows*) signal skin invasion by local extension. Skin thickening without enhancement in the medial breast (*three long arrows*) reflects lymph edema without invasion. (**b**) Axial post contrast fat-saturated T1 MR image more superiorly reveals three abnormal level I axillary nodes lying lateral to the pectoralis muscles. The two lateral nodes are matted to each other, while the medial node adheres to the pectoralis minor muscle. Note the loss of hilar fat in the nodes. Spiculated margins of the nodes suggest extracapsular tumor extension, which was confirmed by core biopsy

alone, without the above mentioned skin changes, does not meet the criteria of a T4 tumor (Table 4.1). On MRI, direct invasion of the skin appears as localized skin thickening and enhancement, which is contiguous with an underlying malignancy, with or without skin retraction (Fig. 4.11a). Skin edema, seen as areas of non-enhancing skin thickening (>3 mm) on MRI, may occur as a result of lymphatic obstruction, with or without malignant involvement (Fig. 4.11a). In later stages, enhancing skin nodules, masses, and ulceration are well demonstrated on MRI (Fig. 4.10b). When skin involvement by a locally advanced tumor is extensive, differentiating it from inflammatory carcinoma on clinical examination and MRI is difficult without a skin punch biopsy [34].

Preoperative evaluation of the nipple-areolar complex (NAC) is important for surgical planning because involvement of the NAC by tumor requires resection of the NAC and precludes patient from nipple-sparing mastectomy. Assessment of the NAC for tumor involvement on MRI may be difficult, because normal nipples may show various patterns of enhancement or no enhancement at all [28]. Sakamoto and colleagues found unilateral nipple enhancement continuous with the underlying index tumor to be highly suggestive of tumor involvement (Figs. 4.2, 4.3, 4.7 and 4.11) [35]. Characteristics of the nipple enhancement include diffuse enhancement, periareolar skin enhancement, and rim or periductal enhancement within the nipple [35]. Nodular enhancement in the involved nipple is occasionally seen (Fig. 4.3b). Tumor size >2 cm and distance from the tumor edge to the NAC < 2 cm on MRI are statistically significant indicators for NAC involvement [36]. However, the tumor to NAC distance indicative of nipple involvement has been reported as <5 mm or <10 mm in other studies (Fig. 4.4) [37, 38]. Moon and associates found enhancement of the NAC itself to have higher predictive value for NAC invasion than short tumor to nipple distance [39].

4.6 Staging of Regional Lymph Nodes

Identification of regional nodal metastases is critical for staging, prognosis and treatment planning in patients with newly diagnosed breast cancer (Table 4.2). Regional lymph nodes include ipsilateral intramammary, axillary, internal mammary, and supraclavicular nodes.

The axilla is divided into 3 levels by the pectoralis minor muscle. Level I nodes are low axillary nodes lateral to pectoralis minor muscle, including the intramammary nodes (Fig. 4.12a). Level II nodes are mid-axillary nodes between the medial and lateral borders of the pectoralis minor muscle, including the Rotter nodes between the pectoralis major and minor muscles (Figs. 4.12b and 4.13a). Level III nodes are apical axillary nodes medial to the pectoralis minor muscle, i.e. the infraclavicular nodes (Fig. 4.12c). The internal mammary nodal chain runs along the margins of the sternum following the course of internal mammary artery and vein (Fig. 4.13b and 4.13c). The internal mammary (IM) nodes are found in the first through sixth intercostal spaces [40]. The supraclavicular nodes are located in the supraclavicular fossa.

The current 7th edition of the AJCC TNM staging system includes clinical and pathologic node staging schemes [1, 41]. The "clinical" scheme classifies "clinically detected" nodes, which are defined as nodes detected by clinical examination and imaging studies. The "pathologic" scheme classifies nodes identified with sentinel node biopsy or axillary node dissection. In the clinical scheme (Table 4.2), ipsilateral level I and II axillary nodes are N1 disease if movable, but become N2 disease when fixed to each other or adjacent structures (i.e. matted), which raises the stage to at least IIIA (Table 4.4). Metastases in the ipsilateral IM nodes in the absence of axillary node metastases are classified as N2 disease, but become N3 disease if the axillary nodes are also involved. Metastasis to the ipsilateral level III axillary (infraclavicular) or supraclavicular nodes indicates N3 disease, which raises the stage to at least IIIC. Metastases to cervical, contralateral internal mammary and contralateral axillary lymph nodes are considered distant metastases (M1 disease) and indicate stage IV disease (Table 4.4) [30]. Metastases to the IM nodes usually occur after a tumor has metastasized to the axilla (N3 disease). Isolated metastasis to the IM nodes is rare, occurring in only 1–5 % of breast cancers, usually from deep or medial lesions [41, 42]. Metastatic involvement of the IM nodes, without or with

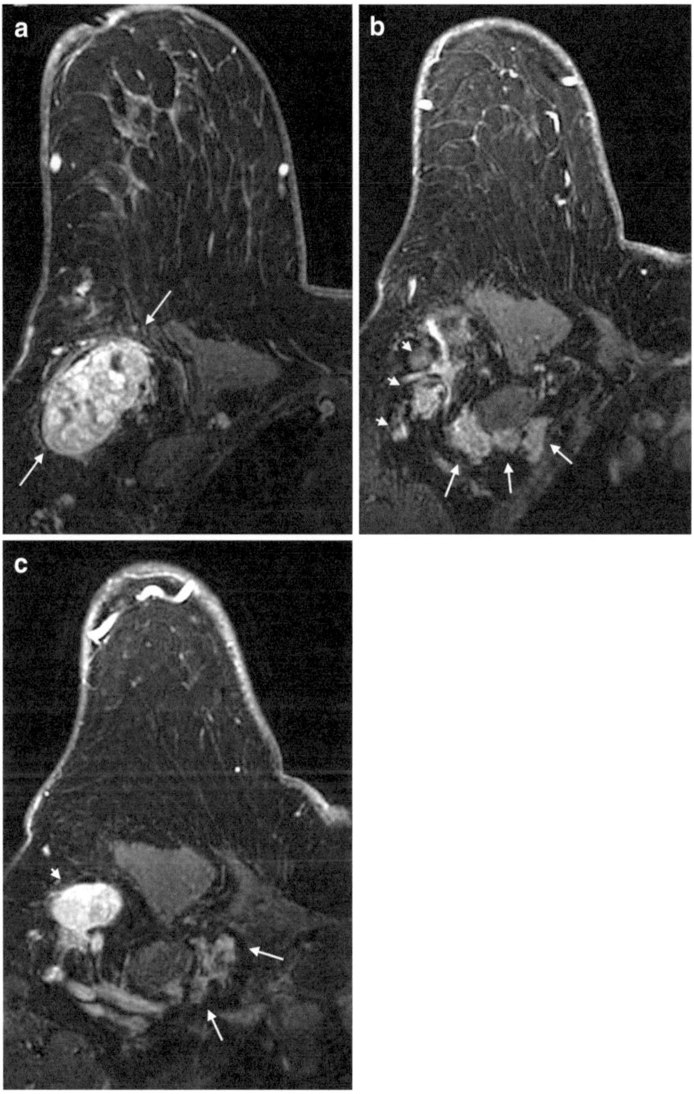

Fig. 4.12 Clinical stage IIIC, TxN3M0 tumor in a 75-year-old woman with right axillary lymphadenopathy and no apparent primary tumor on mammography and ultrasound. (**a**) Axial post contrast T1 fat-saturated MR image shows a large right axillary level I lymph node with heterogeneous enhancement, complete absence of hilar fat and perinodal stranding which may be due to recent biopsy or lymph edema. Biopsy of this node revealed poorly differentiated mammary carcinoma. (**b**) Axial image at a higher level reveals multiple level II nodes posterior to the pectoralis minor muscle (*long arrows*). Some level I nodes lying lateral to the pectoralis minor muscle are seen (*arrowheads*). All nodes show ill-defined margins suspicious for extranodal tumor extension. (**c**) Axial image at the level of infraclavicular fossa demonstrates matted level III lymph nodes medial to the pectoralis minor muscle (between *arrows*). An abnormal level I node is seen (*arrowhead*). No primary tumor is identified in either breast

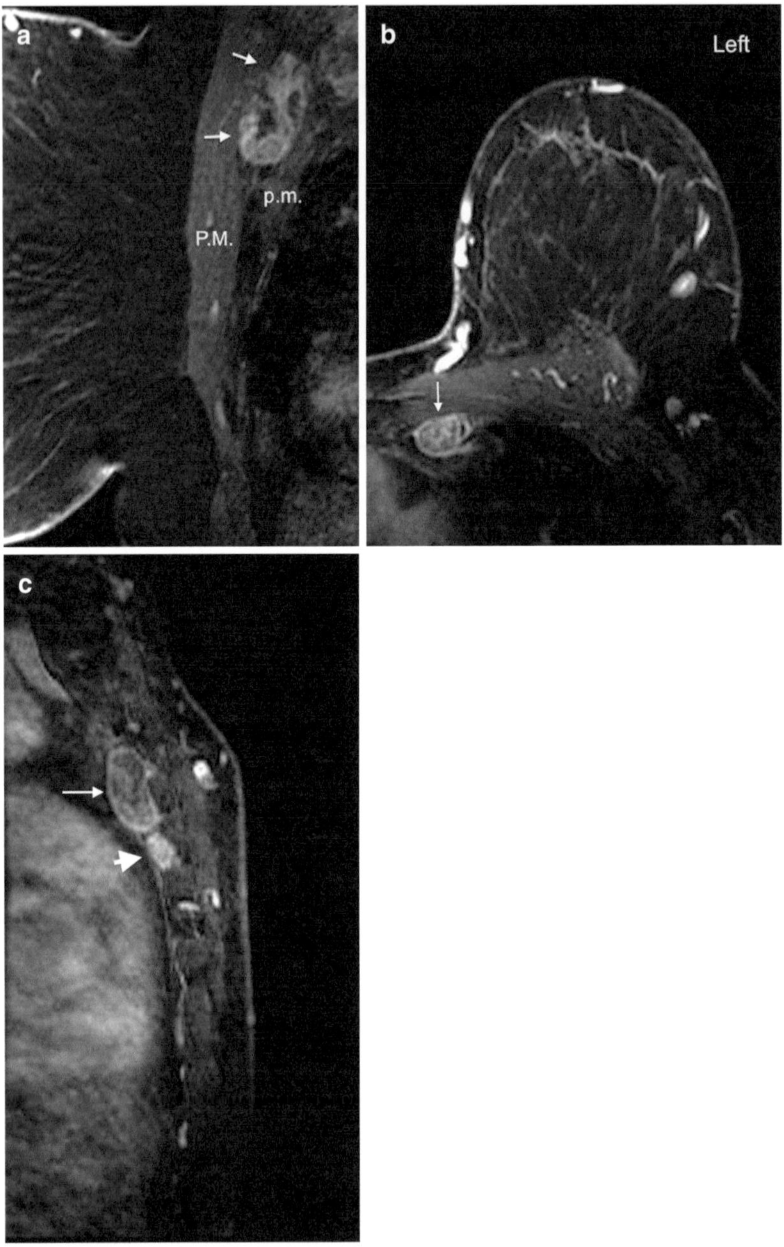

Fig. 4.13 Interpectoral node and internal mammary (IM) nodes. (**a**) Sagittal post contrast fat-saturated T1 image shows an enlarged lymph node (*arrows*) with heterogeneous enhancement between the pectoralis major (P.M.) and pectoralis minor (p.m.) muscles. The interpectoral node is also known as a Rotter node. (**b**) Axial post contrast fat-saturated T1 image of left breast in a different patient demonstrates an enlarged left IM node (*arrow*). (**c**) Sagittal post contrast T1 image of the same patient as in image (**b**) shows the IM node (*arrow*) along the sternal border. A second abnormal IM node is seen inferior to it (*arrowhead*)

axillary disease, carries a small but definite risk of local recurrence and reduced long-term survival [42]. Due to the morbidity involved, dissection of the internal mammary nodes is usually not performed. However, radiation treatment can be utilized to treat these nodes [41, 42].

In most institutions, ultrasound is the primary imaging modality for evaluation of axillary nodes, with moderate sensitivity and high specificity for detection of metastases, especially when morphologic criteria rather than size, are used for diagnosis [41, 43, 44]. However, the results are operator dependent and the evaluation of infraclavicular, supraclavicular and internal mammary nodes is not routinely performed. By contrast, regional lymph nodes, except for supraclavicular nodes, are included in the field of view on most routine breast MRI protocols. The ability of MRI to predict axillary nodal metastases is similar to ultrasound, with reported sensitivity of 36–88 % and specificity of 73–100 % [45–50]. MRI is less operator-dependent than ultrasound and provides a global view of both axillae and internal mammary chains. This may enhance the detection of potentially abnormal nodes and allows comparison with the contralateral axilla [41]. Occasionally, pulsation artifacts through the axilla may limit evaluation of the axillary nodes [41].

On non-contrast MRI, normal lymph nodes are reniform, circumscribed, with low signal intensity on T1-weighted and high signal intensity on T2-weighted sequences. Hilar fat is best seen on a T1-weighted non-contrast sequence without fat saturation, a sequence that should be included in the breast MRI protocol. Upon contrast injection, the normal lymph nodes enhance rapidly and homogeneously with a type III wash out delayed kinetics. Hence, the enhancement kinetics are not useful in differentiating benign and metastatic lymph nodes. Like ultrasound, nodal size alone is not useful for identifying metastatic nodes on MRI [41]. Morphologic features on MRI that suggest a nodal metastasis include: round shape or a long axis to short axis ratio of less than two, loss of the fatty hilum, increased cortical thickness (>3 mm), eccentric or focal cortical thickening, irregular or spiculated margins, edema surrounding the nodes, and asymmetry of morphology of the nodes compared with the contralateral axilla [41, 50–53]. One study described "perifocal edema" (edema surrounding the lymph nodes) and "rim enhancement" (higher signal intensity in the periphery of the nodes) 11 min after contrast injection as the two features with 100 % positive predictive value for the detection of metastases [53]. IM nodes are more likely to contain a metastasis when 5 mm or larger in size [54]. Normal IM nodes are usually not visible on MRI. When visualized, they should be regarded as suspicious and reported [30].

Traditionally, preoperative identification of axillary nodal metastases will spare patients with invasive breast cancer an unnecessary sentinel lymph node biopsy (SLNB) and allow them to proceed directly to axillary lymph node dissection (ALND). In 2011, Giuliano and associates published the results of the American College of Surgeons Oncology Group (ACOSOG) Z0011 randomized trial [55]. This trial suggested that patients with T1 or T2 invasive breast cancer, no palpable nodes, and one or two positive sentinel nodes, who underwent lumpectomy with negative margins, tangential whole-breast radiation, and systemic therapy, might not benefit from ALND [55]. While this finding is potentially practice changing, controversies exist about the relatively short median follow-up interval of 6.3 years and the number of patients enrolled. In light of the Z0011 results, some have questioned the role of imaging for preoperative axillary staging, expressing concerns that preoperative detection of axillary metastasis would prompt ALND for disease that could otherwise have been treated according to Z0011 protocol [56]. Many authors believe that imaging still plays an important role in the axillary staging, especially in identifying patients with N2 and N3 disease. Since nodal disease beyond levels I and II are not routinely included in an axillary dissection, identification of nodes in these higher N categories by imaging may affect initial staging and treatment planning. Two recent studies showed that MRI can predict metastatic disease in more than two sentinel nodes, thereby identifying patients who require further local-regional therapy beyond SLND [57, 58]. In the future, patients may undergo imaging for the purpose of excluding N2 or N3 disease, rather than for diagnosing axillary metastases [41].

4.7 Subsets of Newly Diagnosed Breast Cancer Patients Likely to Benefit from MRI Staging

Because of the ability of MRI to identify lesions that are occult on conventional imaging and to better define extent of disease, it is intuitive that MRI staging is particularly beneficial for a subset of patients with newly diagnosed breast cancer.

Patients with Invasive Lobular Cancer (ILC) ILC tends to present with multiple and bilateral tumor sites and is better detected with MRI than mammography. The reported sensitivity of MRI for detection of ILC, ranging from 93 % to 96 %, is significantly higher than the sensitivity of mammography, which is in the range of 34–81 % [2, 22, 59]. Further more, MRI is more accurate in assessing the extent of ILC than mammography, leading to lower re-excision rates for positive surgical margins [60, 61].

Patients at High-Risk for Developing Breast Cancer A study has shown that patients with genetic alterations (BRCA 1 and BRCA2 mutations) or a history of mantle chest radiation are also at high risk for multiple and bilateral breast cancers [62]. Patients with a family history of breast cancer may also benefit [22].

Patients with Dense Breast Tissue MRI is useful in women with mammographically dense breast, in which an additional cancer tends to be obscured [63]. However, some studies have found MRI staging to be equally beneficial in patients with non-dense breasts [21, 22, 64].

Patients with Posterior Breast Cancer As previously illustrated, MRI is very useful in the detection of pectoral muscle and chest wall invasion, which will impact surgical planning.

Patients with High Grade DCIS or Invasive Cancer with EIC As previously demonstrated, MRI has a higher sensitivity for detection of high grade DCIS, or EIC in an invasive cancer, compared to conventional imaging. Hence the extent of disease in these patients can be better defined with MRI.

Patients with Plans for Partial Breast Irradiation (PBI) PBI is increasingly used for treatment of early stage breast cancers. However, patients with multiple tumors are not fully treated with PBI and are not appropriate candidates. Several studies have demonstrated the benefit of preoperative MRI for appropriate selection of patients to undergo such therapy [65–68].

Patients with Plans for Nipple-Sparing Mastectomy (NSM) NSM is a skin-sparing mastectomy with preservation of the nipple-areolar complex to provide a good cosmetic outcome. Due to the increased cancer recurrence risk, patients with tumors invading the NAC or in close proximity to the NAC on MRI are not appropriate candidates for NSM. Conversely, a negative MRI showing no NAC involvement has a high negative predictive value, as only 2.2 % of these patients were found to have NAC involvement at surgery [69]. MRI is useful in patient selection for this procedure.

4.8 The Utility of MRI in Special Clinical Scenarios

4.8.1 Inflammatory Breast Cancer

Inflammatory breast cancer (IBC) is a rare, aggressive form of breast cancer, accounting for 1–4 % of all breast cancers [34]. As defined by AJCC, the diagnostic criteria for IBC include rapid onset of breast edema; and/or peau d'orange skin changes; and/or erythema of the breast; with or without an underlying palpable mass; duration of the symptoms no more than 6 months; skin edema occupying at least one third of the breast; and pathologic confirmation of invasive carcinoma [70]. The pathologic hallmark of IBC is tumor emboli obstructing the dermal lymphatics of the breast, although this is not a requisite for diagnosis [71].

IBC is classified as a T4d tumor regardless of the primary tumor size (Tables 4.1). The prognosis is poor, with an average survival of 12–36 months [17]. At the time of diagnosis, 55–85 % of patients have regional nodal metastases and 20 % have distant metastases [17]. The treatment for IBC is neoadjuvant chemotherapy, followed by mastectomy and chest wall radiation [71]. The role of breast imaging in IBC is to identify an underlying malignancy, guide biopsy, stage locoregional disease and monitor response to neoadjuvant chemotherapy [72].

MRI has shown superior sensitivity, in the range of 94–98 % for detection of a primary breast tumor in IBC, compared to sensitivities of 43–68 % for mammography and 94–95 % for ultrasound [73, 74]. One study reported the most frequent MRI features of IBC to be: an underlying primary breast lesion (98 %), global skin thickening (93 %), heterogeneous skin enhancement with or without nodular or irregular skin foci (84 %), breast and chest wall edema (78 %), and breast enlargement (68 %). The primary lesion may be a single mass, diffuse nonmass enhancement, or multiple masses that are confluent or interconnected by nonmass enhancement. Multicentric or multifocal disease is more common than a unifocal mass. The majority of the masses exhibited malignant features such as irregular margins, heterogeneous internal enhancement pattern, and delayed washout kinetics. In 79 % of the cases, the enhancing skin lesion showed persistent kinetics [74]. Two examples of these features are shown in Figs. 4.7 and 4.10. The most common histologic type involved in IBC is invasive ductal carcinoma (84 %), although poorly differentiated carcinoma (6 %) and invasive lobular carcinoma (5 %) are also found [74].

It is important to differentiate IBC from locally advanced breast cancer, because the treatments are different. While IBC is treated with mastectomy, patients with locally advanced breast cancer may be candidates for breast conservation after neoadjuvant chemotherapy [17]. IBC and locally advanced breast cancer have many overlapping features on MRI [34]. Some potential differentiating features in favor of IBC include: edema of the breast tissue, skin thickening, thickening and pathologic enhancement of Cooper ligaments, and the "punched-out sign" defined as initially strong focal enhancement of dermal or subcutaneous tissue, followed by slow-continuous enhancement of the surrounding skin (Figs. 4.7 and 4.10) [34].

A difficult clinical and imaging differential diagnosis of IBC is acute mastitis. Differentiation of these two entities with MRI remains challenging due to the significant overlap of morphology and enhancement kinetics [28]. Potential differentiating features in favor of IBC are: masses with a greater average size, T2 hypo intensity of masses, blooming phenomenon (decreasing sharpness of lesion borders on delayed images), infiltration or pathological enhancement of the pectoralis major muscle, perifocal edema, prepectoral and intramuscular pectoral edema, central and dorsal location of the malignant mass vs. the usual subareolar location of an abscess (Fig. 4.10) [75]. A histological punch skin biopsy is needed in cases of diagnostic uncertainty if clinical symptoms fail to improve after a trial of antibiotic therapy.

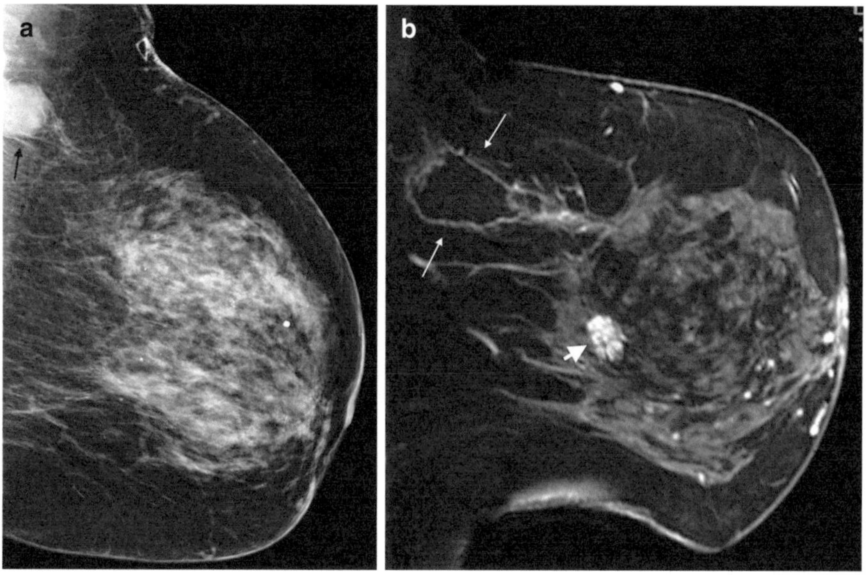

Fig. 4.14 Clinical stage IIA, T1N1M0 tumor in a 68-year-old woman with excisional biopsy of an enlarged left axillary lymph node, yielding metastatic carcinoma suggestive of a breast primary. (**a**) Left MLO view mammogram shows heterogeneously dense breast tissue with a partially visualized large high-density left axillary node (*black arrow*). No visible abnormality is identified in the breast. (**b**) Sagittal post contrast fat-saturated T1 image of left breast demonstrates a seroma at the site of lymph node excision (between *white arrows*). A 1.7 cm enhancing mass (*arrowhead*) is visualized in the central breast. Ultrasound guided biopsy revealed an invasive ductal carcinoma

4.8.2 Metastatic Axillary Lymphadenopathy of Unknown Primary Malignancy

Rarely, breast cancer may present as metastatic axillary lymphadenopathy without a known primary tumor (stage TXN1-2 M0). When a patient presents with unilateral axillary adenopathy, ultrasound guided lymph node sampling is indicated. In the event of nondiagnostic lymph node sampling, a surgical lymph node biopsy should be considered. If a malignant diagnosis suggestive of a breast primary is made, and no primary breast tumor is identified with clinical examination, mammography or ultrasound, breast MRI should be performed. The ability of MRI to identify occult primary breast cancer ranges from 62 to 86 %, with the primary tumor often less than 2 cm in size [76, 77]. The identification of the primary tumor by MRI offers patients the benefit of histologic diagnosis and biomarker evaluation (Fig. 4.14). This will provide information to guide targeted chemotherapy, hormonal treatment, and breast conservation surgery [30]. Otherwise, patients are treated with mastectomy and axillary node dissection if the primary malignancy remains unknown. In one third of cases, a primary tumor may not be identified in the mastectomy specimen (Fig. 4.12). If treated with axillary dissection alone, a high percentage of these patients will develop ipsilateral breast cancer [78]. Recently, some patients are being treated with axillary dissection and whole breast radiation, without mastectomy. The data on the efficacy of this approach are limited, with two small studies showing a 5-year local recurrence rate of 15—16 % and 5-year survival rate of 72—75 %, compared to the rates of 13 and 79 %, respectively, in the mastectomy group [78, 79].

4.8.3 Paget's Disease of the Nipple with Negative Conventional Breast Imaging

Paget's disease of the breast is an uncommon form of breast cancer accounting for 1–3 % of all breast cancers [80, 81]. It is characterized by infiltration of the nipple epidermis by large malignant adenocarcinoma cells (Paget's cells) that contains abundant cytoplasm with large pleomorphic and hyperchromatic nuclei. Patients typically present with symptoms related to the nipple and areola characterized by eczema, scaling, crust formation, erosion or ulceration, without or with a palpable mass [80]. An underlying invasive carcinoma or ductal carcinoma in situ is identified in 82–94 % of cases [81, 82]. The diagnosis is usually suspected on clinical findings, and confirmed by full thickness surgical biopsy of the nipple and areola. Imaging is required to identify an underlying malignancy and assess the extent of disease. However, imaging is normal in 22–50 % of cases with mammography alone and in 13 % of cases when both mammography and ultrasound are performed [30]. Mammography may underestimate the extent of disease in up to 43 % of cases [83]. Breast MRI is both sensitive in detecting the underlying malignancy and accurate in assessing the extent of disease, especially when mammography and ultrasound are negative [82, 83].

The MRI finding of Paget's disease is asymmetric enhancement of the nipple-areolar complex, seen in 100 % of patients with clinically proven Paget's disease in one report [39]. The underlying malignancy may appear as an enhancing mass in the case of invasive cancer or nonmass enhancement, typical of DCIS. Traditionally, Paget's disease is treated with mastectomy. Since the underlying tumors are confined to the central breast in two thirds of patients, central lumpectomy combined with resection of the NAC and radiation therapy has been adopted recently, with similar survival rates [30]. MRI can delineate the location and extent of the underlying malignancy. It can also identify the presence of multifocal or multicentric disease. This is very important, especially for patients planning breast conservation surgery [84]. A negative MRI, however, does not exclude an underlying malignancy [82].

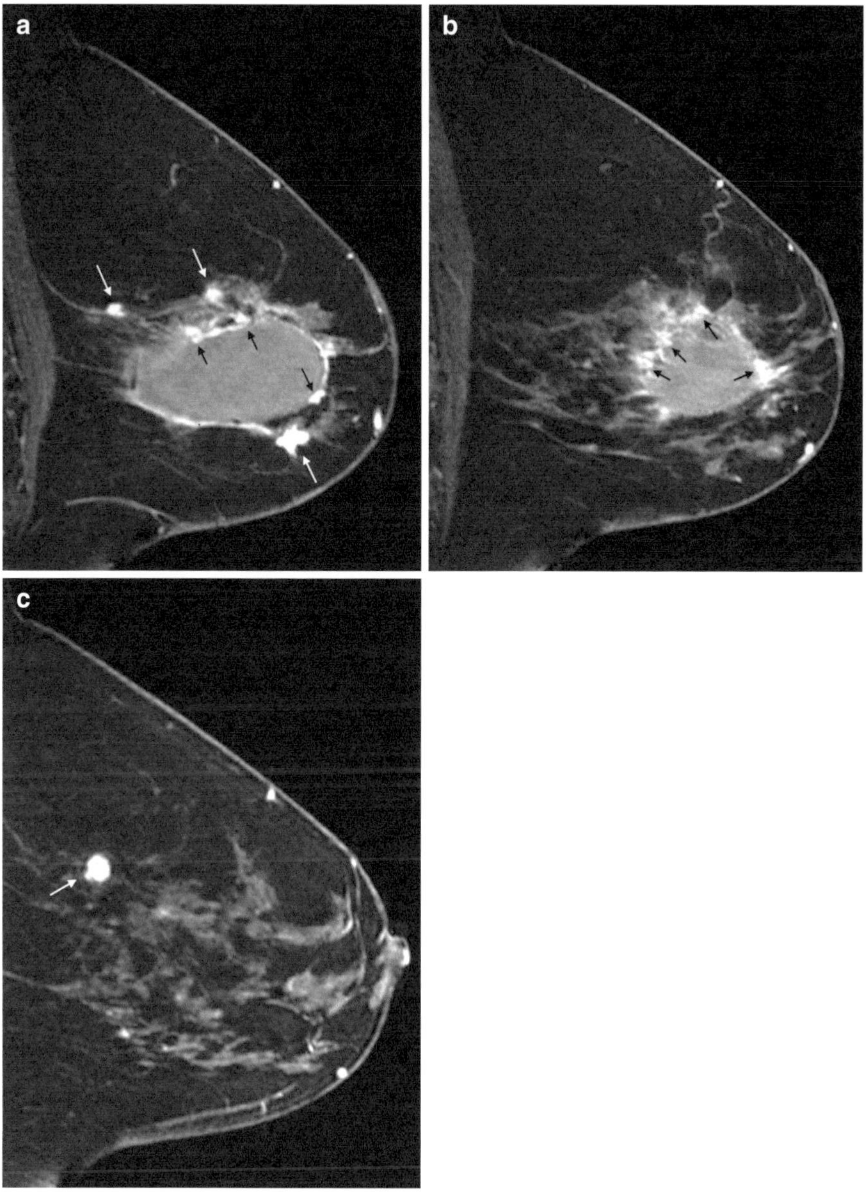

Fig. 4.15 Clinical stage II or higher, TxN1M0 tumor in a 62-year-old woman. The patient underwent a surgical biopsy at another institution for architectural distortion. Pathology yielded ILC and lobular carcinoma in situ with positive resection margins that persisted upon re-excision. Sentinel node biopsy yielded three positive metastatic nodes. (**a**) Sagittal post contrast fat-saturated T1 MR image reveals a large seroma with areas of lumpy enhancement (*black arrows*) at its margins suggestive of residual tumor. Three small enhancing masses (*white arrows*) away from the surgical cavity are concerning for multicentric tumors. (**b**) A more lateral sagittal image shows additional lumpy enhancement at the superior, posterior and anterior margins of the seroma (*black arrows*), suggestive of residual tumor. (**c**) A more medial sagittal image reveals an additional tumor focus (*arrow*)

4.8.4 Positive Surgical Margins After Initial Lumpectomy

Positive surgical margins denote the situation in which malignancy is found at the margins of the lumpectomy specimen after breast conservation surgery for breast cancer. This indicates potential residual malignancy in the breast. Patients are typically treated with repeat excision of the involved margins and may eventually require mastectomy if clear margins cannot be achieved after repeated surgery. Breast MRI has a reported sensitivity of 61–86 % for detection of residual malignancy [85–87]. It is useful in identifying bulky residual tumor at the lumpectomy site or multifocal/multicentric disease elsewhere in the breast (Fig. 4.15). This will guide the repeat excision or identify patients with extensive residual disease that would ultimately require mastectomy.

4.8.5 Known Multifocal, Multicentric or Bilateral Disease

Patients with known multifocal, multicentric or bilateral breast cancers on conventional breast imaging can benefit from MRI staging to determine the true extent of disease. This guides appropriate decision-making regarding breast conservation surgery vs. mastectomy.

4.8.6 Discordant Findings Between Clinical Examination and Imaging or Between Imaging Modalities

When the tumor size on clinical examination differs significant from the size on mammography or ultrasound, the extent of disease is uncertain. A discrepancy in tumor size between mammography and ultrasound greater than 1 cm also raises question about the true size of the tumor [14]. With its superior accuracy in determining tumor size and extent of disease, MRI should be considered in these scenarios (Fig. 4.1).

4.8.7 Planned Neoadjuvant Chemotherapy

Adjuvant chemotherapy is used to decrease the risk of recurrence and improve survival from invasive breast cancer. Neoadjuvant chemotherapy prior to surgery and radiation for local regional control has become widely adopted. It is found to be as effective as adjuvant chemotherapy, but has the added benefit of predicting patient outcome based on tumor response, and helping more patients achieve breast conservation [30]. This will be discussed in detail in the next chapter entitled "*MRI and neoadjuvant chemotherapy*".

4.9 Controversies on MRI Staging of Newly Diagnosed Breast Cancer

Improved staging with breast MRI should lead to decreased positive margins/re-excision rates, and better stratification of patients between breast conserving surgery and mastectomy due to improved surgical planning. There should be decreased local recurrence rates by identification and resection of otherwise occult multifocal or multicentric tumors. The metachronous contralateral cancer rates should also decrease, due to the simultaneous detection and treatment of contralateral tumors. However, the literature regarding the benefit of MRI staging is showing conflicting results. Therefore, the use of preoperative MRI to evaluate breast cancer remains controversial. The recent debates over the use of MRI staging are focused on the issues of *delay in definitive therapy, conflicting data on re-excision rates, increased mastectomy rates, and lack of long- term survival impact.*

4.9.1 Delay in Definitive Therapy

Two retrospective studies reported a mean treatment delay of 12.2–22.4 days in the group of patients undergoing preoperative breast MRI [88, 89]. However, Hollingsworth and associates, who routinely use preoperative MRI, asserted that all of their patients completed MRI workup within 2 weeks of diagnosis, before the surgeon's first available clinic date to see the patient. Hence, there is no delay in treatment among their patients [90]. The detection of additional lesions by MRI, necessitating additional imaging and biopsy is the downside of preoperative MRI and a potential source of delay. While unlikely to affect long-term outcome, it may contribute to patient anxiety and cost. To minimize delay, the facilities that offer breast MRI should have the capability and commitment to complete ultrasound- or MRI- guided biopsy of MRI-detected lesions promptly, or they should at least have an established referral arrangement with an experienced breast center to provide these services in a timely fashion.

4.9.2 Conflicting Data on Re-excision Rates

There are conflicting data on the impact of MRI staging on re-excision rates [60, 61, 89–98]. A meta-analysis of nine studies published between 2009 and 2012, including two randomized controlled trials and seven comparative studies (n = 3112) showed that preoperative MRI staging had no effect on re-excision rates, 11.6 % for the MRI group and 11.4 % for the non-MRI group [99]. The two prospective trials in the meta-analysis were the COMICE (Comparative Effectiveness of MRI in Breast Cancer) and MONET (MR Mammography of Nonpalpable Breast Tumors)

Table 4.5 The impact of preoperative staging MRI on re-excision rates

Lead author	Year published	Type of study	Number of patients	MRI group	No MRI group	P value
Grady	2012	Retrospective	184	11 %	26 %	0.04
Obdeijn	2013	Retrospective	123	18.9 %	37.4 %	<0.01
Sung	2014	Retrospective	174	29 %	45 %	0.02
Gonzalez	2014	Prospective	440	5 %	15 %	<0.001

Sources: Refs. [93, 100–102]

trials [97, 98]. The COMICE trial conducted in UK found no difference in re-excision rates between patients with or without MRI, both at 19 % [97]. However, because UK national health policy mandates reduction of reoperation rate for positive margins to under 10 %, surgeons routinely performed very wide excisions which could have negated the benefit of MRI. The MONET trial found a paradoxical increase in re-excision rates in patients with MRI (34 %) vs. patients without MRI (12 %). The critics of this study noted that the volume of the excised tissue in the MRI group (69.1 cm^3) was much smaller than the volume in the no MRI group (90.2 cm^3). It was even smaller in patients with DCIS and negative MRI (40.3 cm^3). Such bias in surgical approach resulted in the paradoxically higher rate of positive margins and re-excision rate in the MRI group [98].

The recent data on re-excision rates are more promising. Table 4.5 summarizes recently published studies demonstrating decreased rates of re-excision by the use of MRI staging [93, 100–102]. The data regarding ILC are particularly compelling. Although the meta-analysis by Houssami et al. showed only weak evidence that MRI reduced re-excision rate in patients with ILC, numerous studies have found significantly lower re-operation rates with the use of preoperative MRI in these patients [60, 61, 103, 104]. A recent population based study by Fortune-Greeley found a 40 % reduction in re-operation rate by MRI staging in patients with ILC (n = 1928), without increasing mastectomy [104].

4.9.3 *Increased Mastectomy Rates*

There has been a dramatic increase in the use of MRI staging among patients newly diagnosed with breast cancer, with a concurrent rise in the number of unilateral and bilateral mastectomies [105–107]. Many studies identified preoperative MRI as a predictor of mastectomy [88, 91, 99, 108, 109]. However, it is not clear whether the relationship is one of cause and effect [106]. A meta-analysis of 26 studies on the surgical impact of MRI staging found pathologically justified conversion from BCT to mastectomy in 8.3 % of cases [23]. This 8.3 % conversion rate roughly equals the 10-year local recurrence rate for breast cancer. It is probable that MRI identifies the patients with otherwise occult additional tumor burden and high likelihood for recurrence and converts their treatment to mastectomy at initial surgery. On the other hand, false positive MRI findings caused inappropriate conversion to mastectomy in only 1.7 % of cases [23]. These inappropriate mastectomies should decrease by the confirmation of more extensive disease with MRI-guided biopsy before changing the surgical plan, which was not done in all of the prior studies.

Several studies evaluated the rates of mastectomy before and after the widespread use of preoperative MRI. One study found that the mastectomy rate in the United States increased from 29 to 41 % between 2004 and 2006, predominantly among patients without MRI [105]. Another study compared the mastectomy rate before and after installation of MRI scanner at the authors' institution and found the mastectomy rate decreased from 29.9 to 24.5 %, despite sharply increased use of preoperative MRI in breast cancer patients from 17.2 to 78.7 % [107]. Hollingsworth and associates reported increased BCT rate from 48 to 60 % with the use of preoperative MRI, due to its high negative predictive value [110]. Killelea and colleagues also found that the highest BCT rate (66 %) of any group in their study was among patients with a normal MRI, even greater than in those patients without MRI [106].

A study by McGuire et al. showed three strong predictors of mastectomy to be age <40 years, large tumor size, and lymphovascular invasion. Fear of recurrence and fear of radiation are additional factors, while MRI had no impact on mastectomy rates [111]. There are several reports on the increasing rates of contralateral prophylactic mastectomy, especially among younger, highly educated patients, those with a lower stage of breast cancer, and those with a positive family history [106, 107, 112, 113]. One author observed that the rise in contralateral mastectomy is independent of increased MRI use [107].

It is clear that MRI is not the sole cause of rising ipsilateral and contralateral preventive mastectomy rates nationwide. The trend is likely multi-factorial and driven by patients [111–113]. The availability of skin and nipple sparing mastectomy and breast reconstruction surgery with good cosmetic results, the ability to identify women at high risk for in-breast recurrence, the clearer understanding of the late effects of breast irradiation, and patients' increasing knowledge about their disease and options are all contributing factors to this trend [113].

4.9.4 No Demonstrated Long-Term Survival Impact

The impact of MRI staging on long-term survival after BCT is uncertain due to the lack of long-term outcome data. Since long-term survival is directly linked to local control, study of local recurrence rates may provide some clues. However, few reports are available. A meta-analysis of four studies showed no significant effect of MRI on local or distant recurrence-free survival [114]. This analysis did not include a study by Fischer et al. that demonstrated benefits of MRI in reducing local recurrence rates (1.2 % with MRI, 6.8 % without MRI) and contralateral breast cancer rates (1.7 % with MRI, 4 % without MRI) [115]. However, the authors asserted that inclusion of Fischer's data would not have changed their conclusion [114]. A recent study by Yi et al. showed that preoperative bilateral breast MRI was associated with a reduced risk of contralateral breast recurrence [116]. Another study by Bae et al. showed the absence of preoperative MRI to be associated with an increased risk of recurrence in patients with triple-negative breast cancer [117]. This provides indirect evidence of the benefit of MRI in reducing local recurrence rates.

Given the current low rates of local recurrence after BCT and whole breast radiation (4.8–10.1 % over 10 years) and the low rate of contralateral breast cancer (4.1–5.5 %), the opponents of preoperative MRI question the benefit of finding additional cancer foci, since these foci are likely effectively treated with whole breast radiation and systemic therapy and are clinically insignificant [118, 119]. However, this may not be the case for patients undergoing partial breast irradiation. Furthermore, the International Breast MRI Consortium (IBMC) 6883 study showed that cancers detected only on MRI were similar in size and histology to cancers detected on mammography, but had a higher likelihood of being higher grade [21]. Hence, there is no basis to assume that the additional MRI-detected cancers are biologically inert or clinically irrelevant.

4.10 Conclusion

Breast MRI demonstrates superior accuracy for assessment of breast tumor size and extent of disease. Identification of multifocal/multicentric and contralateral tumors helps guide surgical planning and adjuvant therapy. While there is no consensus on the routine use of MRI in staging of all newly diagnosed breast cancers, it is proven to be beneficial in certain subsets of women. There is emerging evidence of decreases in re-excision or re-operation rates with MRI staging. No survival benefit has been demonstrated so far. A well-designed prospective randomized controlled trial on the short- and long- term benefits and cost analysis of preoperative MRI staging is needed. This is currently under development by the American College of Radiology Imaging Network (ACRIN) [120].

References

1. Breast. In: Edge S, Byrd D, Compton CC, editors. AJCC cancer staging manual. 7th ed. New York: Springer; 2010. p. 347–76.
2. Berg WA, Gutierrez L, NessAiver MS, Carter WB, Bhargavan M, Lewis RS, Ioffe OB. Diagnostic accuracy of mammography, clinical examination, US, and MR imaging in preoperative assessment of breast cancer. Radiology. 2004;233(3):830–49. doi:10.1148/radiol.2333031484.
3. Boetes C, Mus RD, Holland R, Barentsz JO, Strijk SP, Wobbes T, Hendriks JH, Ruys SH. Breast tumors: comparative accuracy of MR imaging relative to mammography and US for demonstrating extent. Radiology. 1995;197(3):743–7. doi:10.1148/radiology. 197.3.7480749.
4. Kuhl C, Kuhn W, Braun M, Schild H. Pre-operative staging of breast cancer with breast MRI: one step forward, two steps back? Breast. 2007;(16Suppl 2):S34–44.

5. Van Goethem M, Tjalma W, Schelfout K, Verslegers I, Biltjes I, Parizel P. Magnetic resonance imaging in breast cancer. Eur J Surg Oncol. 2006;32(9):901–10. doi:10.1016/j.ejso.2006.06.009.
6. Onesti JK, Mangus BE, Helmer SD, Osland JS. Breast cancer tumor size: correlation between magnetic resonance imaging and pathology measurements. Am J Surg. 2008;196(6):844–8. doi:10.1016/j.amjsurg.2008.07.028.
7. Luparia A, Mariscotti G, Durando M, Ciatto S, Bosco D, Campanino PP, Castellano I, Sapino A, Gandini G. Accuracy of tumor size assessment in the preoperative staging of breast cancer: comparison of digital mammography, tomosynthesis, ultrasound and MRI. Radiol Med. 2013;118(7):1119–36. doi:10.1007/s11547-013-0941-z.
8. Blair S, McElroy M, Middleton MS, Comstock C, Wolfson T, Kamrava M, Wallace A, Mortimer J. The efficacy of breast MRI in predicting breast conservation therapy. J Surg Oncol. 2006;94(3):220–5. doi:10.1002/jso.20561.
9. Kuhl CK, Schrading S, Bieling HB, Wardelmann E, Leutner CC, Koenig R, Kuhn W, Schild HH. MRI for diagnosis of pure ductal carcinoma in situ: a prospective observational study. Lancet. 2007;370(9586):435–92.
10. Jethava A, Ali S, Wakefield D, Crowell R, Sporn J, Vrendenburgh J. Diagnostic accuracy of MRI in predicting breast tumor size: comparative analysis of MRI vs histopathological assessed breast tumor size. Conn Med. 2015;79(5):261–7.
11. Thomassin-Naggara I, Siles P, Trop I, Chopier J, Darai E, Bazot M, Uzan S. How to measure breast cancer tumoral size at MR imaging? Eur J Radiol. 2013;82(12):e790–800. doi:10.1016/j.ejrad.2013.08.002.
12. Ikeda O, Nishimura R, Miyayama H, Yasunaga T, Ozaki Y, Tsuji A, Yamashita Y. Magnetic resonance evaluation of the presence of an extensive intraductal component in breast cancer. Acta Radiol. 2004;45(7):721–5.
13. Van Goethem M, Schelfout K, Kersschot E, Colpaert C, Verslegers I, Biltjes I, WA T, De Schepper A, Weyler J, PM P. MR mammography is useful in the preoperative locoregional staging of breast carcinomas with extensive intraductal component. Eur J Radiol. 2007;62(2):273–82. doi:10.1016/j.ejrad.2006.12.004.
14. Sardanelli F. Overview of the role of pre-operative breast MRI in the absence of evidence on patient outcomes. Breast. 2010;19(1):3–6. doi:10.1016/j.breast.2009.11.003.
15. Van Goethem M, Schelfout K, Kersschot E, Colpaert C, Verslegers I, Biltjes I, Tjalma WA, Weyler J, De Schepper A. Enhancing area surrounding breast carcinoma on MR mammography: comparison with pathological examination. Eur Radiol. 2004;14(8):1363–70. doi:10.1007/s00330-004-2295-3.
16. Lehman CD. Magnetic resonance imaging in the evaluation of ductal carcinoma in situ. J Natl Cancer Inst Monogr. 2010;2010(41):150–1. doi:10.1093/jncimonographs/lgq030.
17. Molleran VM. MRI features of ductal carcinoma in situ. In: Molleran VM, Mahoney MC, editors. Breast MRI. Philadelphia: Elsevier Saunders; 2014.
18. Miyashita M, Amano G, Ishida T, Tamaki K, Uchimura F, Ono T, Yajima M, Kuriya Y, Ohuchi N. The clinical significance of breast MRI in the management of ductal carcinoma in situ diagnosed on needle biopsy. Jpn J Clin Oncol. 2013;43(6):654–63. doi:10.1093/jjco/hyt055.
19. Wisner DJ, Hwang ES, Chang CB, Tso HH, Joe BN, Lessing JN, Lu Y, Hylton NM. Features of occult invasion in biopsy-proven DCIS at breast MRI. Breast J. 2013;19(6):650–8. doi:10.1111/tbj.12201.
20. Mori N, Ota H, Mugikura S, Takasawa C, Tominaga J, Ishida T, Watanabe M, Takase K, Takahashi S. Detection of invasive components in cases of breast ductal carcinoma in situ on biopsy by using apparent diffusion coefficient MR parameters. Eur Radiol. 2013;23(10):2705–12. doi:10.1007/s00330-013-2902-2.
21. Schnall MD, Blume J, Bluemke DA, Deangelis GA, Debruhl N, Harms S, Heywang-Kõbrunner SH, Hylton N, Kuhl CK, Pisano ED, Causer P, Schnitt SJ, Smazal SF, Stelling CB, Lehman C, Weatherall PT, Gatsonis CA. MRI detection of distinct incidental cancer in

women with primary breast cancer studied in IBMC 6883. J Surg Oncol. 2005;92(1):32–8. doi:10.1002/jso.20381.
22. Liberman L, Morris EA, Dershaw DD, Abramson AF, Tan LK. MR imaging of the ipsilateral breast in women with percutaneously proven breast cancer. AJR Am J Roentgenol. 2003;180(4):901–10.
23. Plana MN, Carreira C, Muriel A, Chiva M, Abraira V, Emparanza JI, Bonfill X, Zamora J. Magnetic resonance imaging in the preoperative assessment of patients with primary breast cancer: systematic review of diagnostic accuracy and meta-analysis. Eur Radiol. 2012;22(1):26–38. doi:10.1007/s00330-011-2238-8.
24. Houssami N, Ciatto S, Macaskill P, Lord SJ, Warren RM, Dixon JM, Irwig L. Accuracy and surgical impact of magnetic resonance imaging in breast cancer staging: systematic review and meta-analysis in detection of multifocal and multicentric cancer. J Clin Oncol. 2008;26(19):3248–58. doi:10.1200/JCO.2007.15.2108.
25. Brennan ME, Houssami N, Lord S, Macaskill P, Irwig L, Dixon JM, Warren RM, Ciatto S. Magnetic resonance imaging screening of the contralateral breast in women with newly diagnosed breast cancer: systematic review and meta-analysis of incremental cancer detection and impact on surgical management. J Clin Oncol. 2009;27(33):5640–9. doi:10.1200/JCO.2008.21.5756.
26. Lehman CD, Gatsonis C, Kuhl CK, Hendrick RE, Pisano ED, Hanna L, Peacock S, Smazal SF, Maki DD, Julian TB, DePeri ER, Bluemke DA, MD S, ACRIN Trial 6667 Investigators Group. . MRI evaluation of the contralateral breast in women with recently diagnosed breast cancer. N Engl J Med. 2007;356(13):1295–303. doi:10.1056/NEJMoa065447.
27. Obdeijn IM, Loo CE, Rijnsburger AJ, Wasser MN, Bergers E, Kok T, Klijn JG, Boetes C. Assessment of false-negative cases of breast MR imaging in women with familiar or genetic predisposition. Breast Cancer Res Treat. 2010;119(2):399–407. doi:10.1007/s10549-009-0607-7.
28. Lee SJ, Mahoney MC. Benign findings in breast MRI. In: Molleran VM, Mahoney MC, editors. Breast MRI. Philadelphia: Elsevier Saunders; 2014.
29. Morris EA. Cancer staging with breast MR imaging. In: Schnall MD, Orel SG, editors. Breast MR imaging. Philadelphia: Saunders; 2001. p. 333–44.
30. Argus A, Mahoney MC. MRI evaluation of the patient with breast cancer. In: Molleran VM, Mahoney MC, editors. Breast MRI. Philadelphia: Elsevier Saunders; 2014.
31. D'Aiuto M, Cicalese M, D'Aiuto G, Rocco G. Surgery of the chest wall for involvement by breast cancer. Thorac Surg Clin. 2010;20(4):509–17. doi:10.1016/j.thorsurg.2010.09.001.
32. Morris EA, Schwartz LH, Drotman MB, Kim SJ, Tan LK, Liberman L, Abramson AF, Van Zee KJ, Dershaw DD. Evaluation of pectoralis major muscle in patients with posterior breast tumors on breast MR images: early experience. Radiology. 2000;214(1):67–72. doi:10.1148/radiology.214.1.r00ja1667.
33. Kazama T, Nakamura S, Doi O, Suzuki K, Hirose M, Ito H. Prospective evaluation of pectoralis muscle invasion of breast cancer by MR imaging. Breast Cancer. 2005;12(4):312–6.
34. Renz DM, Baltzer PA, Bottcher J, Thaher F, Gajda M, Camara O, Runnebaum IB, Kaiser WA. Inflammatory breast carcinoma in magnetic resonance imaging: a comparison with locally advanced breast cancer. Acad Radiol. 2008;15(2):209–21. doi:10.1016/j.acra.2007.09.011.
35. Sakamoto N, Tozaki M, Hoshi K, Fukuma E. Is MRI useful for the prediction of nipple involvement? Breast Cancer. 2013;20(4):316–22. doi:10.1007/s12282-012-0338-1.
36. Steen ST, Chung AP, Han SH, Vinstein AL, Yoon JL, Giuliano AE. Predicting nipple-areolar involvement using preoperative breast MRI and primary tumor characteristics. Ann Surg Oncol. 2013;20(2):633–9. doi:10.1245/s10434-012-2641-7.
37. Ponzone R, Maggiorotto F, Carabalona S, Rivolin A, Pisacane A, Kubatzki F, Renditore S, Carlucci S, Sgandurra P, Marocco F, Magistris A, Regge D, Martincich L. MRI and intraoperative pathology to predict nipple-areola complex (NAC) involvement in patients undergo-

ing NAC-sparing mastectomy. Eur J Cancer. 2015;51(14):1882–9. doi:10.1016/j.ejca.2015.07.001.

38. D'Alonzo M, Martinchich L, Biglia N, Pisacane A, Maggiorotto F, Rosa GD, Montemurro F, Kubatzki F, Sismondi P, Ponzone R. Clinical and radiological predictors of nipple-areola complex involvement in breast cancer patients. Eur J Cancer. 2012;48(15):2311–8. doi:10.1016/j.ejca.2012.04.017.
39. Moon JY, Chang YW, Lee EH, Seo DY. Malignant invasion of the nipple-areolar complex of the breast: Usefulness of breast MRI. AJR Am J Roentgenol. 2013;201(2):448–55. doi:10.2214/AJR.12.9186.
40. Scatarige JC, Boxen IB, Smathers RL. Internal mammary lymphadenopathy: imaging of a vital lymphatic pathway in breast cancer. Radiographics. 1990;10(5):857–70. doi:10.1148/radiographics.10.5.2217975.
41. Ecanow FS, Abe H, Newstead GM, Ecanow DB, Jeske JM. Axillary staging of breast cancer: what the radiologist should know. Radiographics. 2013;33(6):1589–612. doi:10.1148/rg.336125060.
42. Chen L, Gu Y, Leaw S, Wang Z, Wang P, Hu X, Chen J, Lu J, Shao Z. Internal mammary lymph node recurrence: rare but characteristic metastasis site in breast cancer. BMC Cancer. 2010;10:479. doi:10.1186/1471-2407-10-479.
43. Alvarez S, Anõrbe E, Alcorta P, López F, Alonso I, Cortés J. Role of sonography in the diagnosis of axillary lymph node metastases in breast cancer: a systemic review. AJR Am J Roentgenol. 2006;186(5):1342–8. doi:10.2214/AJR.05.0936.
44. Mainiero MB, Cinelli CM, Koelliker SL, Graves TA, Chung MA. Axillary ultrasound and fine-needle aspiration in the preoperative evaluation of the breast cancer patient: an algorithm based on tumor size and lymph node appearance. AJR Am J Roentgenol. 2010;195(5):1261–7. doi:10.2214/AJR.10.4414.
45. Hwang SO, Lee SW, Kim HJ, Kim WW, Park HY, Jung JH. The comparative study of ultrasonography, contrast-enhanced MRI, and ^{18}F-FDG PET/CT for detecting axillary lymph node metastasis in T1 breast cancer. J Breast Cancer. 2013;16(3):315–21. doi:10.4048/jbc.2013.16.3.315.
46. Mumtaz H, Hall-Craggs MA, Davidson T, Walmsley K, Thurell W, Kissin MW, Taylor I. Staging of symptomatic primary breast cancer with MR imaging. AJR Am J Roentgenol. 1997;169(2):417–24. doi:10.2214/ajr.169.2.9242745.
47. Yoshimura G, Sakurai T, Oura S, Suzuma T, Tamaki T, Umemura T, Kokawa Y, Yang Q. Evaluation of axillary lymph node status in breast cancer with MRI. Breast Cancer. 1999;6(3):249–58.
48. Garcia Fernández A, Fraile M, Giménez N, Reñe A, Torras M, Canales L, Torres J, Barco I, González S, Veloso E, González C, Cirera L, Pessarrodona A. Use of axillary ultrasound, ultrasound-fine needle aspiration biopsy and magnetic resonance imaging in the preoperative triage of breast cancer patients considered for sentinel node biopsy. Ultrasound Med Biol. 2011;37(1):16–22. doi:10.1016/j.ultrasmedbio.2010.10.011.
49. Harnan SE, Cooper KI, Meng Y, Ward SE, Fitzgerald P, Papaioannou D, Ingram C, Lorenz E, Wilkinson ID, Wyld L. Magnetic resonance for assessment of axillary lymph node status in early breast cancer: a systematic review and meta-analysis. Eur J Surg Oncol. 2011;37(11):928–36. doi:10.1016/j.ejso.2011.07.007.
50. Valente SA, Levine GM, Silverstein MJ, Rayhanabad JA, Weng-Grumley JG, Ji L, Holmes DR, Sposto R, Sener SF. Accuracy of predicting axillary lymph node positivity by physical examination, mammography, ultrasonography and magnetic resonance imaging. Ann Surg Oncol. 2012;19(6):1825–30. doi:10.1245/s10434-011-2200-7.
51. Scaranelo AM, Eiada R, Jacks LM, Kulkarni S, Crystal P. Accuracy of unenhanced MRI imaging in the detection of axillary lymph node metastasis: study of reproducibility and reliability. Radiology. 2012;262(2):425–34. doi:10.1148/radiol.11110639.
52. Mortellaro VE, Marshall J, Singer L, Hochwald SN, Chang M, Copeland EM, Grobmyer SR. Magnetic resonance imaging for axillary staging in patients with breast cancer. J Magn Reson Imaging. 2009;30(2):309–12. doi:10.1002/jmri.21802.

53. Balzer PA, Dietzel M, Burmeister HP, Zoubi R, Gajda M, Camara O, Kaiser WA. Application of MR mammography beyond local staging: is there a potential to accurately assess axillary lymph nodes? Evaluation of an extended protocol in an initial prospective study. AJR Am J Roentgenol. 2011;196(5):W641–7.
54. Kinoshita T, Odagiri K, Andoh K, Doiuchi T, Sugimura K, Shiotani S, Asaga T. Evaluation of small internal mammary lymph node metastases in breast cancer by MRI. Radiat Med. 1999;17(3):189–93.
55. Giuliano AE, Hunt KK, Ballman KV, Beitsch PD, Whitworth PW, Blumencranz PW, Leitch AM, Saha S, McCall LM, Morrow M. Axillary dissection vs. no axillary dissection in women with invasive breast cancer and sentinel node metastasis: a randomized clinical trial. JAMA. 2011;305(6):569–75. doi:10.1001/jama.2011.90.
56. Lane DL, Adeyefa MM, Yang WT. Role of sonography for the locoregional staging of breast cancer. AJR Am J Roentgenol. 2014;203(5):1132–41. doi:10.2214/AJR.13.12311.
57. Hieken TJ, Trull BC, Boughey JC, Jones KN, Reynolds CA, Shah SS, Glazebrook KN. Preoperative axillary imaging with percutaneous lymph node biopsy is valuable in the contemporary management of patients with breast cancer. Surgery. 2013;154(4):831–8. doi:10.1016/j.surg.2013.07.017.
58. Loiselle C, Eby PR, Kim JN, Calhoun KE, Allison KH, Gadi VK, Peacock S, Storer BE, Mankoff DA, Partridge SC, Lehman CD. Preoperative MRI improves prediction of extensive occult axillary lymph node metastases in breast cancer patients with a positive sentinel lymph node biopsy. Acad Radiol. 2014;21(1):92–8. doi:10.1016/j.acra.2013.10.001.
59. Mann RM, Hoogeveeri YL, Blickman JG, Boetes C. MRI compared to conventional diagnostic work-up in the detection and evaluation of invasive lobular carcinoma of the breast: a review of existing literature. Breast Cancer Res Treat. 2008;107(1):1–14. doi:10.1007/s10549-007-9528-5.
60. Mann RM, Loo CE, Wobbes T, Bult P, Barentsz JO, Gilhuijs KG, Boetes C. The impact of preoperative breast MRI on the re-excision rate in invasive lobular carcinoma of the breast. Breast Cancer Res Treat. 2010;119(2):415–22. doi:10.1007/s10549-009-0616-6.
61. McGhan LJ, Wasif N, Gray RJ, Giurescu ME, Pizzitola VJ, Lorans R, Ocal IT, Stucky CC, Pockaj BA. Use of preoperative magnetic resonance imaging for invasive lobular cancer: good, better, but maybe not the best. Ann Surg Oncol. 2010;17(Suppl 3):255–62. doi:10.1245/s10434-010-1266-y.
62. Bergthorsson JT, Ejlertsen B, Olsen JH, Borg A, Nielsen KV, Barkardottir RB, Klausen S, Mouridsen HT, Winther K, Fenger K, Niebuhr A, Harboe TL, Niebuhr E. BRCA1 and BRCA2 mutation status and cancer family history of Danish women affected with multifocal or bilateral breast cancer at a young age. J Med Genet. 2001;38(6):361–8.
63. Sardanelli R, Giuseppetti GM, Panizza P, Bazzocchi M, Fausto A, Simonetti G, Lattanzio V, Del Maschio A, Italian Trial for Breast MR in Multifocal/Multicentric Cancer. Sensitivity of MRI versus mammography for detecting foci of multifocal, multicentric breast cancer in fatty and dense breasts using the whole-breast pathologic examination as a gold standard. AJR Am J Roentgenol. 2004;183(4):1149–57. doi:10.2214/ajr.183.4.1831149.
64. Gutierrez RL, DeMartini WB, Silbergeld JJ, Eby PR, Peacock S, Javid SH, Lehman CD. High cancer yield and positive predictive value: outcomes at a center routinely using preoperative breast MRI for staging. AJR Am J Roentgenol. 2011;196(1):W93–9. doi:10.2214/AJR.10.4804.
65. Al-Hallaq HA, Mell LK, Bradley JA, Chen LF, Ali AN, Weichselbaum RR, Newstead GM, Chmura SJ. Magnetic resonance imaging identifies multifocal and multicentric disease in breast cancer patients who are eligible for partial breast irradiation. Cancer. 2008;113(9):2408–14. doi:10.1002/cncr.23872.
66. Godinez J, Combos EC, Chikarmane SA, Griffin GK, Birdwell RL. Breast MRI in the evaluation of eligibility for accelerated partial breast irradiation. AJR Am J Roentgenol. 2008;191(1):272–7. doi:10.2214/AJR.07.3465.

67. Tendulkar RD, Chellman-Jeffers M, Rybicki LA, Rim A, Kotwal A, Macklis R, BB O. Preoperative breast magnetic resonance imaging in early breast cancer: implications for partial breast irradiation. Cancer. 2009;115(8):1621–30. doi:10.1002/cncr.24172.
68. Di Leo G, Trimboli RM, Benedek A, Jereczek-Fossa BA, Fossati P, Leonardi MC, Carbonaro LA, Orecchia R, Sardanelli F. MR imaging for selection of patients for partial breast irradiation: a systematic review and meta-analysis. Radiology. 2015;277(3):716–26. doi:10.1148/radiol.2015142508.
69. Sakamoto N, Fukuma E, Higa K, Ozaki S, Sakamoto M, Abe S, Kurihara T, Tozaki M. Early results of an endoscopic nipple-sparing mastectomy for breast cancer. Ann Surg Oncol. 2009;16(12):3406–13. doi:10.1245/s10434-009-0661-8.
70. Dawood S, Merajver SD, Viens P, Vermeulen PB, Swain SM, Buchholz TA, Dirix LY, Levine PH, Lucci A, Krishnamurthy S, Robertson FM, Woodward WA, Yang WT, Ueno NT, Cristofanilli M. International expert panel on inflammatory breast cancer: consensus statement for standardized diagnosis and treatment. Ann Oncol. 2011;22(3):515–23. doi:10.1093/annonc/mdq345.
71. Robertson FM, Bondy M, Yang W, Yamauchi H, Wiggins S, Kamrudin S, Krishnamurthy S, Le-Petross H, Bidaut L, Player AN, Barsky SH, Woodward WA, Buchholz T, Lucci A, Ueno NT, Cristofanilli M. Inflammatory breast cancer: the disease, the biology, the treatment. CA Cancer J Clin. 2010;60(6):351–75. doi:10.3322/caac.20082.
72. Le-Petross CH, Bidaut L, Yang WT. Evolving role of imaging modalities in inflammatory breast cancer. Semin Oncol. 2008;35(1):51–63. doi:10.1053/j.seminoncol.2007.11.016.
73. Yang WT, Le-Petross HT, Macapinlac H, Carkaci S, Gonzalez-Angulo AM, Dawood S, Resetkova E, Hortobagyi GN, Cristofanilli M. Inflammatory breast cancer: PET/CT, MRI, mammography and sonography findings. Breast Cancer Res Treat. 2008;109(3):417–26. doi:10.1007/s10549-007-9671-z.
74. Le-Petross HT, Cristofanilli M, Carkaci S, Krishnamurthy S, Jackson EF, Harrell RK, Reed BJ, Yang WT. MRI features of inflammatory breast cancer. AJR Am J Roentgenol. 2011;197(4):W769–76.
75. Renz DM, Baltzer PA, Böttcher J, Thaher F, Gajda M, Camara O, Runnebaum IB, Kaiser WA. Magnetic resonance imaging of inflammatory breast carcinoma and acute mastitis. A comparative study. Eur Radiol. 2008;18(11):2370–80. doi:10.1007/s00330-008-1029-3.
76. Orel SG, Weinstein SP, Schnall MD, Reynolds CA, Schuchter LM, Fraker DL, Solin LJ. Breast MR imaging in patients with axillary node metastases and unknown primary malignancy. Radiology. 1999;212(2):543–9. doi:10.1148/radiology.212.2.r99au40543.
77. Buchanan CL, Morris EA, Dorn PL, Borgen PI, Van Zee KJ. Utility of breast magnetic resonance imaging in patients with occult primary breast cancer. Ann Surg Oncol. 2005;12(12):1045–53. doi:10.1245/ASO.2005.03.520.
78. Masinghe SP, Faluyi OO, Kerr GR, Kunkler IH. Breast radiotherapy for occult breast cancer with axillary nodal metastases – does it reduce the local recurrence rate and increase overall survival? Clin Oncol (R Coll Radiol). 2011;23(2):95–100.
79. Vlastos G, Jean ME, Mirza AN, Mirza NQ, Kuerer HM, Ames FC, Hunt KK, Ross MI, Buchholz TA, Buzdar AU, Sigletary SE. Feasibility of breast preservation in the treatment of occult primary carcinoma presenting with axillary metastases. Ann Surg Oncol. 2001;8(5):425–31.
80. Ashikari R, Park K, Huvos A, Urban JA. Paget's disease of the breast. Cancer. 1970;26(3):680–5.
81. Kollmorgen DR, Varanasi JS, Edge SB, Carson 3rd WE. Paget's disease of the breast: a 33 year experience. J Am Coll Surg. 1998;187(2):171–7.
82. Morrogh M, Morris EA, Liberman L, Van Zee K, Cody 3rd HS, King TA. MRI identifies otherwise occult disease in select patients with Paget disease of the nipple. J Am Coll Surg. 2008;206(2):316–21. doi:10.1016/j.jamcollsurg.2007.07.046.

83. Kothari AS, Beechey-Newman N, Hamed H, Fentiman IS, D'Arrigo C, Hanby AM, Ryder K. Paget disease of the nipple: a multifocal manifestation of higher-risk disease. Cancer. 2002;95(1):1–7. doi:10.1002/cncr.10638.
84. Corsi F, Sartani A, Galli D, Alineri S, Uccelli M, Fontana A, Foschi D. Usefulness of preoperative diagnosis with magnetic resonance imaging for conservative surgery in Paget's disease of the breast. Breast Care. 2010;5(1):26–8. doi:10.1159/000272304.
85. Frei KA, Kinkel K, Bonel HM, Lu Y, Esserman LJ, Hylton NM. MR imaging of the breast in patients with positive margins after lumpectomy. Influence of the time interval between lumpectomy and MR imaging. AJR Am J Roentgenol. 2000;175(6):1577–84. doi:10.2214/ajr.175.6.1751577.
86. Orel SG, Reynolds C, Schnall MD, Solin LJ, Fraker DL, Sullivan DC. Breast carcinoma MR imaging before re-excisional biopsy. Radiology. 1997;205(2):429–36. doi:10.1148/radiology.205.2.9356624.
87. Lee JM, Orel SG, Czerniecki BJ, Solin LJ, Schnall MD. MRI before re-excision surgery in patients with breast cancer. AJR Am J Roentgenol. 2004;182(2):473–80. doi:10.2214/ajr.182.2.1820473.
88. Bleicher RJ, Ciocca RM, Egleston BL, Sesa L, Evers K, Sigurdson ER, Morrow M. Association of routine pretreatment magnetic resonance imaging with time to surgery, mastectomy rate, and margin status. J Am Coll Surg. 2009;209(2):180–7. doi:10.1016/j.jamcollsurg.2009.04.010.
89. Chandwani S, George PA, Azu M, Bandera EV, Ambrosone CB, Rhoads GG, Demissie K. Role of preoperative magnetic resonance imaging in the surgical management of early-stage breast cancer. Ann Surg Oncol. 2014;21(11):3473–80. doi:10.1245/s10434-014-3748-9.
90. Hollingsworth AB, Stough RG, O'Dell CA, Brekke CE. Breast magnetic resonance imaging for preoperative locoregional staging. Am J Surg. 2008;196(3):389–97. doi:10.1016/j.amjsurg.2007.10.009.
91. Pengel KE, Loo CE, Teertstra HJ, Muller SH, Wesseling J, Peterse JL, Bartelink H, Rutgers EJ, Gilhuijs KG. The impact of preoperative MRI on breast-conserving surgery of invasive cancer: a comparative cohort study. Breast Cancer Res Treat. 2009;116(1):161–9. doi:10.1007/s10549-008-0182-3.
92. Allen LR, Lago-Toro CE, Hughes JH, Careaga E, Brown AT, Chernick M, Barrio AV, Frazier TG. Is there a role for MRI in the preoperative assessment of patients with DCIS? Ann Surg Oncol. 2010;17(9):2395–400. doi:10.1245/s10434-010-1000-9.
93. Obdeijn IM, Tilaanus-Linthorst MM, Spronk S, van Deurzen CH, de Monye C, Hunink MG, Menke MB. Preoperative breast MRI can reduce the rate of tumor-positive resection margins and reoperatations in patients undergoing breast-conserving surgery. AJR Am J Roentgenol. 2013;200(2):304–10. doi:10.2214/AJR.12.9185.
94. Hwang N, Schiller DE, Crystal P, Maki E, McCready DR. Magnetic resonance imaging in the planning of initial lumpectomy for invasive breast carcinoma: its effect on ipsilateral breast tumor recurrence after breast-conservation therapy. Ann Surg Oncol. 2009;16(11):3000–9. doi:10.1245/s10434-009-0607-1.
95. Weber JJ, Bellin LS, Milbourn DE, Verbanac KM, Wong JH. Selective preoperative magnetic resonance imaging in women with breast cancer: no reduction in the reoperation rate. Arch Surg. 2010;147(9):834–9.
96. Wang SY, Kuntz KM, Tuttle TM, Jacobs Jr DR, Kane RL, Virnig BA. The association of preoperative breast magnetic resonance imaging and multiple breast surgeries among older women with early stage breast cancer. Breast Cancer Res Treat. 2013;138(1):137–47. doi:10.1007/s10549-013-2420-6.
97. Turnbull L, Brown S, Harvey I, Olivier C, Drew P, Napp V, Hanby A, Brown J. Comparative effectiveness of MRI in breast cancer (COMICE) trial: a randomized controlled trial. Lancet. 2010;375(9714):563–71. doi:10.1016/S0140-6736(09)62070-5.
98. Peter NH, van Esser S, van den Bosch MA, et al. Preoperative MRI and surgical management in patients with nonpalpable breast cancer: the MONET – randomized controlled trial. Eur J Cancer. 2011;47(6):879–86.

99. Houssami N, Turner R, Morrow M. Preoperative magnetic resonance imaging in breast cancer: meta-analysis of surgical outcomes. Ann Surg. 2013;257(2):249–55. doi:10.1097/SLA.0b013e31827a8d17.
100. Grady I, Gorsuch-Rafferty H, Hadley P. Preoperative staging with magnetic resonance imaging, with confirmatory biopsy, improves surgical outcomes in women with breast cancer without increasing rates of mastectomy. Breast J. 2012;18(3):214–8. doi:10.1111/j.1524-4741.2012.01227.x.
101. Sung JS, Li J, DaCosta G, Patil S, Van Zee K, Dershaw DD, Morris EA. Preoperative breast MRI for early stage breast cancer: effect on surgical and long-term outcomes. AJR Am J Roentgenol. 2014;202:1376–82. doi:10.2214/AJR.13.11355.
102. Gonzalez V, Sandelin K, Karlsson A, Aberg W, Löfgren L, Iliescu G, Eriksson S, Arver B. Preoperative MRI of the breast (POMB) influences primary treatment in breast cancer: a prospective randomized multicenter study. World J Surg. 2014;38(7):1685–93. doi:10.1007/s00268-014-2605-0.
103. Rodenko GN, Harms SE, Pruneda JM, Farrell Jr RS, Evans WP, Copit DS, Krakos PA, Flamig DP. MR imaging in the management before surgery of lobular carcinoma of the breast: correlation with pathology. AJR Am J Roentgenol. 1996;167(6):1415–9. doi:10.2214/ajr.167.6.8956569.
104. Fortune-Greeley AK, Wheeler SB, Meyer AM, Reeder-Hayes KE, Biddle AK, Muss HB, Carpenter WR. Preoperative breast MRI and surgical outcomes in elderly women with invasive ductal and lobular carcinoma: a population-based study. Breast Cancer Res Treat. 2014;143(1):203–12. doi:10.1007/s10549-013-2787-4.
105. Katipamula R, Degnim AC, Hoskin T, Boughey JC, Loprinzi C, Grant CS, Brandt KR, Pruthi S, Chute CG, Olson JE, Couch FJ, Ingle JN, Goetz MP. Trends in mastectomy rates at the Mayo Clinic Rochester: effect of surgical years and preoperative MRI. J Clin Oncol. 2009;27(25):4082–8. doi:10.1200/JCO.2008.19.4225.
106. Killelea BK, Grube BJ, Rishi M, Philpotts L, Tran EJ, Lannin DR. Is the use of preoperative breast MRI predictive of mastectomy? World J Surg Oncol. 2013;11:154. doi:10.1186/1477-7819-11-154.
107. Guilfoyle C, Christoudias M, Collett A, Gracely EJ, Frazier TG, Barrio AV. Effect of preoperative MRI on mastectomy and contralateral prophylactic mastectomy rates at a community hospital by a single surgeon. Breast J. 2014;20(1):79–83. doi:10.1111/tbj.12204.
108. Feigelson HS, James TA, Single RM, Onitilo AA, Aiello Bowles EJ, Barney T, Bakerman JE, McCahill LE. Factors associated with the frequency of initial total mastectomy: results of a multi-institutional study. J Am Coll Surg. 2013;216(5):966–75. doi:10.1016/j.jamcollsurg.2013.01.011.
109. Heil J, Rauch G, Szabo AZ, Garcia-Etienne CA, Golatta M, Domschke C, Badiian M, Kern P, Schuetz F, Wallwiener M, Sohn C, Fries H, von Minckwitz G, Schneeweiss A, Rezai M. Breast cancer mastectomy trends between 2006 and 2010: association with magnetic resonance imaging, immediate breast reconstruction and hospital volume. Ann Surg Oncol. 2013;20(12):3839–46. doi:10.1245/s10434-013-3097-0.
110. Hollingsworth AB, Stough RG. Conflicting outcomes with preoperative breast MRI: differences in technology or methodology? Breast Dis Year Book Quarterly. 2010;21(2):109–12.
111. McGuire KP, Santillan AA, Kaur P, Meade T, Parbhoo J, Mathias M, Shamehdi C, Davis M, Ramos D, Cox CE. Are mastectomies on the rise? A 13-year trend analysis of the selection of mastectomy versus breast conservation therapy in 5,865 patients. Ann Surg Oncol. 2009;16(10):2682–90. doi:10.1245/s10434-009-0635-x.
112. Jones NB, Wilson J, Kotur L, Stephens J, Farrar WB, Agnese DM. Contralateral prophylactic mastectomy for unilateral breast cancer: an increasing trend at a single institution. Ann Surg Oncol. 2009;16(10):2691–6. doi:10.1245/s10434-009-0547-9.
113. Balch CM, Jacobs LK. Mastectomies on the rise for breast cancer: the tide is changing. Ann Surg Oncol. 2009;16(10):2669–72. doi:10.1245/s10434-009-0634-y.
114. Houssami N, Turner R, Macaskill P, Turnbull LW, McCready DR, Tuttle TM, Vapiwala N, Solin LJ. An individual person data meta-analysis of preoperative magnetic resonance imag-

ing and breast cancer recurrence. J Clin Oncol. 2014;32(5):392–402. doi:10.1200/JCO.2013.52.7515.
115. Fischer U, Zachariae O, Baum F, von Heyden D, Funke M, Liersch T. The influence of preoperative MRI of the breasts on recurrence rate in patients with breast cancer. Eur Radiol. 2004;14(10):1725–31. doi:10.1007/s00330-004-2351-z.
116. Yi A, Cho N, Yang KS, Han W, Noh DY, Moon WK. Breast cancer recurrence in patients with newly diagnosed breast cancer without and with preoperative MR imaging: A matched cohort study. Radiology. 2015;276(3):695–705. doi:10.1148/radiol.2015142101.
117. Bae MS, Moon HG, Han W, Noh DY, Ryu HS, Park IA, Chang JM, Cho N, Moon WK. Early stage triple-negative breast cancer: imaging and clinical-pathologic factors associated with recurrence. Radiology. 2015;31:150089 doi:10.1148/radiol.2015150089. [Epub ahead of print].
118. Morrow M. Magnetic resonance imaging in the breast cancer patient: curb your enthusiasm. J Clin Oncol. 2008;26(3):352–3. doi:10.1200/JCO.2007.14.7314.
119. Solin LJ. Counterview: pre-operative breast MRI (magnetic resonance imaging) is not recommended for all patients with newly diagnosed breast cancer. Breast. 2010;19(1):7–9. doi:10.1016/j.breast.2009.11.004.
120. ACRIN American College of Radiology Imaging Network website. Protocol 6694: effect of preoperative breast MRI on surgical outcomes, costs and quality of life in women with breast cancer (Alliance A011104/ACRIN 6694). www.acrin.org/protocolsummarytable/protocol6694.aspx. Accessed 20 Nov 2015.

Chapter 5
Magnetic Resonance Imaging and Neoadjuvant Chemotherapy

H.T. Carisa Le-Petross, Bora Lim, and Nola Hylton

Abstract Neoadjuvant chemotherapy (NAC) is now widely used internationally to provide improved surgical outcomes, recurrent free survival, and overall survival in certain subtypes of breast cancer. Therefore, the opportunity to monitor treatment response *in vivo* and as early in the treatment as possible to identify non-responders is critical. Early initiation of systemic therapy can improve overall and disease-free survival for patients with locally advanced breast cancer (LABC) or inflammatory cancer even though these patients usually receive mastectomies despite complete response after NAC. For non-responders, the sooner these patients are identified, the quicker changes to treatment plans can be made to identify a more ideal regimen for them in a timely manner. Physical examination, mammography, and sonography have all been used to assess the response to NAC, primarily by measuring the size of the residual tumor. Internationally, the 'Response Evaluation Criteria in Solid Tumors" (RECIST) is commonly used to standardize the assessment of response to therapy, based on the tumor size. Unfortunately size assessment does not take into account treatment-induced fibrosis or inflammation which can result in overestimation or underestimation of the residual disease. Magnetic resonance imaging (MRI) with intravenous contrast and advanced MRI techniques provide new opportunities for assessing tumor morphologic changes, tumor vascularity, tumor cellularity, and tumor metabolic features. MRI has been shown to be more accurate and reliable than physical examination, mammography, or sonography. The combination of contrast-enhanced MRI with diffusion-weighted imaging (DWI) and better understanding of tumor biology and genomics improve our ability to predict responders

H.T.C. Le-Petross, MD (✉)
Department of Radiology, MD Anderson Cancer Center, Houston, TX, USA
e-mail: hlepetross@mdanderson.org

B. Lim, MD
Breast Medical Oncology, The University of Texas MD Anderson Cancer Center, Houston, TX, USA

N. Hylton, PhD
Department of Radiology, University of California, San Francisco, San Francisco, CA, USA

S.L. Heller, L. Moy (eds.), *Breast Oncology: Techniques, Indications, and Interpretation*, DOI 10.1007/978-3-319-42563-4_5

from non-responders. To date, there is still no consensus on the role of MRI for assessing response to NAC or on a standardized MRI examination in patients receiving NAC.

Keywords Magnetic resonance imaging • Preoperative chemotherapy • Neoadjuvant chemotherapy • Breast cancer • Response • Pathological complete response

Abbreviations

AC	Anthracycline-cyclophosphamide
ACRIN	American College of Radiology Imaging Network
ADC	Apparent diffusion coefficient map
NAC	Neoadjuvant chemotherapy
DCE-MRI	Dynamic contrast-enhanced MRI
DWI	Diffusion-weighted imaging
FTV	Functional tumor volume
HER 2+ tumor	Human epidermal growth factor receptor 2–positive breast cancer
HR	Hormone receptor
I-SPY TRIAL	Investigation of Serial studies to Predict Your Therapeutic Response with Imaging And moLecular analysis Trial
LABC	Locally advanced breast cancer
NCCN	National Comprehensive Cancer Network
OS	Overall survival
pCR	Pathological complete response to therapy
RCB	Residual cancer burden
RECIST	Response Evaluation Criteria in Solid Tumors
RFS	Recurrent free survival
TNBC	Triple negative breast cancer

5.1 Introduction

Neoadjuvant chemotherapy (NAC) or preoperative systemic therapy given prior to surgery is now widely used as an alternative to the traditional approach of postoperative adjuvant chemotherapy in patients with breast cancer. The term 'neoadjuvant' originated from 'adjuvant', which indicates the systemic therapy after the surgery, but in this case to be given before the surgery, which was a new method developed after adjuvant therapy. To avoid confusion, it has been suggested to use 'pre-operative' instead of neoadjuvant; however, neoadjuvant is a more widely used term. NAC is a critical therapeutic approach in breast cancer in the modern era, especially for patients with locally advanced breast cancer, who are not candidates for breast-conserving surgery or who have proven lymph node metastases [1–3]. Current National Comprehensive Cancer Network (NCCN) guidelines recommend stage II and III patients to undergo NAC. For cancers with lymph node involvement, NAC can reduce the patients' risk of exposure to non-oppressed malignant metastatic behavior of cancer cells before the patient is taken to local therapy with surgery. Even without lymph node involvement, patients can benefit from NAC if NAC can successfully reduce tumor burden and result in downgrading of surgery from mastectomy to breast conserving surgery, and increase the chance of clear surgical margins. Recent data supporting better overall clinical outcome with breast conserving surgery compared to mastectomy favor the utilization of NAC [4, 5].

The traditional postoperative adjuvant trial usually has disease relapse or survival as the definitive endpoints. These types of trials are large and expensive with many years of follow-up. Today, NAC has been shown to be as effective as chemotherapy after surgery [6–8]. NAC trials use intermediate endpoints such as pathological complete response to therapy (pCR), and are smaller and less expensive trials. These intermediate endpoints can be achieved in months versus years. Both human epidermal growth factor receptor (HER) 2–positive breast cancer and triple negative breast cancer (TNBC) show a direct correlation between achieving pCR and longer recurrent free survival (RFS) and overall survival (OS) [9]. This enables clinical trials with NAC to have shorter surrogate endpoints, such as response to therapy or residual disease instead of OS, without having to wait for several decades in some clinical settings [10–12].

The combination of NAC and surgery has been shown to offer better local disease control and overall survival than surgery alone, especially for those with LABC [13, 14]. Moreover, NAC may allow the conversion of non-operable to operable disease or permit breast conservation surgery in patients who otherwise would have required mastectomy. However, a complete pathological response to NAC does not occur in all patients. Most studies have shown that pCR is associated with favorable outcomes. In the National Surgical Adjuvant Breast and Bowel Project B-27 neoadjuvant trial, a significant number of patients did achieve a pCR when paclitaxel was added to a doxorubicin-based chemotherapy regimen, but the improvement in the pCR rate was not significantly associated with prolonged RFS or overall survival [15]. Several recent studies have confirmed these observations [16, 17]. In the imaging literature, radiological complete response does not consistently translate to absence of residual disease on final pathology, RFS, or OS [18]. All agree that it is important to identify early in the course of therapy which patients are likely to have a complete response to therapy and which patients are not. However, the best method and which imaging features may be used to predict responders from non-responders is still not clear.

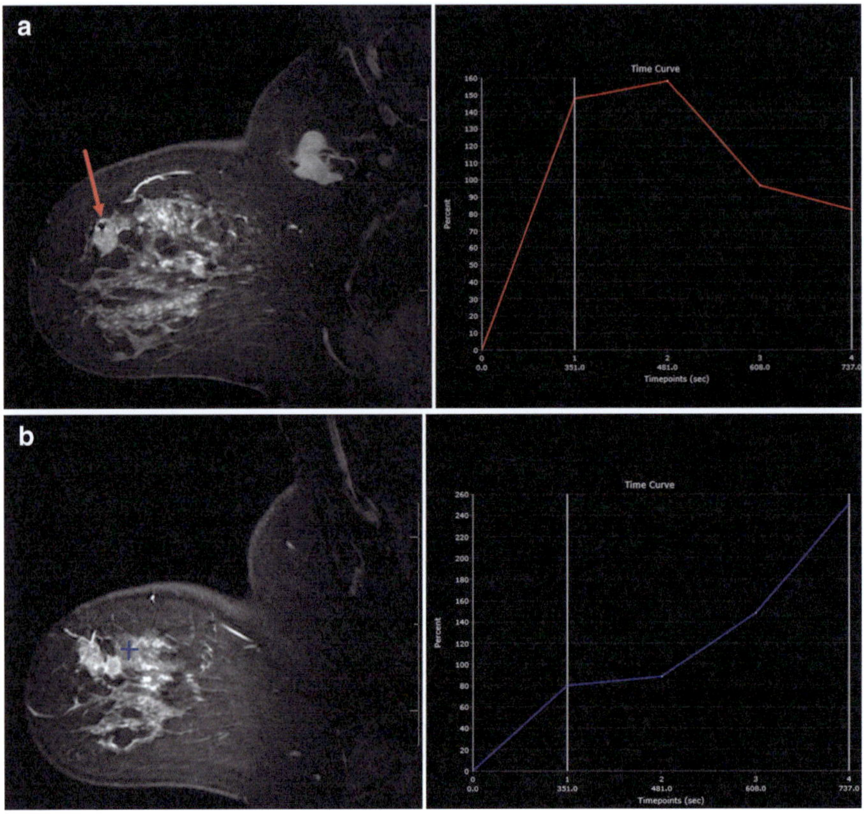

Fig. 5.1 44 year old female with newly diagnosed triple negative invasive ductal carcinoma. (**a**) Sagittal post-contrast fat-saturated MRI nicely differentiates the untreated hypervascular tumor mass (*red arrow*) with delayed washout enhancing pattern (*red curve*) from the (**b**) background glandular tissue with persistent or benign enhancing pattern (*blue cross and blue curve*)

5.2 Assessment of NAC Response

Physical exam, mammography, and sonography (US) have all been used to assess response to NAC (Fig. 5.1). Physical exam is unreliable and subjective, relying on the physician's experience. Post-treatment fibrosis versus residual necrotic tissue from residual viable tumor mass cannot be differentiated on physical exam. Macroscopic tumor at histological examination has been reported in 45% of patients with normal physical exam, while 60% of patients with pCR had an abnormal physical exam [13]. Physical exam has overestimated tumor regression in 23% of cases and underestimated response in 9% [19].

Mammography may overestimate residual disease because of a lack of change in the microcalcifications associated with the tumor. A study of 196 patients with invasive ductal carcinoma and ductal carcinoma-in-situ noted that the extent of microcalcifications on mammography after NAC had lower correlation with residual pathologic tumor than did residual enhancement seen on MRI [20]. Early series evaluating the role of US reported that US tends to underestimate residual tumor size and is less accurate than physical examination [21–23]. MRI is the first breast imaging modality that not only allows detailed visualization of the anatomy but also—when an intravenous contrast agent is administered or advanced sequences, such as DWI or spectroscopy, are used—provides functional information. This article reviews the published data on the role of breast MRI in assessing tumor response in women receiving neoadjuvant chemotherapy.

5.3 Magnetic Resonance Imaging Compared to Other Modalities

Breast MRI traditionally has a high reported sensitivity of up to 97% for the detection of invasive breast cancer, with a wide range between 50 and 100% for the assessment of response to NAC. This high sensitivity is dependent on the ability of MRI to differentiate untreated hypervascular tumor from the background enhancing glandular breast tissue (Fig. 5.1). In patients undergoing NAC, the anti-angiogenic effect of cytotoxic chemotherapy agents reduces tumor vascularity. This decrease in tumor vascularity would be expected to be associated with a decrease in enhancement of that lesion on MRI. This dampening effect of chemotherapy on enhancement of the lesion may compromise the ability to visualize residual viable tumor (Fig. 5.2). However, the alteration of tumor vascularity or other MR characteristics can help identify predictive features to differentiate patients whose cancer is likely to respond to the chemotherapy from those whose cancer would not respond. The dampening effect is not only observed with the tumor but also with the background parenchyma. The average decrease in background enhancement after NAC in cases with complete response was more than in cases with partial response, stable disease, or progressive disease [24].

In the last decade, over 40 studies have been published on the use of MRI in identifying assessing treatment response [3, 10–49]. Many of these studies are single-center trials with small sample sizes, or are meta-analysis of the small sample size studies. The studies vary in many parameters such as the criteria used for distinguishing complete responders from partial responders and non-responders. The MRI examinations performed in each trial are not standardized with regards to the Tesla strength of the scanners, number and type of MRI sequences performed for each examination, number of post-contrast sequences performed, timing of post-contrast sequences, or addition of advanced imaging techniques such as DWI or spectroscopy. Despite these differences, many of the observations from these studies are similar. MRI tends to perform better than clinical exam, mammography, or US and is a more reliable method in assessing tumor size. US was suggested to be more likely underestimate tumor size [24]. A small percentage of investigators

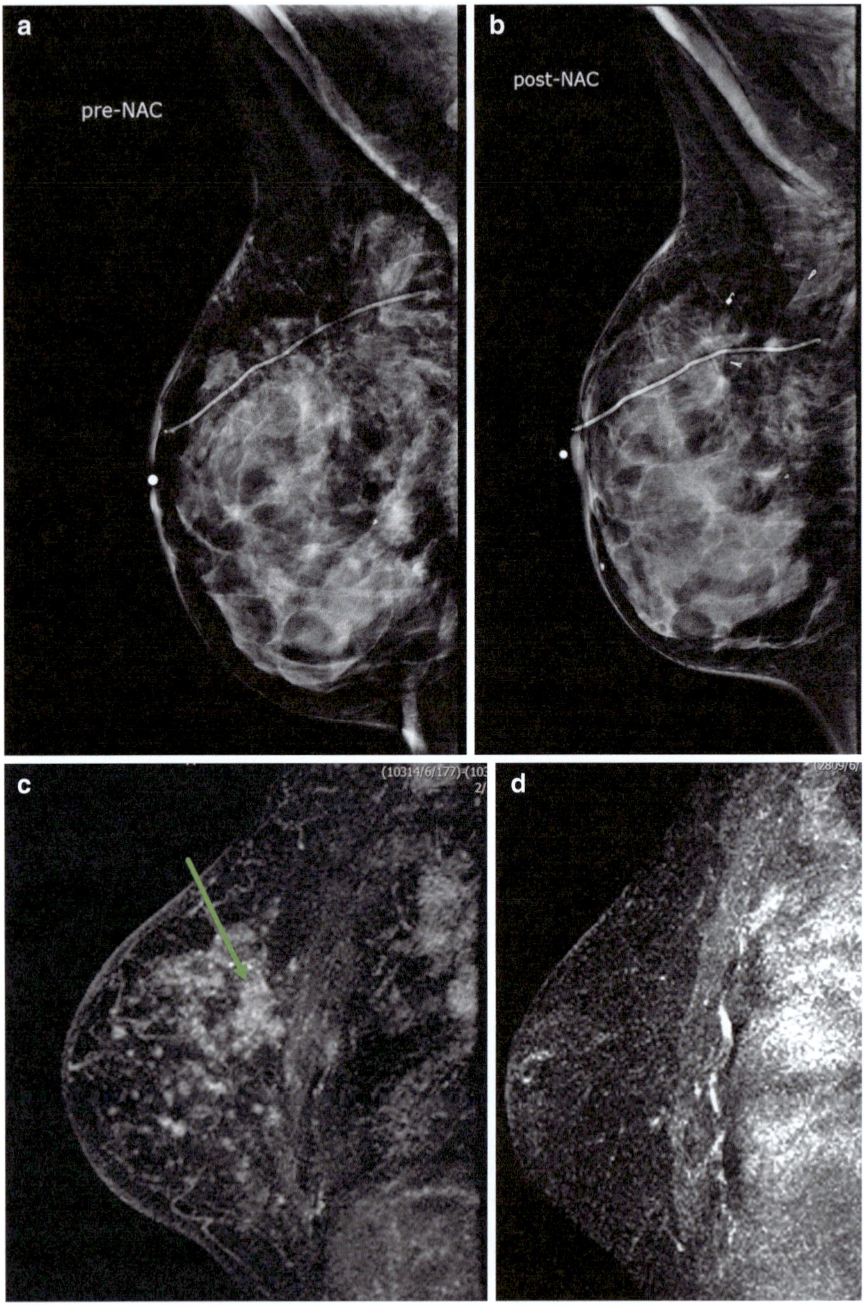

Fig. 5.2 49 year old female with outside excisional biopsy for a palpable finding revealing invasive lobular carcinoma, who received NAC followed by mastectomy. Mammogram prior to NAC (**a**) and after NAC (**b**) show no significant change. Sagittal post-contrast fat-saturated MRI prior to (**c**) and after chemotherapy (**d**) shows complete response by imaging, with no residual suspicious enhancement. Final pathology reveal 10 cm tumor bed with 15% cellularity

noted no difference between the performance of MRI and US [25–29]. Conflicting observations remain with regards to the best modalities for assessing response, even though MRI is favored, with PET/CT emerging as possible better modality. The ability of MRI in assessing specific features is discussed in further details below.

5.4 MRI Assessment of Tumor Size

Accurate measurement of tumor size, before NAC, is important for staging, treatment monitoring and determining prognosis. Tumor size has been known to predict patient survival and is the basis of most disease-staging systems [21]. Studies have shown that imaging-based measurements are superior to clinical palpation in determining tumor size [31–35]. Specifically MRI better reflects true pathological tumor size than does physical examination, mammography, or US and is also superior in predicting the amount of residual disease after NAC [31–35]. Several studies have shown that MRI prediction of tumor response to NAC correlates well with pathology, with the correlation coefficient (r) ranging between 0.6 and 0.9 [31, 37–42]. MRI is not a perfect test and can over estimate or under estimate final pathological tumor size, with a tendency to over-estimate in as many as 6–33% of the cases [35–37, 41]. US, on the other hand, tends to underestimate tumor size [30]. The amount of MRI overestimation is small or within 1 cm of the final tumor size, and may not be statistically significant [36, 37]. The residual tumor that MRI may miss post-NAC is also small, ranging between 0.1 – 1.0 cm with median of 0.6 cm [43, 44]. MRI may also underestimate residual disease in 2–10% of cases, especially if the tumor shrinkage pattern is patchy with areas of necrosis between nests of viable tumor or residual single tumor cell or tiny foci scattered over a large area [37, 39, 42–44]. Underestimation by MRI may be more frequently seen with some chemotherapy agents than others. For example, underestimation was seen more frequently in locally advanced breast cancer patients treated with docetaxel-based chemotherapy, than in those treated with 5-fluoro-uraci-epirubicin regimens [44]. These contradicting observations of underestimation and overestimation by MRI are derived from single institutional trials with small sample sizes. Therefore, validation studies are needed with larger sample sizes and standardization chemotherapy regimens.

Tumor volume calculations, in combination with largest tumor diameter, have been proposed as a better parameter to assess response to NAC. Partridge et al. [40] reports that a change in the final tumor volume measurements by MRI had a stronger association with RFS compared to other prognostic indicators such as largest tumor diameter [40]. This volume change can be observed after only one cycle chemotherapy, and is suggested to be associated with RFS. Martincich and colleagues also compared largest tumor size with tumor volume as possible predictors for response to therapy; the authors noted that a tumor volume reduction of more than 65% after two cycles of chemotherapy was the most predictive value for predicting histological response [41]. The findings from these single center trials are confirmed in the multicenter I-Spy trials, discussed in further detail later in this chapter. Regardless whether maximum size or volume calculation is performed, defining the margins of the residual tumor burden can be challenging during and after NAC due to the dampening effect of chemotherapy on the contrast enhancement [15, 40, 41]. Still, MRI is more accurate for estimating size and extent of residual disease than conventional imaging when there are multifocal cancers but less sensitive when there is minimal residual disease. This suggests that when assessing for response, the different tumor biology, the genomic information of breast cancer, and the type of chemotherapy need to be taken into account and not just the size of tumor or stage [45–48]. MRI does provide additional information on tumor vascularity and enhancing pattern of tumor may be relevant to evaluation of response when combined with morphologic assessment and size or volume change from NAC.

5.5 MRI Assessment of Tumor Enhancement

Even though the widely used RECISTS criteria is based on the largest diameter of the cancer, alteration of enhancement pattern and change in the internal enhancement may also provide prognostic information to aid in predicting response to therapy. Tumor enhancement is subjectively characterized as early phase (0–60 s), initial enhancement (60–120 s) of the dynamic series, or delayed phase (more than 120 s) after injection of a gadolinium-based intravenous contrast. Balu-Maestro and colleagues reported the disappearance of early or initial abnormal enhancement in five cases of complete histological response [32]. Rieber et al. found that flattening of the time-intensity curve or disappearance of the washout segment of the kinetic curve after one course of chemotherapy and absence of contrast uptake after four courses of NAC predicts complete pathological response [48]. Other investigators observed decreases in both the rate and magnitude of contrast enhancement within the tumor mass in patients whose disease responded to chemotherapy (Fig. 5.3), and an increase or no change in patients whose disease responded poorly to therapy (Fig. 5.4) [45, 49]. Loo et al. reported the change in the largest diameter of late enhancement after 2 cycles of chemotherapy was the most predictive MRI characteristic for tumor response: a decrease less than 25% in largest diameter of late enhancement was indicative of residual tumor at final pathological examination [50]. A feasibility study in 19 women of tumor washout volume during the late enhancement phase demonstrated a significant reduction of the washout volume, after two cycles of chemotherapy [51]. The tumor volume reduction by more than 65% after two cycles of chemotherapy was reported as a stronger predictor of histopathological response than early enhancement ratio [41]. The change in the internal enhancement from heterogeneous to homogenous was also observed in responders compared to non-responders [52]. Indirectly, the changes in contrast enhancement time curves and internal tumoral

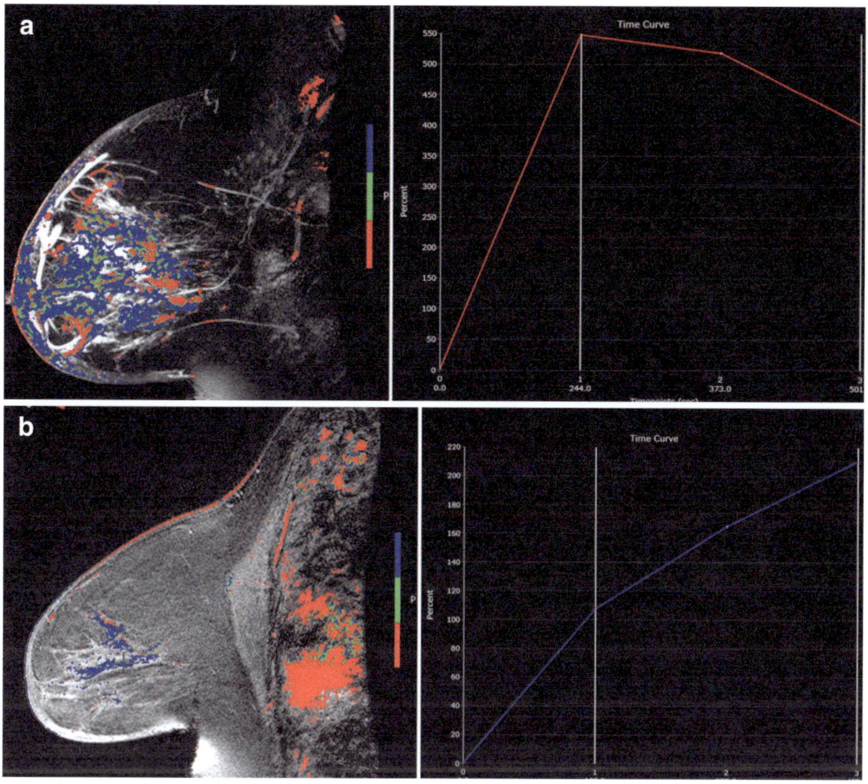

Fig. 5.3 60 year old female with diagnosis of inflammatory breast carcinoma who received NAC. (**a**) Pretreatment sagittal post-contrast fat-saturated MRI with color-overlayed angiogenic map revealed multicentric breast carcinoma with diffuse skin thickening and kinetic curve demonstrates rapid initial enhancement with delayed washout curve. (**b**) After NAC, MRI revealed near normalization of the left breast size with residual skin thickening. The enhancement is markedly decreased and the kinetic curve demonstrates more benign enhancement similar to normal breast tissue. MRI finding suggest response to therapy and reflects final pathology with only residual isolated tumor cells measuring 0.5mm and post-therapy effect

heterogeneous enhancement may produce biological information such permeability and vascularity in combination with genomic information to predict resistance to therapy.

5.6 Functional MRI Assessment: Diffusion-Weighted MRI

DWI can provide additional information to contrast enhanced MRI since DWI uses motion-sensitizing gradient techniques to assess the movement of water molecules and can characterize cell density, membrane integrity, viscosity, and microscopic cellular environment. DWI technique requires little time for image acquisition and

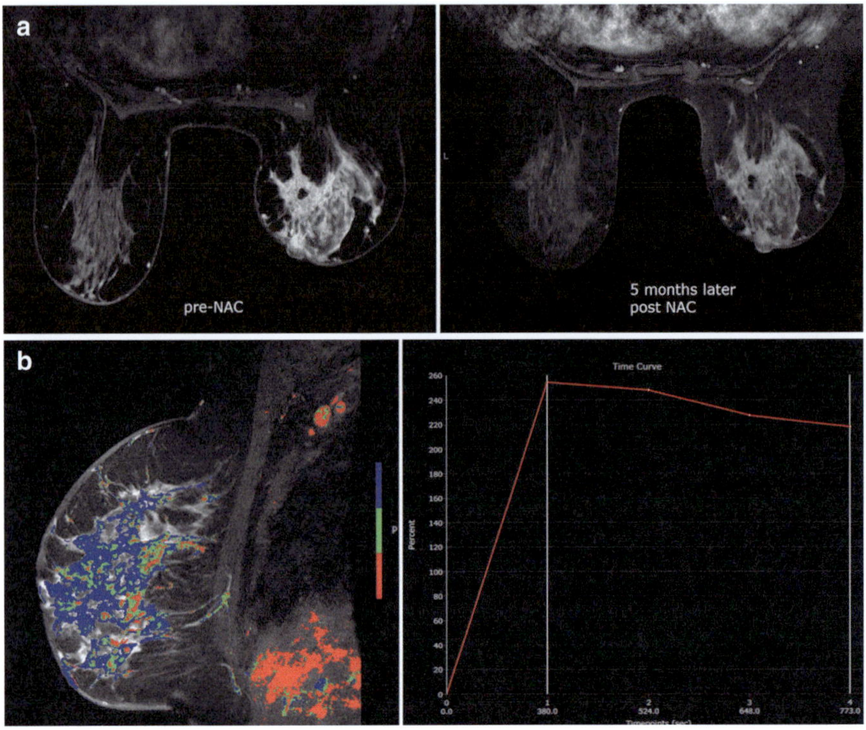

Fig. 5.4 58 year old female with hormonal positive right breast invasive lobular carcinoma treated with 8 cycles of weekly Taxol and Fluorouracil, Epirubicin and Cyclophosphamide (FEC) for 5 cycles. Physical exam suggested clinical response. (**a**) Axial post-contrast fat-saturated MRI revealed diffuse non-mass enhancement with delayed washout curve, compatible with multicentric disease. (**b**) Axial post-contrast fat-saturated MRI after NAC showed little change with persistent diffuse enhancement. Patient had mastectomy revealing residual 13 cm tumor with 10% viable tumor cellularity

evaluation, between 2 and 5 min. The concept behind DWI is that diffusion of water molecules is restricted or decreased in tissues with high cellularity such as malignant tumors, compared to benign lesions or normal breast tissue. Breast tumor, with restricted diffusion, appears bright on DWI and dark on parametric apparent diffusion coefficient map (ADC). The ADC map is created to compensate for the T2 shine-through artifact that occurs with diffusion weighted images. ADC values correlate inversely with the tissue cellularity i.e. tumor has lower ADC than benign breast lesions, and benign breast lesions have lower ADC than normal breast tissue. Quantitative analyses are employed to distinguish between zones of viable cells, edema, and necrosis for treatment planning. Serial changes in tissue cellularity in response to therapy are measurable by diffusion using various quantitative methods that include whole-tumor ADC average, histogram analysis, and pre-treatment versus post-treatment voxel-based differences.

NAC is cytotoxic and damage or kill cells, altering the cell membrane and integrity. This change is hypothesized to cause an increase in water mobility and is demonstrated on imaging as an increase in ADC on DWI. The increase in ADC may allow detection of earlier therapy changes or response to therapy, with the hope of predicting treatment outcome. However, the practice and techniques for DWI are not standardized and its role in response assessment remains an active area of research. Small sample-size single center studies have reported that an increase in tumor ADC or a change in tumor ADC after the first cycle of therapy or early treatment time point is predictive of response to therapy, and is observed even before a change in tumor size or vascularity is detected [53–55]. The ADC measurements from pretreatment DWI did not predict response to therapy in breast cancer [56–59]. The combination of contrast enhanced breast MRI with DWI had the best diagnostic performance than the individual techniques [59]. When compared to tumor size prediction on MRI, ADC performed better in predicting responders from non-responders with reported sensitivity of 100% compared to 50% for volume and 70% for diameter measurements [60]. The preliminary results on DWI from these single centers are promising for ADC as a prognostic indicator of treatment response. Multicenter trials are needed to standardize this technique as well as verify the findings of single center studies.

5.7 Multicenter Clinical Trials: I-SPY Trials

The I-SPY TRIAL (**I**nvestigation of **S**erial studies to **P**redict **Y**our **T**herapeutic **R**esponse with **I**maging **A**nd mo**L**ecular analysis) is a clinical trials platform integrating molecular and imaging biomarkers to evaluate treatment response for women receiving NAC for breast cancer [60–62]. As part of the first phase of I-SPY (I-SPY "1"), American College of Radiology Imaging Network (ACRIN) trial 6657 was performed to test dynamic contrast-enhanced (DCE) MRI for ability to predict response to treatment and risk of recurrence in patients with stage 2 or 3 breast cancer. Women with T3 tumors measuring at least 3 cm in diameter by clinical exam or imaging and receiving NAC with an anthracycline-cyclophosphamide (AC) regimen alone or followed by a taxane were eligible to enroll. MRI were performed within 4 weeks prior to starting AC chemotherapy (MRI_1), at least 2 weeks after the first cycle of AC and prior to the second cycle of AC (MRI_2), between AC treatment and taxane therapy if taxane was administered (MRI_3), and after the final chemotherapy treatment and prior to surgery (MRI_4). The study schema is shown in Fig. 5.5. 237 patients were enrolled between May 2002 and March 2006, of which 230 met eligibility criteria. In an initial analysis MRI was found to be strongly associated with both pCR and residual cancer burden (RCB), with the greatest advantage over clinical assessment found early in treatment using a volumetric measurement of tumor response [63]. In further analysis of the volumetric approach, functional tumor volume (FTV), a metric measured by applying contrast-enhancement thresholds

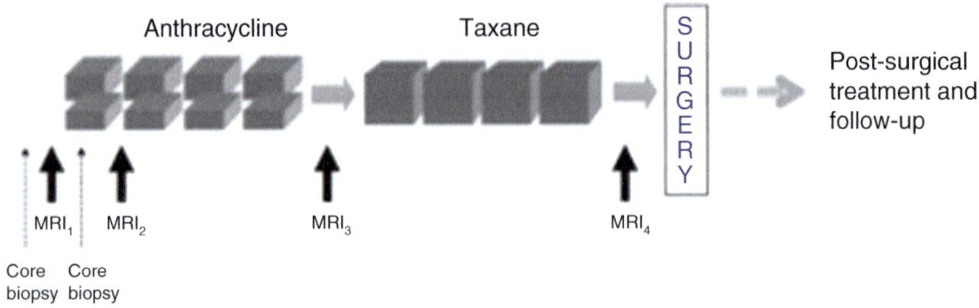

Fig. 5.5 I-SPY 1 TRIAL/ACRIN 6657 trial schema. MRI exams were performed prior to starting AC chemotherapy (MRI_1), prior to the second cycle of AC (MRI_2), between AC treatment and taxane therapy (MRI_3), and after the final chemotherapy treatment (MRI_4)

to MR images, was evaluated for prediction of RFS. FTV was found to be highly associated with RFS and a stronger predictor than pCR. Predictive performance was highest when FTV was combined with histopathologic variables (pCR and RCB) and tumor subtype (HR/HER2) [64]. FTV predicted RFS as early as after one cycle of AC chemotherapy and exploratory Kaplan-Meier analyses suggested that both the optimal timing and predictive performance were different among subtypes defined by HR/HER2 status.

The second phase of I-SPY (I-SPY "2"), is an adaptive, phase II clinical trial designed to identify promising new agents for breast cancer with a high probability of success in a subsequent phase III trial. In I-SPY 2, patients are screened to identify those with high risk of recurrence according to the Mammaprint 70-gene signature, ER and PR hormone receptor status (HR) and HER2 receptor status. The MammaPrint test is a genomic test that analyzes the activity of certain genes in early-stage breast cancer. Low risk patients, defined as Mammaprint low, HR+ and HER2-, do not continue to the experimental treatment phase of the trial. Included patients are randomized to one of several sub-arms testing either paclitaxel alone or paclitaxel in combination with an investigational new drug, selected on the basis of phase I safety data and preliminary evidence of efficacy in the HER2+ and/or HER2- population. Following the taxol-based regimen, all patients continue to standard chemotherapy with doxorubicin and cyclophosphamide. As part of the adaptive design of I-SPY 2, change in MRI FTV measured at serial time-points during chemotherapy is used to adjust the randomization schema as the trial proceeds. Drugs "graduate" from I-SPY 2 when they reach a Bayesian predictive probability of achieving 80% success in a subsequent phase III study, but can be dropped for futility if statistical significance is not reached after a predetermined number of patients have been assigned to that drug arm. Drugs graduate within subtypes defined by hormone receptor (HR) status, HER2 status and Mammaprint score. I-SPY 2 opened in March 2010 at 20 clinical sites. As of January 2016, 3 agents have graduated from I-SPY 2. In addition to incorporating MRI for FTV measurement in I-SPY 2, an imaging science component was added to test DWI. Similarly to the earlier ACRIN 6657 trial, ACRIN 6698 was designed to prospectively test ADC measurements from DWI for ability to predict response to treatment. ACRIN 6698 opened as an imaging sub-study of I-SPY 2 in 2012 and reached its accrual target in January 2015. The results from ACRIN 6698 are currently being analyzed.

5.8 Conclusion

For larger size tumor, such as in locally advanced HER2 positive or triple negative breast cancers, neoadjuvant chemotherapy is a standard of care. The role of neoadjuvant in TNBC subtype cancers is somewhat mixed, and non-linear while the benefit on survival with hormonal receptor positive breast cancer remains unclear. Further investigation is needed to assess tumor response to NAC and potential benefit on recurrent free survival or survival rate among all molecular subtypes of breast cancers. The ability to predict response, accurately assess residual disease, and correlation with biology of different cancers as well as tumor genomics remain a challenge. The techniques related to breast MRI exams have standardized in the last few years. However, the MR imaging features that best predict response remain unclear. Trying to identify specific features that consistently predict outcome is difficult since the available published trials either have small sample size, use different chemotherapy agents between trials, different contrast agents, different parameters measured, or different patient population with different tumor biology and unknown tumor genetics. The two I-SPY trials use consistent MRI techniques and confirmed that volume assessment best predicts response. DWI is now widely performed as a part of breast MRI exam, and has promising preliminary results. Since the ultimate outcome of a successful chemotherapy regimen is destruction of the tumor, including its neovascular system and internal composition, dynamic contrast-enhanced breast MRI coupled with DWI or other functional imaging MR techniques remain the best modality for visualizing the exquisite anatomic change within a tumor. Combining MRI with PET/CT or molecular imaging are promising frontiers for future research to assess residual disease after NAC.

References

1. Belli P, Costantini M, Malaspina C, Magistrelli A, Latorre G, Bonomo L. MRI accuracy in residual disease evaluation in breast cancer patients treated with neoadjuvant chemotherapy. Clin Radiol. 2006;61(11):946–53.
2. Bear HD, Anderson S, Brown A, Smith R, Mamounas EP, Fisher B, Margolese R, Theoret H, Soran A, Wickerham DL, Wolmark N. The effect on tumor response of adding sequential preoperative docetaxel to preoperative doxorubicin and cyclophosphamide: preliminary results from National Surgical Adjuvant Breast and Bowel Project Protocol B-27. J Clin Oncol. 2003;21(22):4165–74.
3. Fisher B, Brown A, Mamounas E, Wieand S, Robidoux A, Margolese RG, Cruz Jr AB, Fisher ER, Wickerham DL, Wolmark N, DeCillis A, Hoehn JL, Lees AW, Dimitrov NV. Effect of preoperative chemotherapy on local-regional disease in women with operable breast

cancer: findings from National Surgical Adjuvant Breast and Bowel Project B-18. J Clin Oncol. 1997;15(7):2483–93.

4. Kurian AW, Lichtensztajn DY, Keegan TH, Nelson DO, Clarke CA, Gomez SL. Use of and mortality after bilateral mastectomy compared with other surgical treatments for breast cancer in California, 1998-2011. Jama. 2014;312(9):902–14.
5. Hwang ES, Lichtensztajn DY, Gomez SL, Fowble B, Clarke CA. Survival after lumpectomy and mastectomy for early stage invasive breast cancer: the effect of age and hormone receptor status. Cancer. 2013;119(7):1402–11.
6. Fisher B, Bryant J, Wolmark N, Mamounas E, Brown A, Fisher ER, Wickerham DL, Begovic M, DeCillis A, Robidoux A, Margolese RG, Cruz Jr AB, Hoehn JL, Lees AW, Dimitrov NV, Bear HD. Effect of preoperative chemotherapy on the outcome of women with operable breast cancer. J Clin Oncol. 1998;16:2672–85.
7. Fisher ER, Wang J, Bryant J, Fisher B, Mamounas E, Wolmark N. Pathobiology of preoperative chemotherapy: findings from the National Surgical Adjuvant Breast and Bowel (NSABP) protocol B-18. Cancer. 2002;95:681–95.
8. Wolmark N, Wang J, Mamounas E, Bryant J, Fisher B. Preoperative chemotherapy in patients with operable breast cancer: nine-year results from National Surgical Adjuvant Breast and Bowel Project B-18. J Natl Cancer Inst Monogr. 2001;30:96–102.
9. Kaufmann M, Hortobagyi GN, Goldhirsch A, Scholl S, Makris A, Valagussa P, Blohmer JU, Eiermann W, Jackesz R, Jonat W, Lebeau A, Loibl S, Miller W, Seeber S, Semiglazov V, Smith R, Souchon R, Stearns V, Untch M, von Minckwitz G. Recommendations from an international expert panel on the use of neoadjuvant (primary) systemic treatment of operable breast cancer: an update. J Clin Oncol Off J Am Soc Clin Oncol. 2006;24(12):1940–9.
10. Ogston KN, Miller ID, Payne S, Hutcheon AW, Sarkar TK, Smith I, Schofield A, Heys SD. A new histological grading system to assess response of breast cancers to primary chemotherapy: prognostic significance and survival. Breast. 2003;12(5):320–7.
11. Abrial SC, Penault-Llorca F, Delva R, Bougnoux P, Leduc B, Mouret-Reynier MA, Mery-Mignard D, Bleuse JP, Dauplat J, Curé H, Chollet P. High prognostic significance of residual disease after neoadjuvant chemotherapy: a retrospective study in 710 patients with operable breast cancer. Breast Cancer Res Treatment. 2005;94(3):255–63.
12. Symmans WF, Peintinger F, Hatzis C, Rajan R, Kuerer H, Valero V, Assad L, Poniecka A, Hennessy B, Green M, Buzdar AU, Singletary SE, Hortobagyi GN, Pusztai L. Measurement of residual breast cancer burden to predict survival after neoadjuvant chemotherapy. J Clin Oncol Off J Am Soc Clin Oncol. 2007;25(28):4414–22.
13. Feldman LD, Hortobagyi GN, Budzar AU, Ames FC, Blumenschein GR. Pathologic assessment of response to induction chemotherapy in breast cancer. Breast Cancer Res Treat. 1986;46:2578–81.
14. Heys SD, Eremin JM, Sarkar TK, Hutcheon AW, Ah-See A, Eremin O. Role of multimodality therapy in the management of locally advanced carcinoma of the breast. J Am Coll Surg. 1994;179(4):493–504.
15. Lorenzon M, Zuiani C, Londero V, Linda A, Furlan A, Bazzocchi M. Assessment of breast cancer response to neoadjuvant chemotherapy: is volumetric MRI a reliable tool? Eur J Radiol. 2009;71(1):82–8.
16. Cortazar P, Zhang L, Untch M, Mehta K, Costantino JP, Wolmark N, et al. Pathological complete response and long-term clinical benefit in breast cancer: the CTNeoBC pooled analysis. Lancet. 2014;384:164–72.
17. Yi A, Cho N, Im SA, Chang JM, Kim SJ, Moon HG, Han W, Park IA, Noh DY, Moon WK. Survival outcomes of breast cancer patients who receive neoadjuvant chemotherapy: association with dynamic contrast-enhanced MR imaging with computer-aided evaluation. Radiology. 2013;268(3):662–72.
18. Ko ES, Han H, Han B-K, Kim SM, Kim RB, Lee G-W, Park YH, Nam SJ. Prognostic Significance of a Complete Response on Breast MRI in Patients Who Received Neoadjuvant Chemotherapy According to the Molecular Subtype. Korean J Radiol. 2015;16(5):986.

19. Cocconi G, Di Blasio B, Alberti G, Bisagni G, Botti E, Peracchia G. Problems in evaluating response of primary breast cancer to systemic therapy. Breast Cancer Res Treat. 1984;4:309–13.
20. Kim YS, Chang JM, Moon HG, Lee J, Shin SU, Moon WK. Residual Mammographic Microcalcifications and Enhancing Lesions on MRI After Neoadjuvant Systemic Chemotherapy for Locally Advanced Breast Cancer: Correlation with Histopathologic Residual Tumor Size. Ann Surg Oncol. 2015. [Epub ahead of print] PMID:26628432
21. Herrada J, Iyer RB, Atkinson EN, Sneige N, Buzdar AU, Hortobagyi GN. Relative value of physical examination, mammography, and breast sonography in evaluating the size of the primary tumor and regional lymph node metastases in women receiving neoadjuvant chemotherapy for locally advanced breast carcinoma. Clin Cancer Res. 1997;3:1565–9.
22. Finlayson CA, MacDermott TA. Ultrasound can estimate the pathologic size of infiltrating ductal carcinoma. Arch Surg. 2000;135(2):158–9.
23. Peintinger F, Kuerer HM, Anderson K, Boughey JC, Meric-Bernstam F, Singletary SE, Hunt KK, Whitman GJ, Stephens T, Buzdar AU, Green MC, Symmans WF. Accuracy of the combination of mammography and sonography in predicting tumor response in breast cancer patients after neoadjuvant chemotherapy. Ann Surg Oncol. 2006;13(11):1443–9.
24. Therasse P, Arbuck SG, Eisenhauer EA, Wanders J, Kaplan RS, Rubinstein L, Verweij J, Van Glabbeke M, van Oosterom AT, Christian MC, Gwyther SG. New guidelines to evaluate the response to treatment in solid tumors. European Organization for Research and Treatment of Cancer, National Cancer Institute of the United States, National Cancer Institute of Canada. J Natl Cancer Inst. 2000;92(3):205–16.
25. Vriens BE, de Vries B, Lobbes MB, van Gastel SM, van den Berkmortel FW, Smilde TJ, van Warmerdam LJ, de Boer M, van Spronsen DJ, Smidt ML, Peer PG, Aarts MJ, Tjan-Heijnen VC; INTENS Study Group. Ultrasound is at least as good as magnetic resonance imaging in predicting tumour size post-neoadjuvant chemotherapy in breast cancer. Eur J Cancer. 2016; 52:67–76.
26. Lobbes MB, Prevos R, Smidt M, Tjan-Heijnen VC, van Goethem M, Schipper R, Beets-Tan RG, Wildberger JE. The role of magnetic resonance imaging in assessing residual disease and pathologic complete response in breast cancer patients receiving neoadjuvant chemotherapy: a systematic review. Insights Imag. 2013;4(2):163–75.
27. Marinovich ML, Houssami N, Macaskill P, Sardanelli F, Irwig L, Mamounas EP, von Minckwitz G, Brennan ME, Ciatto S. Meta-analysis of magnetic resonance imaging in detecting residual breast cancer after neoadjuvant therapy. J Natl Cancer Inst. 2013;105(5):321–33.
28. Marinovich ML, Macaskill P, Irwig L, Sardanelli F, von Minckwitz G, Mamounas E, Brennan M, Ciatto S, Houssami N. Meta-analysis of agreement between MRI and pathologic breast tumour size after neoadjuvant chemotherapy. Br J Cancer. 2013;109(6):1528–36.
29. Segara D, Krop IE, Garber JE, Winer E, Harris L, Bellon JR, Birdwell R, Lester S, Lipsitz S, Iglehart JD, Golshan M. Does MRI predict pathologic tumor response in women with breast cancer undergoing preoperative chemotherapy? J Surg Oncol. 2007;96(6):474–80.
30. Marinovich ML, Macaskill P, Irwig L, Sardanelli F, Mamounas E, von Minckwitz G, Guarneri V, Partridge SC, Wright FC, Choi JH, Bhattacharyya M, Martincich L, Yeh E, Londero V, Houssami N. Agreement between MRI and pathologic breast tumor size after neoadjuvant chemotherapy, and comparison with alternative tests: individual patient data meta-analysis. BMC Cancer. 2015;15:662.
31. Akazawa K, Tamaki Y, Taguchi T, Tanji Y, Miyoshi Y, Kim SJ, Ueda S, Yanagisawa T, Sato Y, Noguchi S. Preoperative evaluation of residual tumor extent by three-dimensional magnetic resonance imaging in breast cancer patients treated with neoadjuvant chemotherapy. Breast J. 2006;12(2):130–7.
32. Balu-Maestro C, Chapellier C, Bleuse A, Chanalet I, Chauvel C, Largillier R. Imaging in evaluation of response to neoadjuvant breast cancer treatment benefits of MRI. Breast Cancer Res Treat. 2002;72(2):145–52.
33. Cheung YC, Chen SC, Su MY, See LC, Hsueh S, Chang HK, Lin YC, Tsai CS. Monitoring the Size and Response of Locally Advanced Breast Cancers to Neoadjuvant Chemotherapy

(Weekly Paclitaxel and Epirubicin) with Serial Enhanced MRI. Breast Cancer Res Treat. 2003;78(1):51–8.
34. Gilles R, Guinebretière JM, Toussaint C, Spielman M, Rietjens M, Petit JY, Contesso G, Masselot J, Vanel D. Locally advanced breast cancer: contrast-enhanced subtraction MR imaging of response to preoperative chemotherapy. Radiology. 1994;191(3):633–8.
35. Yeh E, Slanetz P, Kopans DB, Rafferty E, Georgian-Smith D, Moy L, Halpern E, Moore R, Kuter I, Taghian A. Prospective Comparison of Mammography, Sonography, and MRI in Patients Undergoing Neoadjuvant Chemotherapy for Palpable Breast Cancer. AJR. 2005;184(3):868–77.
36. Lorenzon M, Zuiani C, Londero V, Linda A, Furlan A, Bazzocchi M. Assessment of breast cancer response to neoadjuvant chemotherapy: is volumetric MRI a reliable tool? Eur J Radiol. 2009;71(1):82–8.
37. Rosen EL, Blackwell KL, Baker JA, Soo MS, Bentley RC, Yu D, Samulski TV, Dewhirst MW. Accuracy of MRI in the Detection of Residual Breast Cancer After Neoadjuvant Chemotherapy. AJR. 2003;181(5):1275–82.
38. Prati PR, Minami CA, Gornbein JA, Debruhl N, Chung D, Chang HR. Accuracy of clinical evaluation of locally advanced breast cancer in patients receiving neoadjuvant chemotherapy. Cancer. 2009;115(6):1194–202.
39. Wasser K, Sinn HP, Fink C, Klein SK, Junkermann H, Lüdemann HP, Zuna I, Delorme S. Accuracy of tumor size measurement in breast cancer using MRI is influenced by histological regression induced by neoadjuvant chemotherapy. EUR Radiol. 2003;13:1213–23.
40. Partridge SC, Gibbs JE, Lu Y, Esserman LJ, Tripathy D, Wolverton DS, Rugo HS, Hwang ES, Ewing CA, Hylton NM. MRI Measurements of Breast Tumor Volume Predict Response to Neoadjuvant Chemotherapy and Recurrence-Free Survival. AJR. 2005;184(6):1774–81.
41. Martincich L, Montemurro F, Rosa GD, Marra V, Ponzone R, Cirillo S, Gatti M, Biglia N, Sarotto I, Sismondi P, Regge D, Aglietta M. Monitoring Response to Primary Chemotherapy in Breast Cancer using Dynamic Contrast-enhanced Magnetic Resonance Imaging. Breast Cancer Res Treat. 2004;83(1):67–76.
42. Warren RM, Bobrow LG, Earl HM, Britton PD, Gopalan D, Purushotham AD, Wishart GC, Benson JR, Hollingworth W. Can breast MRI help in the management of women with breast cancer treated by neoadjuvant chemotherapy? Br J Cancer. 2004;90(7):1349–60.
43. Johansen R, Jensen LR, Rydland J, Goa PE, Kvistad KA, Bathen TF, Axelson DE, Lundgren S, Gribbestad I. Predicting survival and early clinical response to primary chemotherapy for patients with locally advanced breast cancer using DCE-MRI. J Magnet Res Imag. 2009;29(6):1300–7.
44. Loo CE, Straver ME, Rodenhuis S, Muller SH, Wesseling J, Vrancken Peeters MJ, Gilhuijs KG. Magnetic resonance imaging response monitoring of breast cancer during neoadjuvant chemotherapy: relevance of breast cancer subtype. J Clin Oncol Off J Am Soc Clin Oncol. 2011;29(6):660–6.
45. Kim HJ, Im YH, Han BK, Choi N, Lee J, Kim JH, Choi YL, Ahn JS, Nam SJ, Park YS, Choe YH, Ko YH, Yang JH. Accuracy of MRI for estimating residual tumor size after neoadjuvant chemotherapy in locally advanced breast cancer: Relation to response patterns on MRI. Acta Oncol. 2007;46(7):996–1003.
46. Chen JH, Feig B, Agrawal G, Yu H, Carpenter PM, Mehta RS, Nalcioglu O, Su MY. MRI evaluation of pathologically complete response and residual tumors in breast cancer after neoadjuvant chemotherapy. Cancer. 2008;112(1):17–26.
47. McGuire KP, Toro-Burguete J, Dang H, Young J, Soran A, Zuley M, Bhargava R, Bonaventura M, Johnson R, Ahrendt G. MRI staging after neoadjuvant chemotherapy for breast cancer: does tumor biology affect accuracy? Ann Surg Oncol. 2011;18(11):3149–54.
48. Rieber A, Bambs HJ, Gabelmann A, Heilmann V, Kreienberg R, Kuhn T. Breast MRI for monitoring response of primary breast cancer to neoadjuvant chemotherapy. Eur Radiol. 2002;12:1711–9.
49. Denis F, Desbiez-Bourcier A, Chapiron C, Arbion F, Body G, Brunereau L. Contrast enhanced magnetic resonance imaging underestimates residual disease following neoadjuvant docetaxel based chemotherapy for breast cancer. Eur J Surg Oncol. 2004;30(10):1069–76.

50. Loo CE, Teertstra HJ, Rodenhuis S, Vijver MJVD, Hannemann J, Muller SH, Peeters MJ, Gilhuijs KG. Dynamic Contrast-Enhanced MRI for Prediction of Breast Cancer Response to Neoadjuvant Chemotherapy: Initial Results. AJR. 2008;191(5):1331–8.
51. Khoury CE, Servois V, Thibault F, Tardivon A, Ollivier L, Meunier M, Allonier C, Neuenschwander S. MR Quantification of the Washout Changes in Breast Tumors Under Preoperative Chemotherapy: Feasibility and Preliminary Results. AJR. 2005;184(5): 1499–504.
52. Chang Y-C, Huang C-S, Liu Y-J, Chen J-H, Lu Y-S, Tseng W-YI. Angiogenic response of locally advanced breast cancer to neoadjuvant chemotherapy evaluated with parametric histogram from dynamic contrast-enhanced MRI. Phys Med Biol. 2004;49(16):3593–602.
53. Buijs M, Vossen JA, Hong K, Georgiades CS, Geschwind JF, Kamel IR. Assessment of metastatic breast cancer response to chemoembolization with contrast agent enhanced and diffusion-weighted MR imaging. AJR. 2008;191(1):285–9.
54. Kuroki Y, Nasu K. Advances in breast MRI: diffusion-weighted imaging of the breast. Breast Cancer. 2008;15(3):212–7.
55. Sharma SU, Danishada KK, Seenub V, Jagannathan NR. Longitudinal study of the assessment by MRI and diffusion-weighted imaging of tumor response in patients with locally advanced breast cancer undergoing neoadjuvant chemotherapy. NMR Biomed. 2009;22(1):104–13.
56. Fujimoto H, Kazama T, Nagashima T, Sakakibara M, Suzuki TH, Okubo Y, Shiina N, Fujisaki K, Ota S, Miyazaki M. Diffusion-weighted imaging reflects pathological therapeutic response and relapse in breast cancer. Breast Cancer. 2014;21(6):724–31.
57. Woodhams R, Kakita S, Hata H, Iwabuchi K, Kuranami M, Gautam S, Hatabu H, Kan S, Mountford C. Identification of residual breast carcinoma following neoadjuvant chemotherapy: diffusion-weighted imaging – comparison with contrast-enhanced MR imaging and pathologic findings. Radiology. 2010;254(2):357–66.
58. Richard R, Thomassin I, Chapellier M, Scemama A, de Cremoux P, Varna M, Giacchetti S, Espié M, de Kerviler E, de Bazelaire C. Diffusion-weighted MRI in pretreatment prediction of response to neoadjuvant chemotherapy in patients with breast cancer. Eur Radiol. 2013;23(9):2420–31.
59. Hahn SY, Ko EY, Han BK, Shin JH, Ko ES. Role of diffusion-weighted imaging as an adjunct to contrast-enhanced breast MRI in evaluating residual breast cancer following neoadjuvant chemotherapy. Eur J Radiol. 2014;83(2):283–8.
60. Esserman LJ, Berry DA, Cheang MC, Yau C, Perou CM, Carey L, DeMichele A, Gray JW, Conway-Dorsey K, Lenburg ME, Buxton MB, Davis SE, van't Veer LJ, Hudis C, Chin K, Wolf D, Krontiras H, Montgomery L, Tripathy D, Lehman C, Liu MC, Olopade OI, Rugo HS, Carpenter JT, Livasy C, Dressler L, Chhieng D, Singh B, Mies C, Rabban J, Chen YY, Giri D, Au A, Hylton N, I-SPY 1 TRIAL Investigators. Chemotherapy response and recurrence-free survival in neoadjuvant breast cancer depends on biomarker profiles: results from the I-SPY 1 TRIAL (CALGB 150007/150012; ACRIN 6657). Breast Cancer Res Treat. 2012;132(3): 1049–62.
61. Barker AD, Sigman CC, Kelloff GJ, Hylton N, Berry D, Esserman L. I-SPY 2: An Adaptive Breast Cancer Trial Design in the Setting of Neoadjuvant Chemotherapy. Clin Pharmacol Ther. 2009;86(1):97–100.
62. Esserman LJ, Berry DA, Cheang MC, Yau C, Perou CM, Carey L, DeMichele A, Gray JW, Conway-Dorsey K, Lenburg ME, Buxton MB, Davis SE, van't Veer LJ, Hudis C, Chin K, Wolf D, Krontiras H, Montgomery L, Tripathy D, Lehman C, Liu MC, Olopade OI, Rugo HS, Carpenter JT, Livasy C, Dressler L, Chhieng D, Singh B, Mies C, Rabban J, Chen YY, Giri D, Au A, Hylton N; I-SPY 1 TRIAL Investigators. Chemotherapy response and recurrence-free survival in neoadjuvant breast cancer depends on biomarker profiles: results from the I-SPY 1 TRIAL (CALGB 150007/150012; ACRIN 6657). Breast Cancer Res Treat. 2012;132(3): 1049-62.
63. Esserman LJ, Berry DA, DeMichele A, Carey L, Davis SE, Buxton M, Hudis C, Gray JW, Perou C, Yau C, Livasy C, Krontiras H, Montgomery L, Tripathy D, Lehman C, Liu MC, Olopade OI, Rugo HS, Carpenter JT, Dressler L, Chhieng D, Singh B, Mies C, Rabban J, Chen YY, Giri D. van't Veer L, Hylton N. Pathologic complete response predicts recurrence-free

survival more effectively by cancer subset: results from the I-SPY 1 TRIAL--CALGB 150007/150012, ACRIN 6657. J Clin Oncol. 2012;30(26):3242–9.

64. Hylton NM, Blume JD, Bernreuter WK, Pisano ED, Rosen MA, Morris EA, Weatherall PT, Lehman CD, Newstead GM, Polin S, Marques HS, Esserman LJ, Schnall MD. Locally advanced breast cancer: MR imaging for prediction of response to neoadjuvant chemotherapy--results from ACRIN 6657/I-SPY TRIAL. Radiology. 2012;263(3):663–72.
65. Hylton NM, Gatsonis CA, Rosen MA, Lehman CD, Newitt DC, Partridge SC, Bernreuter WK, Pisano ED, Morris EA, Weatherall PT, Polin SM, Newstead GM, Marques HS, Esserman LJ, Schnall MD. Neoadjuvant Chemotherapy for Breast Cancer: Functional Tumor Volume by MR Imaging Predicts Recurrence-free Survival-Results from the ACRIN 6657/CALGB 150007 I-SPY 1 TRIAL. Radiology. 2016;279(1):44–55. doi: 10.1148/radiol.2015150013. Epub 2015.

Chapter 6
Breast MRI and Implants

Claudia Seuss and Samantha L. Heller

Abstract Breast augmentation is the most common cosmetic surgical procedure performed in the United States. Magnetic resonance imaging (MRI) is the most sensitive modality for evaluating implant integrity. MRI also has the potential to detect breast cancer in women with implants. This chapter reviews the use of breast MRI in women with implants for identification of implant rupture and breast cancer detection. Implant imaging pitfalls as well as future MRI techniques and sequences for evaluating breast implants will also be addressed.

Keywords Breast implants • MRI • Silicone • Saline • Intracapsular rupture • Extracapsular rupture • Implant integrity • Radial folds • Breast cancer • Diffusion Weighted Imaging (DWI) • Spatiotemporally encoded (SPEN) • Anaplastic lymphoma

6.1 History of Breast Implants

The history of breast reconstruction dates back to 1895, when Czerny used a lipoma from a patient to augment her breast after removal of an adenoma [1]. After this, in the early 1900s there are reports of paraffin injections used for breast augmentation; however, due to the high incidence of complications including tissue necrosis, inflammatory reactions, draining sinus tracts and hard masses termed 'paraffinomas' its use was discontinued by the 1920s [2]. In the late 1940s surgeons experimented with plastic implants including silicone sponges. Shortly after their development however, many complications including capsular contracture, seroma, fistulation and infection became apparent and their use rapidly declined. In the 1940s and 1950s silicone injections became popular. However it was soon noted that pure liquid silicone tended to migrate away from the injection site. This fueled the idea of adding fibrosing agents such as vegetable oils and fatty acids to silicone;

C. Seuss, MD (✉) • S.L. Heller, MD, PhD
Department of Radiology, New York University School of Medicine,
New York, NY 10016, USA
e-mail: claudia.reuben@gmail.com; Samantha.heller@nyumc.org

S.L. Heller, L. Moy (eds.), *Breast Oncology: Techniques, Indications, and Interpretation*, DOI 10.1007/978-3-319-42563-4_6

however these were not well tolerated and produced painful silicone granulomas, skin sloughing, granulomatous hepatitis, embolism and even death. With such serious complications, these injected substances were banned in many countries.

In 1963, Dr. Thomas Cronin introduced what is now recognized as the modern silicone gel-filled implant, created by placing silicone gel in a bag consisting of rubberlike silicone elastomer [3]. The first generation of silicone gel-filled implants, which were manufactured between the 1960s and 1970s had a thick shell, a peripheral seam and a backing of Dacron mesh, which was meant to promote tissue ingrowth and fixation along the posterior surface. From mid 1970s to the late 1980s a second generation of silicone gel-filled implants were manufactured, which had a thin elastomeric shell, and less viscous silicone gel. The third generation of silicone gel-filled implants, which have been produced since the 1980s have a multilayer shell, with a barrier layer and thick silicone gel. Although saline filled implants never attained the popularity of the silicone-gel filled implant, they have been used since the 1960s in the United States [2].

Concerns about implant related complications led the FDA to place a moratorium on commercially available silicone breast implants in 1992, limiting their use to patients requiring breast reconstruction and replacement of existing implants. Potential feared complications included low birth weights of infants born to women with silicone implants and increased incidence of brain tumors and suicide rates in women with silicone implants. The most widely publicized concern was related to the development of collagen vascular disease in women with silicone implants due to an immunologic response [4]. Eleven years later, following 15 studies involving 34,000 subjects, with 7–15 years of follow-up data and no evidence of the above mentioned complications, the FDA allowed implants back on the market [4].

6.2 Types of Implants

There have been innumerable types, styles and sizes of implants developed over the past century. Different shapes, sizes, components, shell texturing, fixation patches and valves have been developed to provide sufficient variation for women. In their review of breast implant classification, Middleton and McNamara noted over 240 breast implant styles from American manufacturers alone [2].

The most frequently encountered breast implant is the single-lumen silicone gel filled implant, which consists of an outer silicone elastomer semipermeable implant shell filled with silicone gel (Fig. 6.1). The silicone gel is a lightly crosslinked polymer of polydimethylsiloxane (PDMS) [5]. Single-lumen implants also come in an adjustable variety, in which saline can be added to the lumen at the time of placement [2]. Saline implants consist of the same silicone elastomer shell, and are filled centrally with saline. These implants often have a fill valve which is visible on imaging.

Less commonly encountered is the standard double-lumen implant, which consists of a silicone gel filled inner lumen and a saline outer lumen. The primary

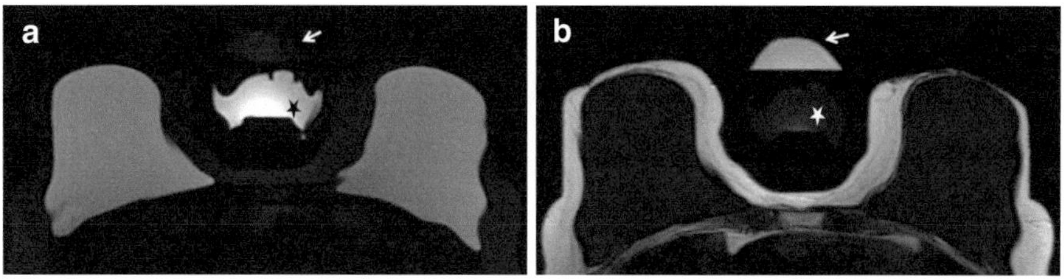

Fig. 6.1 (**a**) Axial STIR with water suppression (silicone sensitive) MRI image showing bilateral intact silicone implants. Signal from the saline component of the phantom (*white arrow*) is suppressed. High intensity signal from the silicone component of the phantom (*black star*) matches the high signal of the silicone implants. (**b**) Axial STIR with silicone suppression MRI image showing bilateral intact silicone implants. There is high intensity signal from the saline component of the phantom (*white arrow*). Suppressed signal from the silicone component of the phantom (*white star*) matches the suppressed signal of the silicone implants

purpose of this implant type is to allow size adjustability at the time of and after implant placement. A reverse double lumen implant, most commonly used after reconstructive surgery, consists of a saline filled inner lumen and silicone gel outer lumen. Size adjustments can be made by adding saline to the inner lumen while preserving the feel of a silicone gel-filled implant. A gel-gel double lumen implant consists of silicone gel within the inner and outer lumens.

Additional more rarely encountered implants on the market include reverse-adjustable, triple-lumen, double lumen Cavon "cast gel", custom, soft pectus, non-adjustable sponge, adjustable sponge and others [2].

Breast implants can be placed behind the glandular tissue but anterior to the pectoralis major muscle (termed subglandular, retroglandular or retromammary position). This position maximizes the augmentation effect of the implant, but obscures more breast tissue on mammogram, limiting evaluation. Alternatively, implants may be placed posterior to the pectoralis muscle (termed subpectoral or retropectoral position); this is the case for all implants placed after total mastectomy [6]. After placement, a thin fibrous capsule of scar tissue normally forms around the implant. On occasion, pronounced fibrous capsule formation can occur with silicone implants, which causes discomfort and alters the shape of the breast. This is known as capsular contracture and can be difficult to diagnose by imaging. Although surgically more challenging to place, advantages of subpectoral implants include lower rate of capsular contracture and easier imaging of the surrounding breast tissue [1].

6.3 Imaging of Implants

Breast augmentation is the most common cosmetic surgical procedure performed in the United States, and has been since the FDA re-approved the use of silicone implants in 2006. In 2014 there were 286,254 cases of breast augmentation with implants reported, a 35 % increase since 2000 [7]. With the widespread prevalence and ever increasing number of women with implants, there is an ongoing need to evaluate breast implant integrity as well as to identify breast cancer in women with implants.

6.4 Mammography

The primary indication for performing mammography in women with implants is to detect breast cancer. Conventional mammography is of little value in the assessment of implant integrity, with sensitivity ranging from 25 to 68 % [8] (Fig. 6.2). The sensitivity of screening mammography for detecting malignancy is also decreased in the presence of implants and has been reported at 45 % versus 67 % in patients without implants [9]. Mammography does however remain useful for the evaluation of the surrounding breast tissue and for the detection of extracapsular silicone rupture. Additionally, mammography can identify periprosthetic calcifications, which are occasionally seen with capsular contracture as well as focal bulges or contour deformity of the implant shell. Given that mammography is the main screening tool to identify breast cancer in women, annual mammography is still recommended in patients with implants.

6.5 Ultrasound

There are conflicting reports on the usefulness of ultrasonography for detecting implant ruptures, which may reflect the variation in exam quality depending on the experience of the operator, type of equipment used, and technical factors [8]. Ultrasound can delineate some of the internal structure of the implant, particularly in the anterior aspect and therefore can detect both intracapsular and extracapsular rupture. Intracapsular rupture is seen as a series of horizontal echogenic straight or curvilinear lines traversing the interior of the implant, commonly known as the stepladder sign [10] (Fig. 6.3). Extracapsular silicone has the characteristic "snowstorm" appearance characterized by a highly echogenic pattern of scattered and reverberating echoes with a well-defined anterior margin and loss of detail posteriorly (Fig. 6.4). Ultrasound is also able to detect small amounts of free silicone within axillary lymph nodes, manifesting as the characteristic echogenic snowstorm appearance.

Ultrasound has proven to be useful in patients who are claustrophobic or unable to undergo MRI because of unsafe implanted devices such as pacemakers. Importantly however, silicone does cause marked attenuation of the ultrasound beam; thus evaluation of the back wall of an implant and the tissue posterior to it is limited. Additionally, previous silicone injections and residual silicone granulomas from extracapsular rupture will significantly limit ultrasound evaluation [11].

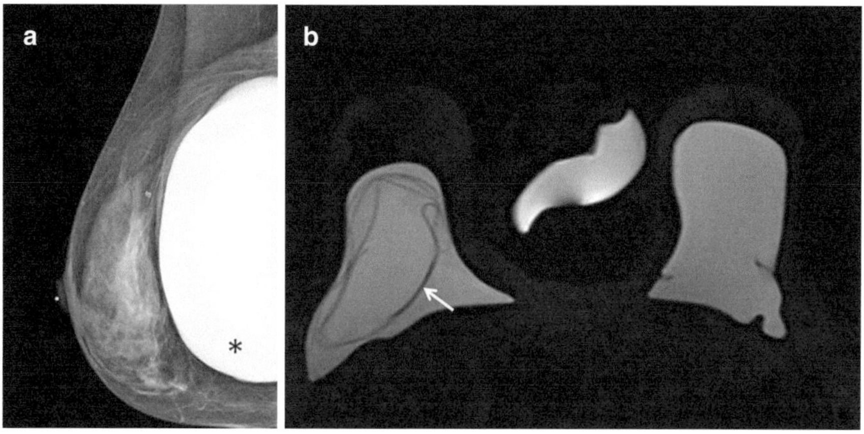

Fig. 6.2 (**a**) Right MLO view mammogram shows a subpectoral silicone implant, which appears intact (*black asterix*). (**b**) Axial STIR with water suppression (silicone sensitive) MRI image from the same patient demonstrates the "linguine sign" (*white arrow*) of intracapsular implant rupture on the right, which was not detected on mammography performed the same day

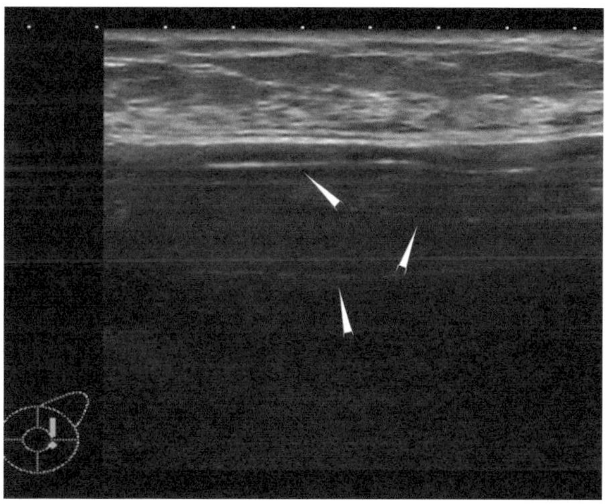

Fig. 6.3 Image from an ultrasound demonstrates the stepladder sign of intracapsular silicone implant rupture (*white arrowheads*). The discontinuous parallel echogenic lines represent the collapsed implant shell within the implant lumen

6.6 Magnetic Resonance Imaging

Magnetic resonance imaging is the most accurate noninvasive method available to evaluate silicone gel-filled implant integrity. The FDA currently recommends that asymptomatic women with silicone implants undergo an MR imaging examination to check for implant rupture 3 years after placement and then every 2 years thereafter. In addition, MR imaging is recommended to evaluate for implant rupture if the patient is having new breast symptoms [12]. This is because although clinical signs of implant rupture may include contour deformity, displacement, and mass formation,

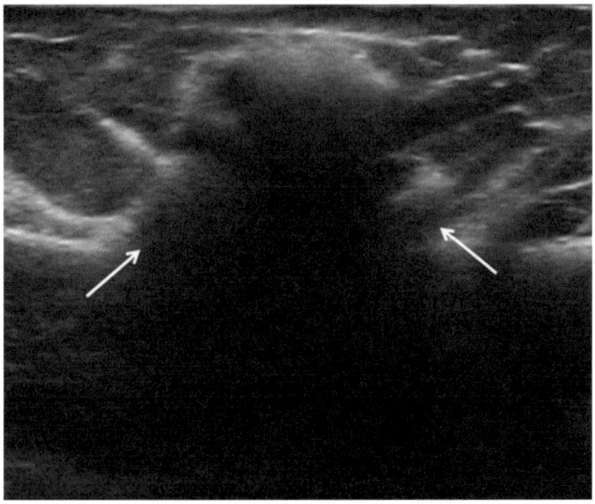

Fig. 6.4 Image from an ultrasound demonstrates the "snowstorm" pattern of extracapsular silicone implant rupture (*white arrows*)

the diagnosis of implant rupture based on physical exam findings is extremely insensitive, with failure to diagnose implant rupture in greater than 50 % of ruptures [13]. The overall sensitivity of MRI for detection of implant rupture is between 80 and 90 % and its specificity is between 90 and 97 % [14].

6.6.1 MRI Sequences

Currently breast implant imaging can be performed on 1.5 and 3 T MR scanners from all major manufacturers using a dedicated breast imaging coil. Studies are performed in the prone position to minimize respiratory artifact and to allow the implant to be imaged in maximum size. The MR sequences that are used in silicone implant imaging are strategically developed to separate three main components: water, silicone and fat [4].

We find imaging of a saline bag/silicone phantom to be helpful both in terms of aiding confirmation of implant material, but also as a quality control measure for signal suppression (Fig. 6.1). Implant sequences can be performed using 5 mm slices and can be performed in under 15 minutes; however, a longer high resolution sequence may be useful for thin shell and some standard double-lumen implants when early rupture detection is difficult.

We suggest that MRI to evaluate for implant rupture should include a scout localizer sequence, to help plan other sequences. The scout sequence is useful for example, in the rare situation when extracapsular silicone has spread outside the normal field of view (FOV), and can be utilized to plan extended FOV studies. A bilateral 2D axial T2-weighted turbo spin-echo sequence is used to differentiate water from silicone in cases of failure of nulling or suppression.

A bilateral 2D axial short tau inversion recovery sequence with water saturation is the main sequence used to detect intracapsular and extracapsular rupture of silicone implants. In this sequence silicone will appear hyperintense against a dark background of fat and water suppressed images. The dark implant shell folds will contrast with the bright silicone gel in cases of intracapsular rupture.

A bilateral 2D axial short tau inversion recovery sequence with silicone saturation is used to increase confidence in detecting extracapsular soft-tissue silicone. In this sequence, water and fat will appear hyperintense, and silicone will be hypointense, and thus extracapsular silicone will appear dark against a bright background. This sequence is not used to detect intracapsular implant rupture because the hypointense implant shell folds are not well seen against the background of suppressed (hypointense) silicone gel.

Additional sequences used to evaluate implant integrity at our institution include a bilateral 2D axial STIR, bilateral 2D axial T2 and a bilateral 2D axial T1-weighted volumetric interpolated breath-hold examination (VIBE) (see Table 6.1).

6.7 Implant Integrity/Complications

The normal silicone implant should have a smooth, well-defined margin with homogeneous appearance of silicone on MRI. Breast silicone implants are designed to approximate the cosmetic ptosis of a normal breast and, thus are not meant to be taut.

Table 6.1 Protocol for implant evaluation (3 T magnet)

Description	Main parameters	Uses
Bilateral 2D axial T2-weighted unsupressed, breast coil	Turbo spin-echo, 5 mm slice thickness, TR 3000 ms, TE 79.0 ms, 384 × 288 matrix, 1 average	Allows differentiation of water from silicone in cases of nulling/suppression failure
Bilateral 2D axial STIR, breast coil	Turbo spin-echo, 5 mm slice thickness, TR 3500 ms, TE 61.0 ms, 320 × 256 matrix, 2 averages	Used in conjunction with unsuppressed T2 to confirm fat signal, which will be hypointense on this sequence
Bilateral 2D axial STIR, silicone saturated, breast coil	Turbo spin-echo, 5 mm slice thickness, TR 4000 ms, TE 61.0 ms, 320 × 256 matrix, 2 averages	Used to confirm the presence of extracapsular silicone, which will appear hypointense
Bilateral 2D axial STIR, water saturated, breast coil	Turbo spin-echo, 5 mm slice thickness, TR 4000 ms, TE 61.0 ms, 320 × 256 matrix, 2 averages	Main sequence to detect intracapsular and extracapsular implant rupture
Bilateral 2D axial T1- weighted VIBE, breast coil	Gradient echo, 0.9 mm slice thickness, TR 3.78 ms, TE 1.11 ms, 448 × 358 matrix, 1 average	High resolution sequence useful for thin shell and some standard double-lumen implants when early rupture detection is difficult. Can also be used to evaluate non-implant related breast findings

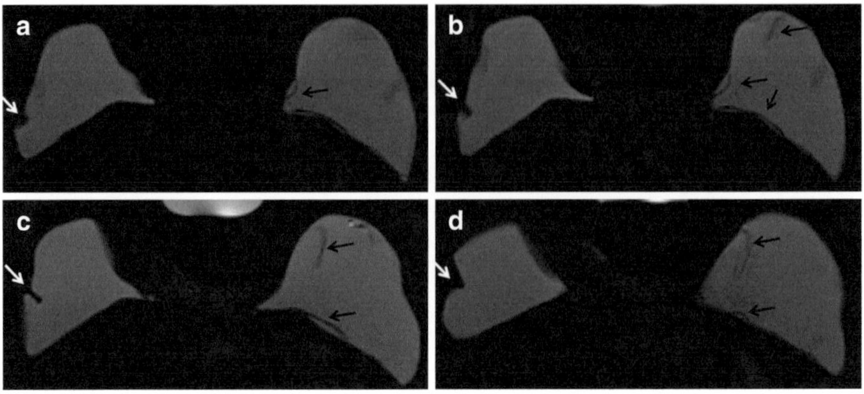

Fig. 6.5 Axial STIR with water suppression (silicone sensitive) MRI image demonstrates a radial fold (*white arrow*) on multiple slices of the right breast implant (**a**–**d**). When scrolling through the entire sequence, the radial fold extends to the surface of the implant shell. This is in contrast to the hypointense curvilinearities signaling intracapsular rupture ("linguine sign") seen in the left implant (*black arrows*) (**a**–**d**)

This means when an under-filled implant is placed into a confined space, it in-folds on itself as needed to conform to the space, and as such minor rippling or undulation is a normal finding on MR imaging. This commonly seen fold pattern can cause confusion as it mimics implant rupture; however normal folds should extend from the edge of the implant shell inward (Fig. 6.5). Additionally, no silicone should ever be seen outside the implant as a whole, along the inner surface of the fibrous capsule or within the folds themselves.

6.7.1 Intracapsular Rupture

When breast implants fail, the most common cause is a small defect or worn area of the implant shell. A large percentage of implant failures occur during surgical implantation; however tears can also occur in-vivo. While trauma can cause an implant to rupture, most implant ruptures have no identifiable cause. The most important factor predisposing an implant to rupture is age of the implant. Historically the prevalence of implant rupture is approximately 30 % at 5 years after implantation, 50 % at 10 years and 70 % at 17 years, with the median age of implants at rupture being around 10.8 years [15]. Additional studies, however, have shown lower rates of implant rupture with later-generation silicone implants [16–18].

When there is a defect in the implant elastomer shell, silicone gel will slowly ooze out, but will be contained in the intracapsular space by the outer fibrous capsule. Over time the escaped silicone contained by the fibrous capsule will surround the implant elastomer shell and cause it to collapse into the pool of remaining silicone.

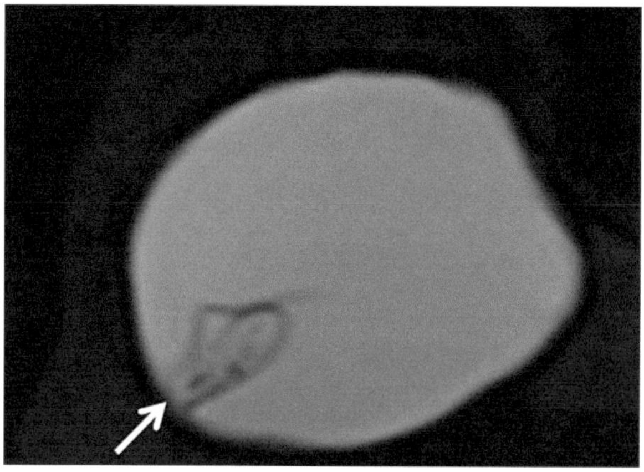

Fig. 6.6 Axial STIR with water suppression (silicone sensitive) MRI image shows the "keyhole" sign (*white arrow*) of intracapsular rupture on the right. At surgical explantation, right intracapsular implant rupture was confirmed

Four categories of implant intracapsular rupture have been described, from early to advanced; these include uncollapsed, minimally collapsed, partially collapsed and fully collapsed [19]. Describing intracapsular rupture by stage using these common terms can be helpful and informative for surgeons and patients when making clinical decisions.

Uncollapsed, or very early implant rupture is seen as silicone gel present in folds outside of the implant shell but contained by the fibrous capsule. This has been referred to by a variety of names including the inverted-loop sign, keyhole sign, teardrop sign or hangnoose sign. This occurs when silicone oil osmotically transgresses the intact elastomer shell and adheres to the fibrous capsule. Later when a tear occurs in the elastomer shell, the liquid silicone will slowly leak out; however it cannot circumferentially extend between the shell and the capsule, as it is confined by the shell-capsule adherence. As a result, the exiting silicone gel accumulates focally and begins to invaginate the otherwise intact regions of the elastomer shell; this has the appearance of a keyhole. This is the most common sign of implant rupture, but it is less specific than other signs described below, especially in cases with motion artifact or suboptimal slice thickness when the keyhole sign can be confused with normal radial folds (Fig. 6.6).

Minimally collapsed intracapsular implant rupture occurs when silicone gel is seen within shell in-foldings as well as between stretches of the implant shell and fibrous capsule. This appearance has been called the 'subcapsular line' or 'back-patch' sign and is seen as dark signal paralleling the dark signal of the fibrous capsule with silicone on both sides.

The 'C-sign' has been used to describe partially collapsed intracapsular implant rupture, and describes a finding seen only with implants from the late 1960s and early 1970s. These implants had thick shells which tended to curl when the implant shell collapsed to the point where there was not enough silicone gel remaining to keep the shell-patches flat. This sign is rarely seen today as these implants are now quite old.

The final and most advanced stage of implant rupture, known as fully collapsed, occurs when the implant shell is completely collapsed within the silicone gel that it used to contain. The elastomer shell which is dark on MR imaging appears as wavy lines within the silicone gel. This curvilinear appearance has been called the "linguine" or 'wavy-line' sign and is the most specific sign of intracapsular implant rupture (Fig. 6.2b).

6.8 Saline Implants

As opposed to silicone implants, saline-filled implants do not rupture, but instead are said to deflate. If there is a defect in the shell or the valve of a saline-filled implant, the saline leaks into the breast parenchyma and will be resorbed within 5 days to 2 weeks. Imaging is not necessary as the clinical exam finding of a deflated implant will be obvious; however if imaging is done for another reason and there is a deflated saline-filled implant in place the appearance is characteristic (Fig. 6.7).

6.8.1 Extracapsular Rupture

If the fibrous capsule is disrupted for any reason, silicone that has escaped the elastomer shell can also escape through the capsule and into the breast, referred to as extracapsular rupture (Figs. 6.8 and 6.9). Extracapsular silicone can be seen as diffusely infiltrating silicone gel collections with or without their own fibrous capsules, silicone granulomas and silicone adenopathy [19].

Diffusely infiltrated silicone gel and silicone gel collections will have the same T2-weighted signal as the silicone contained within intact implants. Silicone granulomas and silicone adenopathy however, will appear less bright on T2-weighted

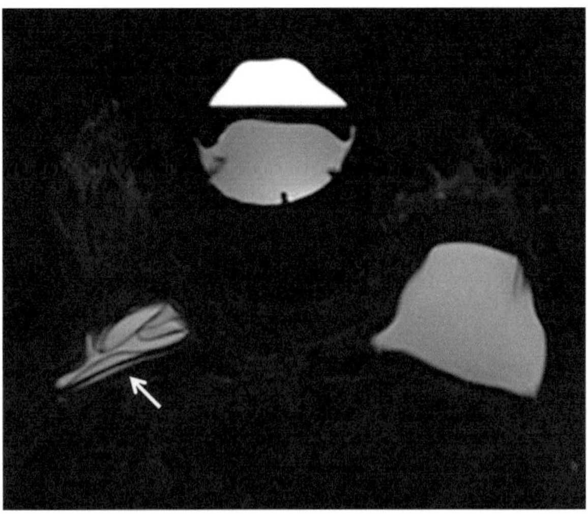

Fig. 6.7 Axial STIR image in a woman with bilateral saline implants demonstrates deflation of the right saline implant (*white arrow*). This patient also had clinical findings compatible with right saline implant rupture

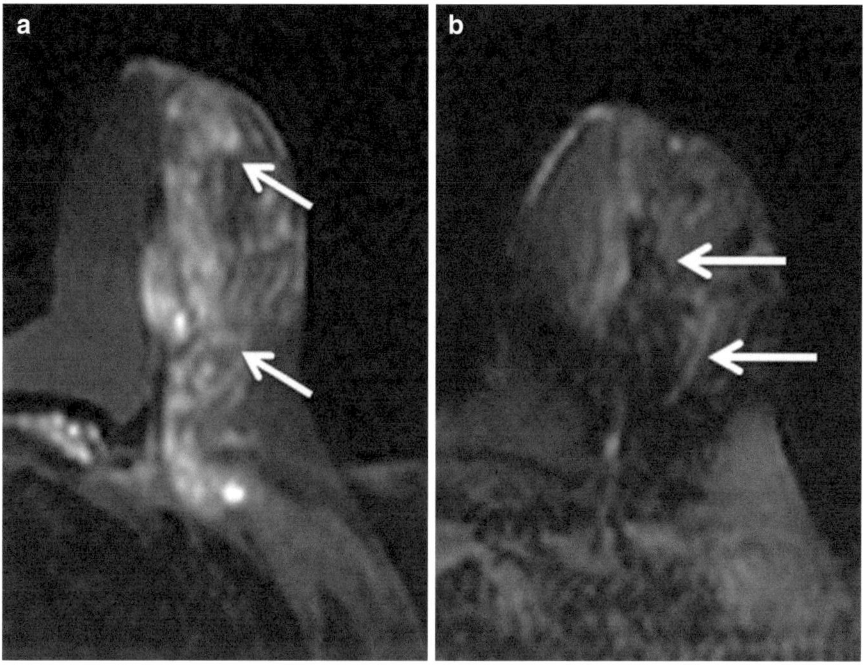

Fig. 6.8 (**a**) Axial STIR with water suppression (silicone sensitive sequence) MRI image demonstrates extensive hyperintense material throughout the left lateral breast (*white arrows*) compatible with extracapsular silicone. (**b**) Axial STIR with silicone suppression (water sensitive sequence) MRI image demonstrates the material in the left lateral breast is hypointense (*white arrows*), compatible with extracapsular silicone

sequences due to fibrosis and have a more heterogeneous appearance with scattered hyperintense T2 foci [19].

When silicone is seen outside the fibrous capsule without signs of intracapsular rupture this should raise the possibility that the current implants are replacements for previously removed implants. Silicone remnants are occasionally inadvertently left in the breast and other times en-bloc removal of the entire implant is not feasible.

6.9 Pitfalls

The most common interpretation pitfall in MR imaging of implants is distinguishing complex folds from the linguine sign of intracapsular implant rupture. The key to differentiating between these entities is to scroll through the images and evaluate whether or not the folds extend all the way to the fibrous capsule surface, a finding which strongly suggests normal folds. Additionally, evaluating the implants in at least two orthogonal planes can be helpful when there is a questionable finding which may be normal folds versus intracapsular rupture.

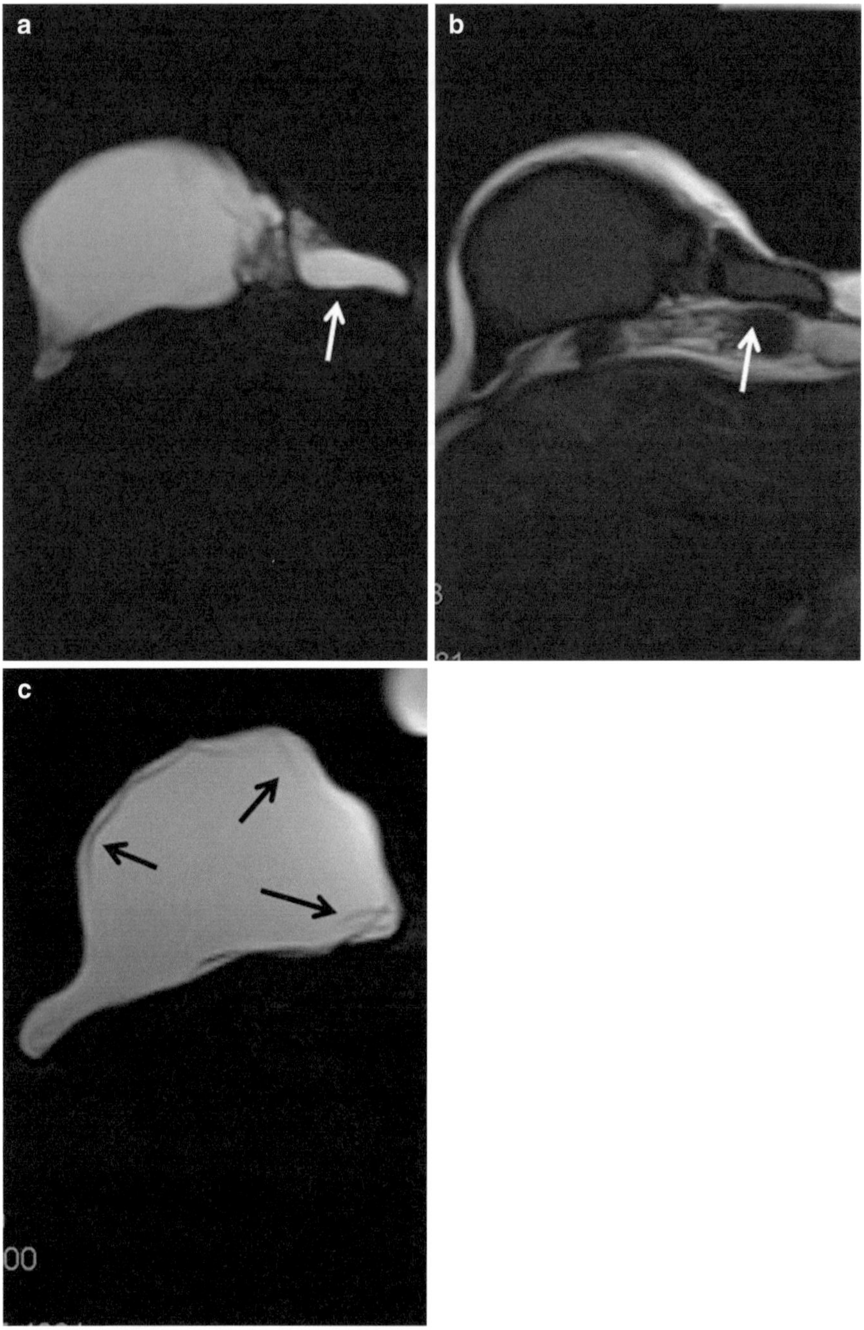

Fig. 6.9 (**a**) Axial water suppressed sequence demonstrates free silicone at the medial aspect of the implant, consistent with extracapsular rupture (*white arrow*). (**b**) This also seen on axial silicone suppression sequence (*white arrow*). (**c**) The implant also demonstrates intrcapsular rupture with multiple curvilinear hypointense lines seen on this axial water suppressed image (*black arrows*)

Another common pitfall occurs when small amounts of silicone oil osmotically transgress the intact elastomer shell and accumulate between the fibrous capsule and shell. Occasionally, because the oils maintain silicone signal, the accumulation of such oils can cause confusion with small inverted-loop appearances.

Sometimes it can be difficult to differentiate between a single lumen implant with intracapsular rupture and a double-lumen implant where no saline was placed in the outer lumen or the outer lumen saline deflated previously. In this situation, medical records and old mammograms can be very useful. Additionally, high resolution implant imaging can sometimes identify both the inner and outer lumen shells [19].

An additional, less frequently encountered pitfall occurs when extracapsular soft-tissue silicone is seen as an enhancing mass within the breast, which can be confused with malignancy. However, silicone granulomas and silicone fluid collections usually enhance with benign enhancement characteristics, and implant specific imaging sequences (silicone-sensitive and silicone-saturated) can also help resolve this dilemma. Breast MRI can be particularly helpful in women with free silicone injections. Mammography and ultrasound have limited sensitivity in this population, but a silicone suppression sequence may be employed in conjunction with a contrast-enhanced study in order to differentiate between concerning lesions and silicone (Fig. 6.10).

6.9.1 Implants and Breast Cancer

There is no direct association between breast implants and breast cancer; however as patients with breast implants age, there is an anticipated increase in the number of breast cancers seen in women with augmented breasts [20]. While mammography is still the primary imaging technique for detecting breast cancer in women with implants, given the decreased sensitivity of screening mammography in this population, there is an increased interest in using MRI to detect breast cancer. Patients who are high-risk will be candidates for dynamic contrast enhanced studies, which involves injecting contrast material and obtaining multiple T1-weighted sequences before and at three time points after the injection (Figs. 6.11 and 6.12).

Studies have examined the features of breast cancers detected in women with implants, and have shown that there is a higher rate of palpable, invasive cancers in women with implants. Importantly however, the stage distribution of cancers in women with implants is similar to screening populations [6]. Mango et al. characterized the MRI features of breast carcinomas detected in the augmented breast [21]. The authors found that the majority of cancers (63 %) appeared as irregular, non-circumscribed, enhancing masses. Most commonly tumors were located in the upper outer quadrant of the breast and frequently (37 % of the time), the tumor abutted the implant. Tumor spread along the implant contour was more likely to be seen with subglandular implants than with subpectoral implants. There was no signifi-

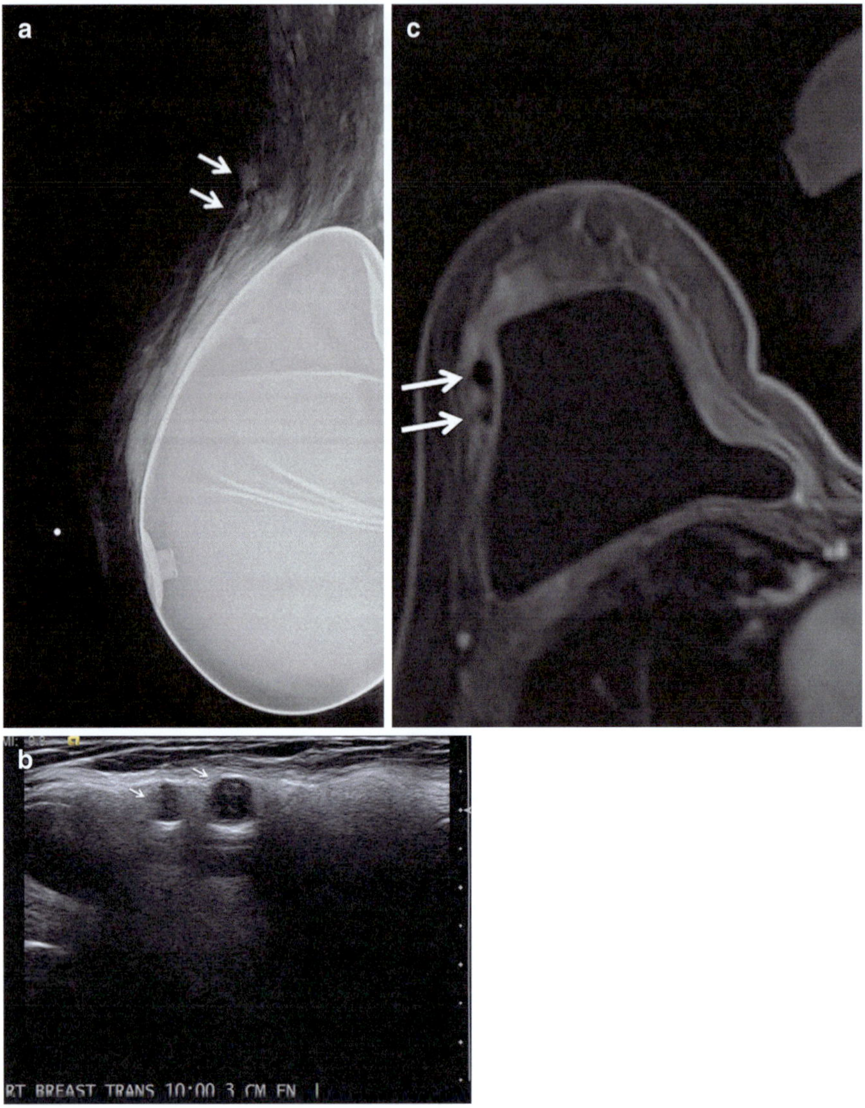

Fig. 6.10 (**a**) 46 year-old woman with previous history of ruptured silicone implant and current saline implants. Right mediolateral oblique mammogram demonstrates the saline implant. At the superior aspect of the breast, abutting the implant, are two asymmetries (*white arrows*). (**b**) Directed ultrasound demonstrates two round circumscribed hypoechoic masses abutting the implant and correlating with mammography (*white arrows*). (**c**) Breast MRI was performed with both contrast-enhanced and implant evaluation sequences. Axial post-contrast T1 demonstrates two adjacent non-enhancing circumscribed masses (*white arrows*) which correlate with mammographic and sonographic findings. (**d**, **e**) The masses follow silicone signal on water suppression and silicone suppression sequences (*white arrows*) and are consistent with silicone granulomas

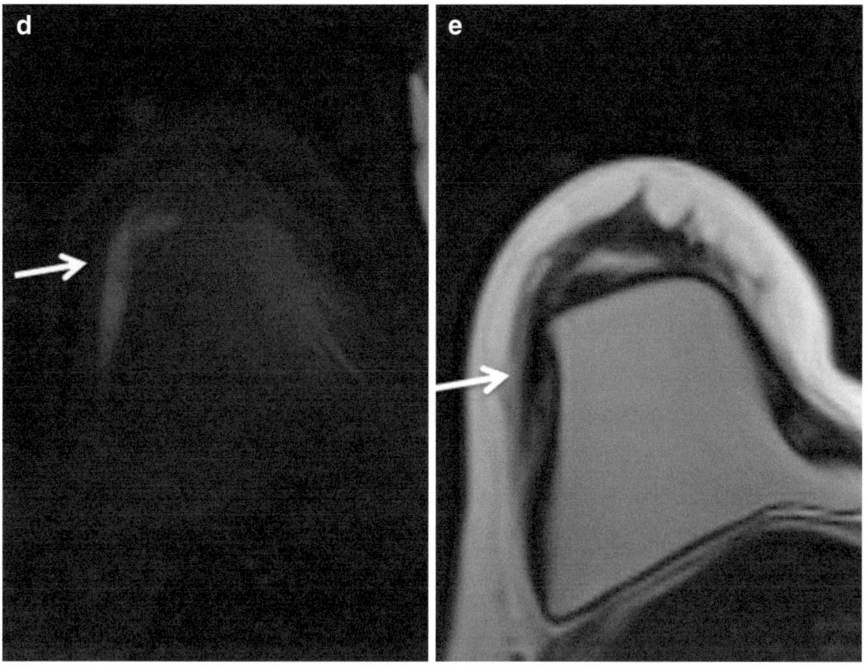

Fig. 6.10 (continued)

cant difference between implant position and lesion morphology or tumor size. In this study, MRI identified mammographically and sonographically occult cancer in 30 % of cases and identified patients with otherwise occult multifocal disease (7 %) and multicentric disease (22 %). While further studies are needed, the results of this study suggest that MRI should be considered to assess extent of disease in women with implants and newly diagnosed cancer before surgery.

For breast cancer patients treated with mastectomy, there is no significant difference in the rate of cancer recurrence in augmented versus non-augmented breasts. A small series has shown MR imaging to be superior to physical exam and mammography for the detection of recurrent cancer in postmastectomy patients with implants, especially when tumor was close to the chest wall [22].

A promising alternative to diagnose breast cancer without the injection of contrast has been proposed using diffusion-weighted MR imaging (DWI) [23]. While still in the process of being validated, the main concept behind DWI is that the high cellular density of proliferating cancers will cause increased restricted diffusion and thus the calculated apparent diffusion coefficient (ADC) maps will be lower when compared with normal fibroglandular tissue or benign lesions. Performing screening MRI based on diffusion measurements would require a fast technique, with reduced sensitivity to motion artifact. Recently, in 2015 Solomon et al evaluated the usefulness of diffusion-weighted spatiotemporally encoded (SPEN) MRI sequences to obtain ADC maps of normal fibroglandular

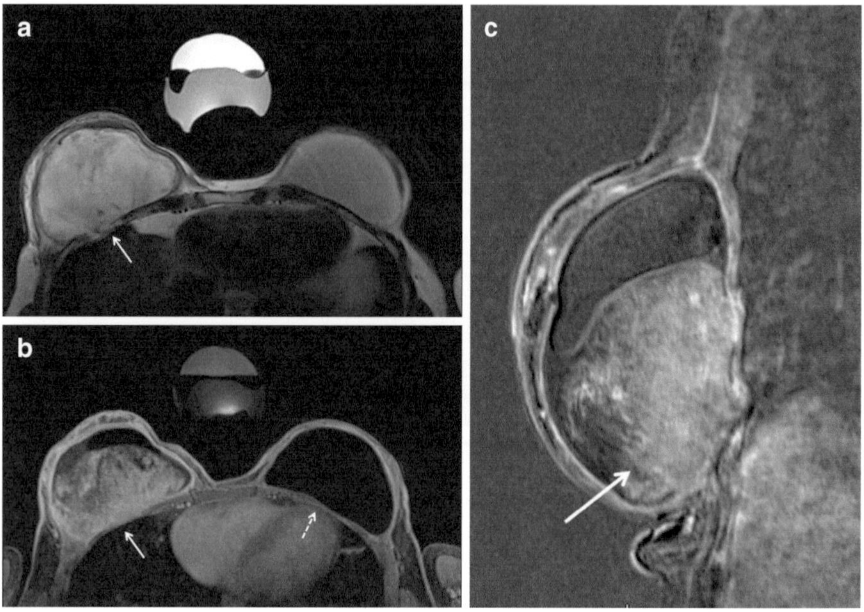

Fig. 6.11 (**a**) 45-year-old woman with history of left mastectomy for LCIS and bilateral silicone implant reconstruction with enlarging right breast mass. Axial nonsuppressed T2 MRI image demonstrates a large heterogeneous right breast mass (*white arrow*) which invades the chest wall and displaces the silicone implant. Note normal appearance of the silicone implant on the left (*white dashed arrow*). Axial (**b**) and sagittal (**c**) post-contrast T1-VIBE with fat-saturation MRI images demonstrates this mass is heterogeneously enhancing (*white arrow* on each figure). Final pathology revealed aggressive fibromatosis

tissue in the presence of silicone implants in seven healthy volunteers [24]. They found that despite dominant signal from silicone implants, they were able to obtain reliable ADC maps of fibroglandular tissue. While additional studies with more patients are needed to validate these results, the findings present promising new MRI screening possibilities for the future.

6.9.2 Other MRI Findings in Patients with Implants

Postoperative seromas are expected following implantation; however the development of a large fluid collection beyond the immediate postoperative period raises the possibility of infection. Occasionally fluid collections are noted following viral syndromes and aspiration of the fluid does not demonstrate a causative organism [25].

Recently a relationship has been described between breast silicone implants and the development of anaplastic large cell lymphoma. This usually manifests as an ill-defined mass, however one of the unexpected imaging findings of anaplastic

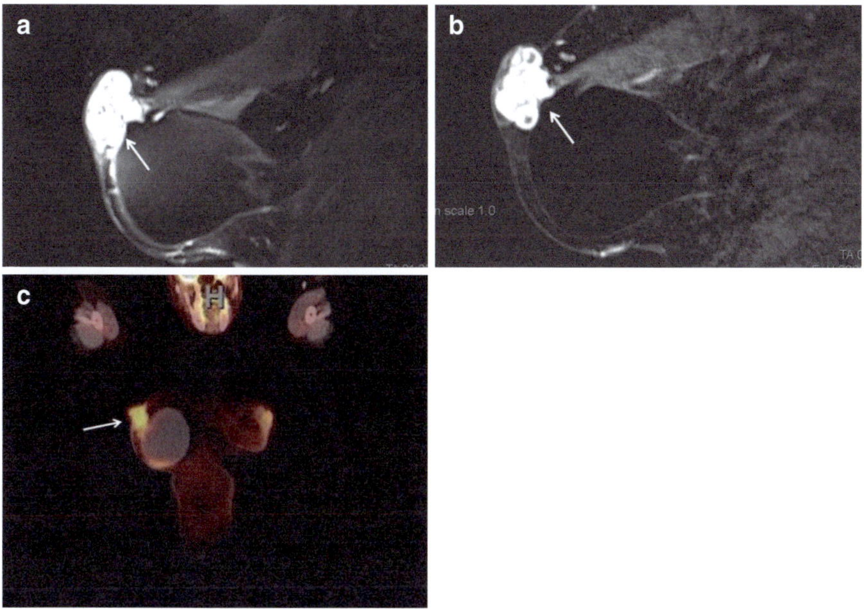

Fig. 6.12 50-year-old woman with a history of benign right phyllodes tumor 3 years ago and status post bilateral mastectomies and reconstruction with silicone implants presents with a new right periareolar mass. (**a**) T2 weighted sagittal MRI image demonstrates T2 hyperintense exophytic mass correlating with palpable lump abutting the superior aspect of the implant (*white arrow*). (**b**) The enhancing mass (*white arrow*) demonstrates Type 1 (persistent) enhancement. (**c**) The mass is FDG-avid on PET-CT (*white arrow*). Ultrasound-guided biopsy demonstrated recurrent phyllodes

large cell lymphoma is that it can mimic a seroma or fluid collection related to infection or post-viral syndrome [26].

After placement of silicone implants, nonspecific inflammation or silicone migration can cause axillary and internal mammary lymph nodes to enlarge. The differential diagnosis of enlarged lymph nodes includes recurrent breast cancer and second primary nodal metastases. In a study of 923 women with breast cancer and silicone implants by Sutton et al in 2015, the authors concluded that intramammary lymph nodes identified on MRI after oncoplastic surgery for breast cancer were overwhelmingly more likely to be benign than malignant [27] (Fig. 6.13).

6.10 Conclusions

Breast implant magnetic resonance imaging is the primary modality used to evaluate implant integrity and to determine the relationship of breast implants to any breast lesions that may be present. Much existing data supports the utility of MRI in

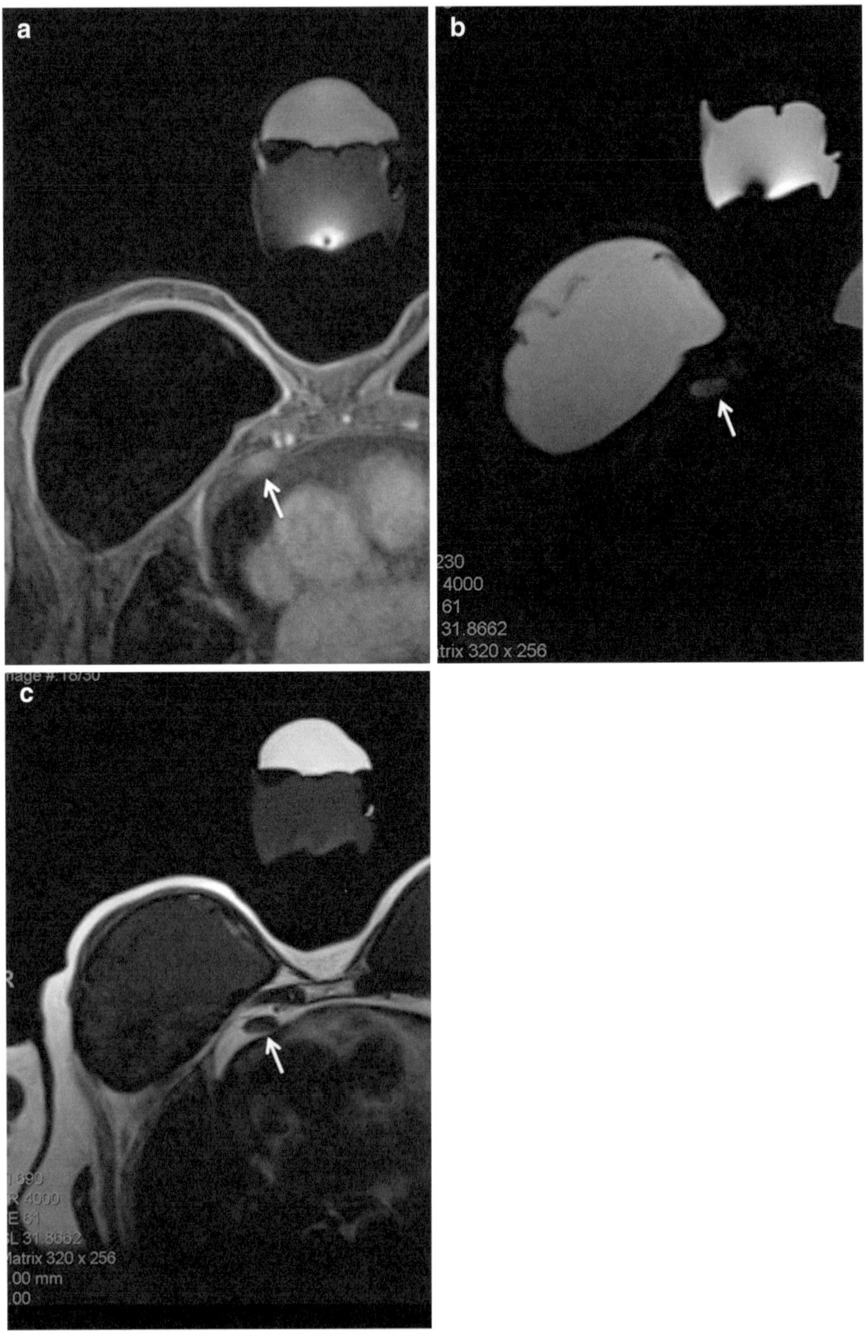

Fig. 6.13 75-year-old woman with history of remote left breast cancer status post bilateral mastectomies and multiple silicone implant revisions. Breast MRI demonstrates an enlarged enhancing anterior mediastinal lymph node (*white arrow*) seen on delayed post contrast T1 weighted axial image (**a**). The lymph node follows silicone signal on water suppression (*white arrow*) (**b**) and silicone suppression (*white arrow*) (**c**) sequences

evaluating women with breast implants. Noncontrast MRI utilizes sequences that are designed to separate water, silicone and fat to evaluate the internal implant structure and assess for extracapsular silicone. Contrast enhanced MRI has been shown to be a useful adjunct to mammography, which has limited sensitivity in detecting breast cancer in women with breast implants. The role of MRI in screening asymptomatic women with breast implants remains to be determined, and future directions include utilizing diffusion weighted imaging, avoiding the need for contrast enhancement.

References

1. Steinbach BG, Hardt NS, Abbitt PL, Lanier L, Caffee HH. Breast implants, common complications, and concurrent breast disease. Radiographics (A Review Publication of the Radiological Society of North America, Inc.). 1993;13(1):95–118. Epub 1993/01/01.
2. Middleton MS, McNamara Jr MP. Breast implant classification with MR imaging correlation: (CME available on RSNA link). Radiographics (A Review Publication of the Radiological Society of North America, Inc.). 2000;20(3):E1. Epub 2000/06/02.
3. Cronin TD, Gerow FJ, editors. Augmentation mammoplasty: a new "natural feel" prosthesis. Transactions of the third international congress of plastic surgery. Excerpta Medica Foundation; Amsterdam, The Netherlands; 1963.
4. Brenner RJ. Evaluation of breast silicone implants. Magn Reson Imaging Clin N Am. 2013;21(3):547–60. Epub 2013/08/10.
5. LeVier RR, Harrison MC, Cook RR, Lane TH. What is silicone? Plast Reconstr Surg. 1993;92(1):163–7. Epub 1993/07/01.
6. Morris EA, Liberman L. Breast MRI. New York: Springer; 2005.
7. Surgeons ASoP. Plastic surgery statistics report. 2014.
8. Juanpere S, Perez E, Huc O, Motos N, Pont J, Pedraza S. Imaging of breast implants – a pictorial review. Insights Imaging. 2011;2(6):653–70. Epub 2012/02/22.
9. Miglioretti DL, Rutter CM, Geller BM, Cutter G, Barlow WE, Rosenberg R, et al. Effect of breast augmentation on the accuracy of mammography and cancer characteristics. JAMA. 2004;291(4):442–50. Epub 2004/01/30.
10. Di Benedetto G, Cecchini S, Grassetti L, Baldassarre S, Valeri G, Leva L, et al. Comparative study of breast implant rupture using mammography, sonography, and magnetic resonance imaging: correlation with surgical findings. Breast J. 2008;14(6):532–7. Epub 2008/12/05.
11. DeBruhl ND, Gorczyca DP, Ahn CY, Shaw WW, Bassett LW. Silicone breast implants: US evaluation. Radiology. 1993;189(1):95–8. Epub 1993/10/01.
12. Administration USFaD. Silicone gel-filled breast implants. 2013.
13. Kreymerman P, Patrick RJ, Rim A, Djohan R, Crowe JP. Guidelines for using breast magnetic resonance imaging to evaluate implant integrity. Ann Plast Surg. 2009;62(4):355–7. Epub 2009/03/28.
14. Holmich LR, Vejborg I, Conrad C, Sletting S, McLaughlin JK. The diagnosis of breast implant rupture: MRI findings compared with findings at explantation. Eur J Radiol. 2005;53(2):213–25. Epub 2005/01/25.
15. Chung KC, Wilkins EG, Beil Jr RJ, Helvie MA, Ikeda DM, Oneal RM, et al. Diagnosis of silicone gel breast implant rupture by ultrasonography. Plast Reconstr Surg. 1996;97(1):104–9. Epub 1996/01/01.
16. Maxwell GP. Discussion. Rupture rate and patterns of shell failure with the McGhan Style 153 double-lumen breast implant. Plast Reconstr Surg. 2011;127(1):54–5. Epub 2011/01/05.
17. Hammond DC. Discussion: prevalence of rupture in poly implant Prothese silicone breast implants, recalled from the European market in 2010. Plast Reconstr Surg. 2012;129(6):1379–80. Epub 2012/05/29.

18. Stevens WG, Pacella SJ, Gear AJ, Freeman ME, McWhorter C, Tenenbaum MJ, et al. Clinical experience with a fourth-generation textured silicone gel breast implant: a review of 1012 Mentor MemoryGel breast implants. Aesthet Surg J (The American Society for Aesthetic Plastic Surgery). 2008;28(6):642–7. Epub 2008/12/17.
19. Middleton MS. MR evaluation of breast implants. Radiol Clin North Am. 2014;52(3):591–608. Epub 2014/05/06.
20. McCarthy CM, Pusic AL, Disa JJ, Cordeiro PG, Cody 3rd HS, Mehrara B. Breast cancer in the previously augmented breast. Plast Reconstr Surg. 2007;119(1):49–58. Epub 2007/01/27.
21. Mango VL, Kaplan J, Sung JS, Moskowitz CS, Dershaw DD, Morris EA. Breast carcinoma in augmented breasts: MRI findings. AJR Am J Roentgenol. 2015;204(5):W599–604. Epub 2015/04/24.
22. Bone B, Aspelin P, Isberg B, Perbeck L, Veress B. Contrast-enhanced MR imaging of the breast in patients with breast implants after cancer surgery. Acta Radiol. 1995;36(2):111–6. Epub 1995/03/01.
23. Sharma U, Danishad KK, Seenu V, Jagannathan NR. Longitudinal study of the assessment by MRI and diffusion-weighted imaging of tumor response in patients with locally advanced breast cancer undergoing neoadjuvant chemotherapy. NMR Biomed. 2009;22(1):104–13. Epub 2008/04/04.
24. Solomon E, Nissan N, Schmidt R, Furman-Haran E, Ben-Aharon U, Frydman L. Removing silicone artifacts in diffusion-weighted breast MRI by means of shift-resolved spatiotemporally encoding. Magn Reson Med. 2015;75(5):2064–71. Epub 2015/06/23.
25. Soo MS, Kornguth PJ, Georgiade GS, Sullivan DC. Seromas in residual fibrous capsules after explantation – mammographic and sonographic appearances. Radiology. 1995;194(3):863–6.
26. de Jong D, Vasmel WLE, de Boer JP, Verhave G, Barbe E, Casparie MK, et al. Anaplastic large-cell lymphoma in women with breast implants. JAMA. 2008;300(17):2030–5.
27. Sutton EJ, Watson EJ, Gibbons G, Goldman DA, Moskowitz CS, Jochelson MS, et al. Incidence of internal mammary lymph nodes with silicone breast implants at MR imaging after oncoplastic surgery. Radiology. 2015;277(2):381–7. Epub 2015/06/23.

Chapter 7
Problem Solving Breast MRI for Mammographic, Sonographic, or Clinical Findings

Eren D. Yeh and Catherine S. Giess

Abstract Because of the high sensitivity of breast MRI in detection of invasive breast cancer, there has been interest in using breast MRI as a problem solving tool for evaluation of mammographic or sonographic findings, or for clinical breast symptoms in which conventional mammographic or ultrasound evaluation is negative. In this chapter, we review and discuss the current literature on problem solving MRI for imaging or clinical findings. Breast MRI does not have sufficient negative predictive value to avoid biopsy of a suspicious mammographic or sonographic finding. It may rarely be indicaed for equivocal or inconclusive findings at diagnostic mammographic and sonographic evaluation and when biopsy cannot be performed. It has not been found to be helpful for most clinical symptoms such as a palpable finding or breast pain when conventional imaging is negative, but may have utility in patients with nipple discharge, or symptoms suggestive of inflammatory breast cancer or Paget's disease.

Keywords Breast MRI • Problem solving MRI • Breast pain • Nipple discharge

7.1 Introduction

Breast MRI is currently considered the most sensitive breast imaging modality for the detection of invasive breast cancer [1, 2] with reported sensitivities of 71–100 % [2]. Because of this high sensitivity of breast MRI in detecting invasive breast cancer, there has been considerable interest in adding breast MRI to imaging algorithms

E.D. Yeh, MD (✉) • C.S. Giess, MD
Department of Radiology, Brigham and Women's Hospital, Section of Breast Imaging, 75 Francis Street, RA Bldg, RA-014, Boston, MA 02115, USA
e-mail: eyeh@partners.org; cgiess@partners.org

S.L. Heller, L. Moy (eds.), *Breast Oncology: Techniques, Indications, and Interpretation*, DOI 10.1007/978-3-319-42563-4_7

for the evaluation of mammographic or ultrasound findings, or for clinical breast symptoms in which standard mammographic or ultrasound evaluation has proved to be unrevealing. In fact, problem solving has been noted to be one of the earliest applications of breast MRI described in the medical literature [3].

The positive predictive value for malignancy of suspicious mammographic or ultrasound findings is approximately 25–40 % [4, 5]; thus, the majority of breast biopsies in the United States are benign. Breast MRI could theoretically improve the specificity of breast biopsy for suspicious imaging findings. Similarly, the use of breast MRI in the further evaluation of suspicious clinical findings such as palpable abnormalities, focal pain, or nipple discharge which have negative mammographic and or ultrasound evaluation could conceivably guide clinical management and reduce delayed cancer diagnosis in patients.

However, problem solving MRI for findings on conventional mammography or ultrasound has been considered a somewhat controversial application of the modality because percutaneous biopsy is so readily available, so easily tolerated, and usually allows a definitive histopathologic diagnosis, while breast MRI is expensive, not universally available, and has moderate specificity [3, 6]. Additionally, MRI for the evaluation of palpable findings for which conventional mammography and ultrasound are unrevealing has been considered to have a limited role [7, 8], since the chance of malignancy for a palpable finding or focal pain with negative conventional imaging is so low [9–11]. The diagnostic evaluation of nipple discharge has been more variable in clinical practice [7], and MRI could perhaps improve diagnosis and management. The current literature on problem solving MRI for imaging or clinical findings will be reviewed and discussed.

7.2 Mammographic and Ultrasound Findings

7.2.1 Suspicious Lesions

Utilizing MRI to downgrade lesions considered suspicious on mammography or ultrasound has been evaluated previously [12–16]. Perhaps the most influential study to date was reported by Bluemke et al. [12], who conducted a prospective multi-institutional study of 821 patients who underwent breast MRI before biopsy of suspicious findings. In their study the majority (84.7 %) of the 821 patients had suspicious mammographic findings, 1.8 % had suspicious ultrasound findings, and the remaining 11.7 % had suspicious clinical findings. Details on the specific mammographic findings were not given, other than the presence or absence of microcalcifications. The sensitivity and specificity of breast MRI were 88.1 % and 67.7 % respectively, and neither sensitivity nor specificity was affected by breast density, tumor type, or menopausal status. Although MRI had a higher positive predictive value (72.4 %) than mammography (52.8 %), its negative predictive value was only 85.4 %, and those authors concluded that MRI should not be used to avoid biopsy of suspicious findings.

Several studies have evaluated breast MRI in the management of suspicious calcifications [13, 14, 17]. Bazzocchi et al. [13] performed a multi-center trial evaluating the use of breast MRI in the evaluation of 112 suspicious (BI-RADS 4 or 5) microcalcifications, 38 with and 74 without an associated mass. Overall, breast MRI had a sensitivity and specificity for malignancy of 87 % and 68 % respectively, with a positive predictive value of 84 % and a negative predictive value of 71 %. Not surprisingly, the sensitivity for malignancy for calcifications associated with a mass (97 %) was significantly higher compared to calcifications alone (80 %); the authors suggested this was likely due to increased neo-angiogenesis when calcifications had an associated mass. These authors concluded that MRI should not be used in the assessment of mammographically suspicious microcalcifications because of the overall 87 % sensitivity. Cilotti et al. [14] also evaluated the use of MRI in evaluating mammographically suspicious microcalcifications, and reported that MRI had a 73 % sensitivity, 76 % specificity, a 73 % positive predictive value and a 76 % negative predictive value. These authors also concluded that MRI had no role in the management algorithm of suspicious microcalcifications. Uematsu et al. [17] used diagnostic MRI to evaluate suspicious calcifications prior to stereotactic vacuum-assisted core biopsy. They suggested that while MRI can offer additional diagnostic information for women who decline biopsy, because of its imperfect positive and negative predictive values, it should not replace stereotactic biopsy.

In a different study by Yau et al. [15] evaluating problem solving MRI, comparison to the aforementioned studies is limited by different study inclusion criteria. The results of 204 clinical and or mammographic findings that underwent problem solving MRI were reported together, with fourteen (6.9 %) malignancies. Eleven (79 %) of the fourteen cancers had mammographic and or sonographic findings considered suspicious; the authors pointed out these cases had already been referred for biopsy regardless of MRI findings. The other three patients with cancers found on MRI had clinical symptoms but negative mammography and US. No details regarding the specific types of imaging findings referred for evaluation with MRI were reported. The premise that breast MRI should not be utilized to determine management of suspicious imaging findings was recently challenged in the radiology literature. Strobel et al. [16] evaluated 353 BI-RADS 4 lesions with breast MRI, 198 (56.1 %) found on screening mammography and 155 (43.9 %) on screening ultrasound, in asymptomatic women and correlated the MRI with either histopathology or imaging surveillance for at least 18 months. In this study, types of mammographic findings were reported and included 71 (35.9 %) masses, 34 (17.2 %) focal asymmetries, 15 (7.6 %) architectural distortions, and 78 (39.4 %) microcalcifications; ultrasound findings were 115 (74.2 %) masses and 40 (25.8 %) non-mass lesions. MRI correctly found no cancer in 92 % of benign BI-RADS 4 lesions, while identifying 95.5 % of malignant BI-RADS 4 lesions. The authors had false negative MRI results in three women with pure clustered microcalcifications, all representing low grade ductal carcinoma in situ (DCIS). Based on their results, the authors concluded that MRI could be used to help avoid biopsy in mammographically or sonographically suspicious lesions (perhaps excepting pure microcalcifications), and proposed that diagnostic breast MRI be accepted instead of tissue diagnosis for BI-RADS 4 lesions. This proposal would be a significant deviation from current clinical practice.

7.2.2 Probably Benign Lesions

Several studies have evaluated the use of problem solving MRI for probably benign (BI-RADS 3) lesions. Cilotti et al. [14] reported 23 cases of microcalcifications assessed as BI-RADS 3, six malignant; MRI identified three of these malignancies. They found no significant difference in the sensitivity of MRI and mammography to diagnose malignancy in BI-RADS 3 calcifications. Uematsu et al. [17] reported the use of MRI before biopsy of 55 screen-detected calcifications assessed as BI-RADS 3. There were four malignancies (7.2 %) in this group, three identified with MRI. Both of these studies reported a higher than 2 % malignancy rate in their BI-RADS 3 mammographic calcifications. Gokalp et al. [18] performed breast MRI in 56 mammographic lesions (85.7 % masses or focal asymmetries, 14.3 % calcifications) assessed as BI-RADS 3, and correlated findings with either biopsy or 2 years of imaging follow up. They reported a malignancy rate of 1.8 % (1 of 56) and concluded that MRI did not add to the diagnostic evaluation or management of BI-RADS 3 lesions. In a meta-analysis of studies on problem solving MRI for BI-RADS 3 lesions, Dorrius et al. [19] noted that the negative predictive value for non-calcified BI-RADS 3 lesions was 100 %, and suggested that MRI might be helpful to exclude further evaluation of non-calcified BI-RADS 3 lesions.

It must be noted that by definition, a probably benign (BI-RADS 3) mammographic lesion should have a less than 2 % chance of malignancy, and such lesions are typically referred for imaging surveillance at 6, 12, and 24 months [5]. Adding problem solving MRI to the diagnostic imaging algorithm for lesions with such a high probability of benignity is unlikely to offer a favorable cost-benefit ratio.

7.2.3 Equivocal Lesions

The American College of Radiology 2014 practice guidelines for breast MRI [20] state that the use of breast MRI for the evaluation of imaging or clinical findings considered inconclusive may *rarely* be indicated when biopsy cannot be performed. In a high quality clinical practice, a very small minority of mammographic or ultrasound lesions should remain "equivocal", or of uncertain clinical significance at diagnostic imaging evaluation. Moy et al. [21] reported that only 0.14 % of diagnostic mammograms at their institution were considered equivocal. At Brigham and Women's Hospital over a recent 4 year period, only 0.7 % of diagnostic mammograms were considered inconclusive or equivocal [22]. Breast MRI might guide management of such equivocal or inconclusive findings at diagnostic evaluation, and improve cancer detection and diagnosis.

There are a number of situations in which an imaging finding at diagnostic evaluation may be considered equivocal, or of uncertain clinical significance [22]. A lesion may be equivocal if it is present on only some but not all diagnostic views (Fig. 7.1). Sometimes there is uncertainty whether a perceived mammographic change is due to true morphologic change or a technical factor affecting conspicuity, such as differences in positioning, compression, or radiographic technique (Fig. 7.2). A lesion may be suspected, but biopsy choices are limited. This can occur when the mammographic finding lacks an ultrasound correlate and targeting for stereotactic biopsy is considered problematic because the mammographic finding is vague, hard to identify in the background parenchyma (Fig. 7.3), or inaccessible to

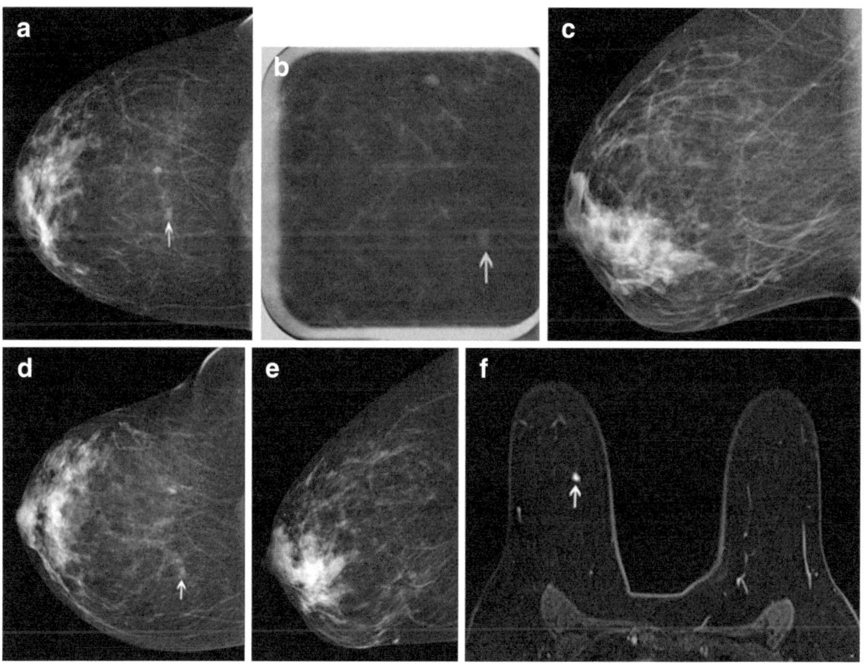

Fig. 7.1 Sixty-four year old with a screen recalled asymmetry (*arrow*) in the medial right breast on the CC view (**a**), persistent (*arrow*) on spot compression CC (**b**), but not evident on ML view (**c**). Rolled CC views show a pliable appearing asymmetry (*arrow*) on the medially rolled CC view (**d**), but no abnormality on the laterally rolled CC view (**e**). The equivocal asymmetry was localized to the upper inner breast (based on its displacement on the medially rolled CC view relative to the full CC view) for diagnostic US evaluation, which was negative. The patient was referred for problem solving MRI. Axial post contrast fat suppressed image (**f**) shows a 5 mm enhancing mass (*arrow*), which represented a stage 1, 0.7 cm invasive ductal cancer

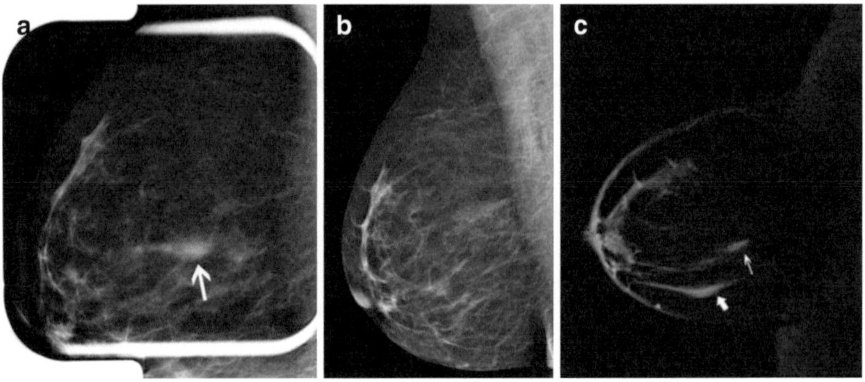

Fig. 7.2 Forty-eight year old recalled for developing focal asymmetry in the right upper outer breast on screening views (not shown). The finding persisted on spot compression MLO view (**a**, *arrow*) and ML view (not shown), and was new since the prior MLO view (**b**). Targeted ultrasound was negative. The patient had undergone a twenty pound weight loss since the prior imaging and it was uncertain if the developing asymmetry was due to differences in tissue composition and mammographic compression versus a true lesion. MRI was performed, and sagittal post contrast fat suppressed image (**c**) showed normally enhancing fibroglandular tissue (*thin arrow*), which appeared similar to other areas of normally enhancing fibroglandular tissue (*thick arrow*). The patient underwent mammographic surveillance, and has been without evidence of disease for greater than 3 years

needle biopsy. Further, sometimes in this setting biopsy has already been attempted unsuccessfully or biopsy results are considered possibly discordant [22]. When there is underlying diagnostic uncertainty about whether the lesion is even real, the diagnostic radiologist may be hesitant to proceed to surgical excision without additional diagnostic testing such as MRI.

A number of studies have evaluated the use of MRI for problem solving of equivocal mammographic lesions [21, 23–25]. In 1998, Sardanelli et al. [23] published results on 19 mammographic findings considered equivocal that underwent diagnostic MRI. Lesions included questionable change in the appearance of lumpectomy scar (N = 11), questionable distortions (N = 2), "nodular opacities" (N = 5), or calcifications (N = 1). There were five (26.3 %) malignancies, one with negative MRI. The following year, Lee et al. [24] described the use of problem solving MRI for 86 equivocal mammographic findings in their institution. These 86 lesions included lesions that demonstrated questionable/uncertain change (N = 26), questioned lesions that could not be localized (N = 16) or persisted on only some views (N = 20), or questioned change in the appearance of a benign surgical site (N = 9) or lumpectomy scar (N = 15). They had 9 (10.5 %) malignancies, and one additional malignant lesion incidentally detected by MRI. Moy and colleagues [21] had 115 equivocal mammographic lesions referred for problem solving MRI, including asymmetries (N = 55), focal asymmetries (N = 43), architectural distortions (N = 12), and change in appearance of a benign surgical scar (N = 5), with 6 (5.2 %) malignancies. Spick et al. [25] reported 111 patients with inconclusive findings on conventional mammographic or

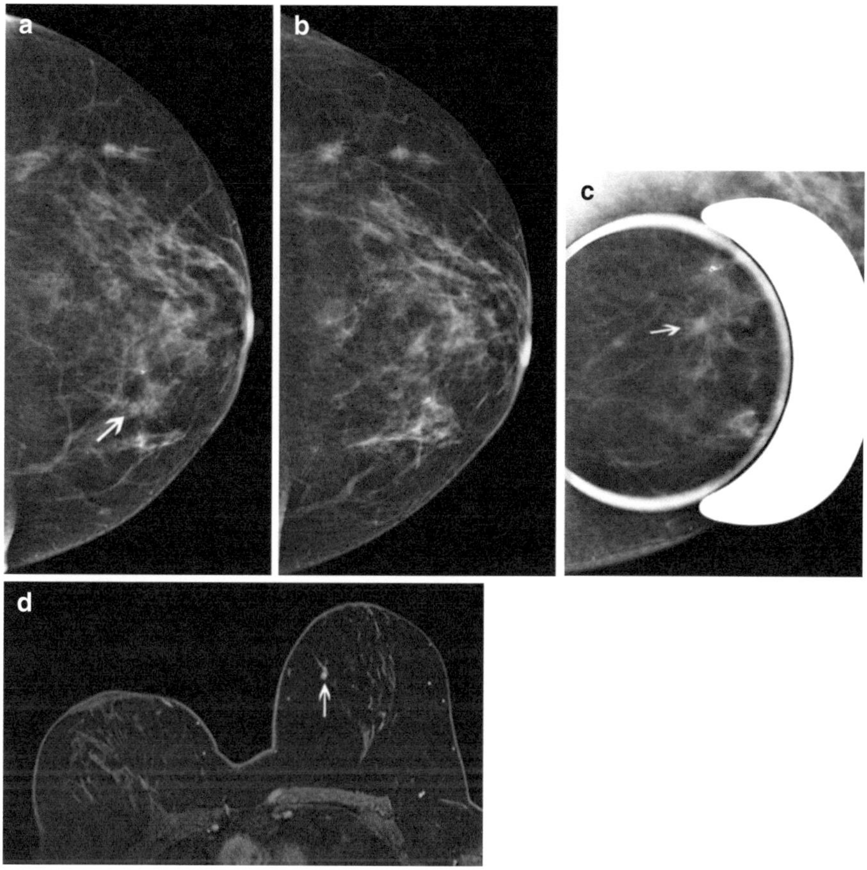

Fig. 7.3 Fifty-five year old with prior right lumpectomy and questionable subtle asymmetry (*arrow*) in the medial left breast on the CC view (**a**) only, apparently new since the prior CC view (**b**). Biopsy clip lateral to the finding was from a prior benign biopsy. The one view finding was subtle and equivocal on spot compression CC view (**c**, *arrow*), and felt to be difficult to identify in a background of heterogeneously dense tissue for an attempted stereotactic biopsy. US evaluation of the medial left breast was negative. Problem solving MRI was performed for further evaluation. Axial fat suppressed post contrast image (**d**) showed a correlative 4 mm enhancing mass in the medial left breast, which represented an invasive lobular cancer, stage 2

ultrasound imaging assessed as BI-RADS 0 who underwent problem solving MRI, with 15 (13.5 %) malignancies. At our institution (unpublished data) over a 4 year period, we had 294 equivocal mammographic lesions (including 89 focal asymmetries, 76 asymmetries, 64 masses, 44 architectural distortions, 17 scars versus malignancy, and 4 miscellaneous) referred for problem solving MRI, with 40 (13.6 %) malignancies (Fig. 7.4). Other studies [15, 26] did not specify lesion types considered equivocal, and reported equivocal clinical and imaging findings together, making direct comparison of their results to the aforementioned studies challenging.

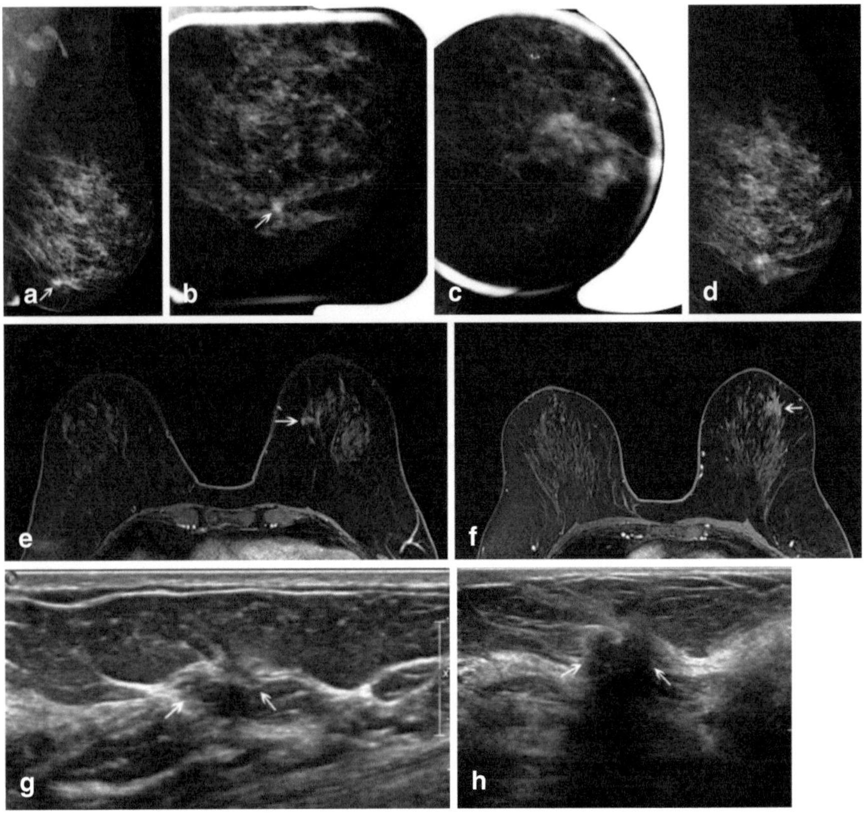

Fig. 7.4 Sixty-eight year old with a one view asymmetry (*arrow*) with questionable associated distortion on screening left MLO view (**a**). The finding persisted on one spot MLO view (**b**) but was not persistent on another spot MLO view (**c**), nor on an LM view (**d**), which both showed heterogeneously dense tissue but no discrete finding. The questioned finding was not seen on the CC view (not shown) and targeted US evaluation was negative. The finding was considered equivocal, and problem solving MRI was performed. Axial fat suppressed post contrast enhanced images (**e**, **f**) showed an area of non-mass enhancement (*arrow*, **e**) in the left lower inner quadrant corresponding to the mammographic equivocal asymmetry, as well as an incidentally detected, mammographically occult spiculated mass in the upper outer quadrant (*arrow*, **f**). Both findings demonstrated slow early and persistent late kinetics. Repeat targeted ultrasound (**g**, **h**) showed a subtle area of architectural distortion (**g**, *arrows*) corresponding to the mammographic asymmetry, and a hypoechoic ill-defined mass with posterior acoustic shadowing (**h**, *arrows*) corresponding to the incidentally detected spiculated mass. Findings represented multi-centric invasive lobular cancer, stage 2, with positive sentinel node

The possibility of detecting otherwise unsuspected, incidental findings in patients undergoing MRI is not at all uncommon [27]. This is an important consideration, since otherwise unsuspected but ultimately benign findings detected solely on MRI generate additional costs with either biopsy or follow up imaging surveillance. An otherwise unsuspected occult malignancy detected by MRI is even less common. However, only a few of the studies on the use of MRI for equivocal mammographic lesions reported their incidental MRI findings [21, 24]. Lee et al. [24] found 12 incidental enhancing lesions on MRI, with one (8.3 %) malignancy. Moy et al. [21] had 18 incidental enhancing lesions on MRI, all benign on either follow up or biopsy. At our institution (unpublished data), out of 294 problem solving MRIs over a 4 year period, we had 44 incidental enhancing lesions, 41 had biopsy or at least 1 year of stable follow up imaging, and 7 (17.0 %) were malignant (Fig. 7.4).

7.2.4 Recurrence Versus Scarring After Breast Conservation Therapy

A type of equivocal situation on mammography which deserves individual discussion is that of breast cancer recurrence versus post treatment change after breast conservation therapy. This was an early utilization of breast MRI for problem solving, because it is well known that mammography has reduced sensitivity for malignancy after breast conservation therapy [28]. Sometimes it may be unclear whether an apparent mammographic change in the lumpectomy scar's appearance (such as increased density) is due to technical factors or a subtle recurrence.

Several studies have reported that MRI was able to distinguish recurrent breast cancer from scar [29–33]. Heywang et al. [29] found that the performance of MRI less than 18 months following definitive surgery was unhelpful due to post-surgical enhancement, but that after 18 months treatment related enhancement was rare. They concluded that after 18 months MRI allowed both early detection of, and reliable exclusion of recurrent tumor. In 1998 Viehweg et al. [30] performed MRI in 207 women with a history of breast conservation therapy, 80 of whom had suspicious clinical or conventional imaging findings. Similarly to Heywang et al. [29], they found that MRI performed within 12 months of definitive surgery was of limited value because of enhancement due to benign post-treatment changes, but that after 12 months MRI had a sensitivity of 100 % and a specificity of 91 % in the detection of recurrent tumor. Gilles et al. [31] performed MRI in 26 patients with suspected recurrence based on clinical or mammographic findings, and found that all 14 surgically proven recurrences demonstrated enhancement on MRI, while 11 of 12 without recurrence showed no enhancement. There was one false positive MRI due to fat necrosis. Preda and colleagues [32] performed breast MRI in 93 patients suspected of local recurrence after breast conservation based on mammographic and ultrasound findings. In their series, MRI had a 90 % sensitivity, 91.6 % specificity, 56.3 % positive predictive value, and 98.7 % negative predictive value for the detection of recurrence at the lumpectomy bed, and they suggested that MRI could be useful to avoid unnecessary biopsy. In a meta-analysis of studies using breast MRI to distinguish post treatment changes from recurrence [33], Quinn et al. found the sensitivity of MRI in detecting recurrence to range from 75 to 100 % with a specificity of 66.6 to 100 %, with both sensitivity and specificity improving with a longer interval between definitive surgery and MRI. The authors noted however, that the studies evaluated in the meta-analysis were case series with heterogeneous populations, and suggested that while MRI could be helpful as a second line investigative tool for possible recurrence, it should not be performed routinely in this setting.

7.3 Clinical Findings

7.3.1 *Nipple Discharge*

Nipple discharge is a relatively common symptom in women presenting for diagnostic imaging evaluation. In Leis's series of 8,703 breast surgeries, nipple discharge was the presenting symptom in 7.4 % of cases [34]. Pathologically significant discharge is often described as unilateral, spontaneous, arising from a single duct, and bloody, clear or serous. Benign etiologies are the most common causes of nipple discharge. In one study reporting 586 patients who had surgery for clear (watery), serous (yellow), serosanguineous (pink), or bloody discharge, the majority had a benign etiology, including 48 % with intraductal papilloma, 33 % with fibrocystic changes, 14 % with cancer, and 7 % with precancerous lesions [34]. Patients with a bloody nipple discharge had a markedly higher breast cancer risk (404 of 1632, OR 2.27), compared with patients with non-bloody nipple discharge (179 of 1478) in Chen's meta-analysis [35].

In patients with a clinically concerning discharge, conventional imaging with mammography, ultrasound, and galactography may fail to identify an underlying lesion. Conventional galactography with cannulation of the discharging duct and injection of iodinated contrast is invasive and may be painful for the patient or unsuccessful. The gold standard in management of patients with a clinically suspicious nipple discharge and negative imaging findings has been surgical duct excision. Nipple discharge cytology has a high false positive rate; negative cytology with negative imaging has not been found to have a sufficiently high negative predictive value to avoid surgery in patients with a clinically suspicious discharge [36].

In patients with negative conventional imaging, MRI may have potential to identify both malignant and benign lesions. In one study of 15 patients who underwent excisional biopsy for nipple discharge, MRI findings correlated with histology in eleven patients [37]. MRI correctly identified four of six papillomas and one of two fibroadenomas as circumscribed masses and six of seven malignancies as peripherally enhancing irregular masses or regional or ductal enhancement. In a different retrospective study of 55 patients with bloody nipple discharge, MRI demonstrated all malignancies [38].

MRI shows superior performance in the evaluation of nipple discharge compared to ductography [39]. Morrogh et al. [39] retrospectively reviewed 306 patients with nipple discharge and negative standard imaging evaluation, 186 patients who underwent ductography (N = 163), MRI (N = 52) or both (N = 29) before surgery. They found a higher predictive value for malignancy for MRI compared with ductography. They reported that MRI had a positive predictive value of 56 % and a negative predictive value of 87 %. Nakahara et al. [38] found that MRI most clearly demon-

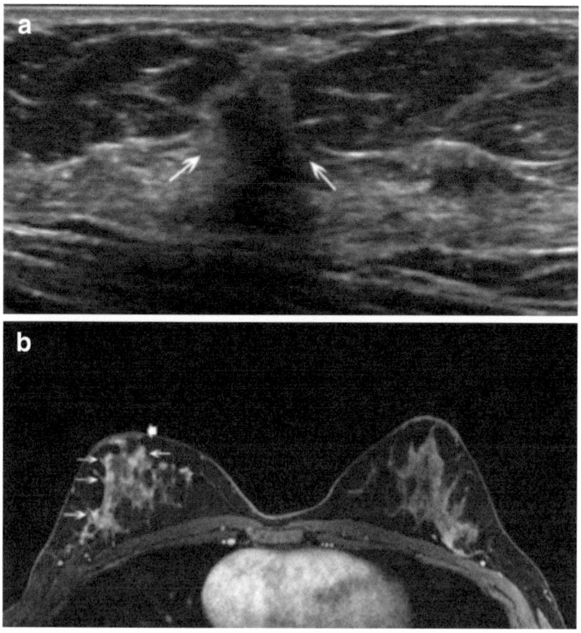

Fig. 7.5 Forty-three year old woman with 3 weeks of bloody nipple discharge, possible nipple retraction, and retraction of the breast. Mammogram (not shown) from an outside institution showed dense breast tissue but was negative. Ultrasound (**a**) of a focal area of concern in the right breast at 10:00 demonstrated a 6 mm hypoechoic mass (*arrows*) with irregular margins and posterior shadowing. Ultrasound-guided core biopsy was performed with pathology of invasive ductal carcinoma, grade II, ER/PR positive, Her-2 neu negative. Because the mammographic and sonographic imaging underestimated the clinical extent of disease, breast MRI was performed. Axial fat suppressed post contrast MRI (**b**) shows extensive diffuse clumped non mass enhancement (*arrows*) throughout the right breast with persistent kinetics and mild nipple retraction (*thick arrow*). The patient was treated with preoperative chemotherapy followed by mastectomy and implant reconstruction. The mastectomy specimen showed residual invasive ductal carcinoma microscopically in all four quadrants and in 2/7 lymph nodes. The MRI was helpful in confirming clinically suspicious more extensive disease than demonstrated on conventional imaging

strated the location and distribution of lesions, especially DCIS, compared with galactography and sonography, in 55 patients with bloody nipple discharge. MRI demonstrates extent of disease better than the other modalities (Fig. 7.5) [38].

Investigators have attempted to find other methods for evaluating the ductal system in the setting of nipple discharge. Direct MR-galactography, T1 and T2-weighted sequences after injection of gadolinium into the discharging duct, was compared with indirect MR-galactography, a T2-weighted sequence, in 23 patients with pathologic discharge and pathologic conventional galactogram [40]. Indirect MR-galactography has the advantage of being non-invasive and does not require radiation or contrast. Eight of the 23 women showed additional findings at direct MR-galactography in comparison with standard imaging sequences, indicating that the non-invasive T2-weighted sequences were suboptimal.

One study compared direct MR-galactography and conventional galactography in 30 patients and found no significant difference, suggesting that there is no additional advantage to MRI after galactogram [41]. Direct MRI-galactogram has disadvantages such as additional cost and the need to schedule magnet time compared with conventional galactogram. Both techniques may show a lesion as an intraductal filling defect, irregular duct wall, or ductal obstruction. Neither technique may specifically differentiate benign from malignant pathologies. In addition, a failed study may result if the radiologist is unable to cannulate the discharging duct and introduce contrast, or if multiple ducts have discharge.

Several studies have shown that MRI has the highest sensitivity in detecting benign or malignant etiologies for nipple discharge compared with other imaging modalities Nicholson et al. [42] found that MRI had the highest sensitivity, PPV, and NPV compared with conventional galactogram or indirect MR-galactogram, a heavily T2-weighted sequence, in 21 patients. Lorenzon et al. [43] retrospectively compared the sensitivity of MRI, mammography and ultrasound in 38 patients with nipple discharge and found MRI had statistically significant higher overall sensitivity. They concluded that MRI should be recommended when conventional imaging is negative. Advantages to MRI are that it is non-invasive and can image the ducts, subareolar area adjacent to the ducts, remainder of the breast and contralateral breast, whereas galactogram images a single ductal system.

In 2011, Yau et al. [15] reviewed 204 MRIs at their institution that had a clinical indication of problem solving. One hundred twelve of these had a problem identified by clinical breast examination. Two cancers were detected in patients with suspicious nipple discharge, negative mammogram and ultrasound, and failed or negative ductography. One of these two patients had prior lumpectomy for DCIS, the other is not further detailed in the report. They found one incidental cancer and one false negative MRI. They reported that at their institution, the patients with the suspicious nipple discharge and negative conventional imaging would have undergone surgical duct excision regardless of the MRI findings. However, they suggested that the utility of MRI for suspicious nipple discharge needs to be further investigated.

Sanders et al. [44] compared outcomes of 200 patients who had central duct excision for bloody nipple discharge following negative conventional imaging, 115 without and 85 with preoperative MRI. In their retrospective review, of 115 patients without pre-operative MRI, duct excision showed 8 (7 %) malignancies, including 7 DCIS and one invasive ductal cancer. In the 85 patients with pre-operative MRI, there were 8 (9.4 %) malignancies, all DCIS, and 7 were detected at MRI (true positives). The one falsely negative MRI represented Paget's disease on nipple biopsy. Fifty-six patients had a benign or negative MRI; central duct excision was negative for malignancy in all with the exception of the false negative MRI. The sensitivity and specificity were 88 and 71 %, and PPV and NPV were 24 and 98 %. Their conclusion was that the extremely high negative predictive value of MRI suggests that a negative study could obviate surgical duct excision in most patients, unless overriding clinical factors prevail.

In the surgical literature, Morrogh et al. [45] reported 416 cases of nipple discharge, 287 that underwent definitive biopsy or surgery, and 56 that had pre-operative

MRI. Of 13 malignancies found in the group that had pre-operative MRI, 10 (77 %) had a suspicious MRI correlate. Unpublished review of diagnostic breast MRIs at our institution performed for nipple discharge over a 3 year period revealed 83 patients, 40 of whom underwent biopsy, yielding 6 malignancies, 16 papillomas, and 18 miscellaneous benign histologies. MRI was positive in 5 of 6 malignancies and 13 of 16 papillomas; the sensitivity of MRI for detecting papilloma or malignancy was 82 % and specificity was 67 % for biopsied cases.

In summary, in patients with negative conventional imaging and suspicious clinical nipple discharge, contrast-enhanced MRI has the highest sensitivity compared with other imaging modalities, including conventional galactogram, and indirect- and direct-MR galactography. It has been proposed that the high negative predictive value of MRI suggests that a negative study may obviate surgical duct excision in most patients, unless overriding clinical factors prevail [44]. Other authors have suggested that clinical stratification can reliably identify pathologic discharge [39, 45], and that since MRI did not identify all malignancies and was unable to distinguish benign from malignant etiologies for discharge, that surgical duct excision should remain the gold standard of care. Surgical duct excision serves both a diagnostic as well as a therapeutic role for bloody nipple discharge, and this should be balanced against the cost of breast MRI. However, further investigation is warranted regarding the utility of problem solving MRI in this subset of patients, because a standard imaging algorithm remains elusive.

7.4 Palpable Findings with Negative Mammogram and Ultrasound

In patients with a suspicious palpable clinical finding, a complete evaluation with diagnostic mammography and ultrasound is the initial imaging recommendation by the American College of Radiology (ACR) recommendations and National Comprehensive Cancer Network (NCCN) clinical practice guidelines [46, 47].

The majority of patients will either have a negative mammogram and ultrasound, with a sufficiently low clinical suspicion that clinical follow up is recommended rather than further advanced imaging, or a finding prompting biopsy on diagnostic mammography and/or ultrasound. A few will have a probably benign imaging finding for which short interval follow up imaging is recommended. Multiple studies have shown an extremely high negative predictive value of mammography and ultrasound in evaluation of patients with a palpable lump, ranging from 97.4 to 100 % [9–11, 48]. However, negative imaging should not preclude biopsy if there is a suspicious clinical finding.

The 2013 ACR Appropriateness Criteria for Palpable Breast Masses are evidence-based guidelines for specific clinical conditions developed by a multidisciplinary expert panel [46]. Diagnostic mammography is recommended in the initial evaluation in women age ≥40 with a palpable lump, followed by focal ultrasound targeted specifically to the palpable finding. The addition of ultrasound to diagnostic mammography has been shown to increase the true-positive rate [10, 49]. However, MRI is categorized as "usually not appropriate" as the initial imaging evaluation in women age $\geq$ 40 and women < age 30 with a palpable lump.

According to the 2014 ACR practice parameters for contrast-enhanced MRI of the breast, "in rare cases, breast MRI may be indicated when other imaging examinations, such as ultrasound and mammography, and physical examination are inconclusive for the presence of breast cancer, and biopsy cannot be performed." [20] They further state inappropriate uses of MRI: "MRI should not be used in lieu of biopsy of a mammographically, clinically, and/or sonographically suspicious finding."

There are only a few studies in the literature regarding the diagnostic utility of problem solving breast MRI in detection of breast cancer in patients with palpable masses when conventional imaging is negative. Yau et al. retrospectively reviewed 204 MRIs with a clinical indication of problem solving, of which 112 had a problem identified by clinical breast examination [15]. One patient had a false negative MRI but one month later presented with bilateral palpable lumps with mammographic and sonographic findings which prompted biopsy. The bilateral biopsies revealed invasive lobular carcinoma on one breast and invasive ductal carcinoma on the contralateral breast. Two cancers were detected in patients with suspicious nipple discharge and negative conventional imaging. One incidental cancer was detected in a high risk patient. The added malignancy yield in this population for problem solving was low, with only three cancers in 204 patients identified by MRI. They concluded that problem solving breast MRI can be falsely negative in patients with suspicious mammographic and sonographic findings, and that until the benefits and risks of problem-solving MRI are clarified, it should be used judiciously.

Olsen et al. retrospectively reviewed 77 MRIs performed to assess palpable abnormalities with negative mammogram and ultrasound findings in a community health care setting [8]. Of 22 patients who underwent biopsy, two were positive for cancer, both of whom had positive MRI findings. Fifty-five patients with negative MRIs were followed clinically, of whom 27 were lost to follow-up and the remainder had no evidence of cancer on imaging and clinical examination at 1 year. Sensitivity of MRI was 100 %, specificity was 70 %, PPV was 25 % and NPV 100 %. They concluded that in patients with palpable breast mass and negative conventional imaging, breast MRI likely offers low yield of cancer diagnosis and low specificity. A significant limitation of their study was that almost half of the patients with negative imaging were lost to follow up. They concluded that negative MRI results may cause a low compliance rate for recommended follow up. Both patients in this series [8] with negative mammogram/ultrasound and positive MRI/ biopsy had prior malignancy with post treatment changes, mammographic distortion, and non-mass enhancement on MRI. The clinical exam is challenging in patients with prior lumpectomy and radiation; MRI can be helpful in cases of scar vs recurrence if a patient has prior history of breast cancer and suspicion of recurrence when clinical, mammographic, and/or sonographic findings are inconclusive [7].

In patients with palpable breast masses with negative conventional imaging, the diagnostic yield of cancer and cost-benefit ratio of breast MRI is low. Since the patient can point to the area of concern, focal diagnostic mammographic views, targeted ultrasound, and if necessary, targeted fine needle aspiration and/or biopsy can be performed. Breast MRI is expensive, and although has a high sensitivity, has a low specificity, which may lead to false positive biopsies. Negative MRIs may also lead to false reassurance and patients may have a low compliance rate for follow up. In a recent review of the literature including algorithms with recommendations for imaging management of palpable breast abnormalities, the authors state that there is "no evidence to support the utility of breast MRI for patients with palpable masses and no evidence that breast MRI leads to clinical benefit for such patients." [50].

In summary, in patients presenting with a palpable lump, diagnostic mammography and targeted ultrasound are the initial imaging recommendations, with a high negative predictive value of >97 %. If there is a persistent suspicious focal area of concern despite negative conventional imaging, biopsy should be based upon the clinical assessment. There is little evidence in the literature to support a benefit from advanced imaging techniques such as breast MRI in this patient population at this time.

7.5 Focal or Diffuse Pain

In patients with focal or diffuse breast pain and negative conventional imaging, to our knowledge, there are no studies supporting the use of diagnostic breast MRI as a problem solving tool. The negative predictive value of diagnostic mammography and ultrasound for breast pain ranges from 97 to 100 % [51–53], and therefore MRI is unlikely to add significantly to the clinical management of focal breast pain. Further investigation is needed to determine the diagnostic utility of breast MRI in detection of cancer in patients such as patients with pain or other clinical symptoms. MRI may theoretically be more useful when patients have clinically suspicious symptoms but do not have a palpable focal area of concern, therefore precluding a discrete location for evaluation with diagnostic mammographic spot views, targeted ultrasound, or targeted biopsy.

7.6 Skin Changes

Skin changes may be a sign of breast cancer. In patients with skin changes including peau d'orange or erythema and clinical suspicion of inflammatory breast cancer, the NCCN guidelines recommend mammogram and/or ultrasound as the initial imaging evaluation [47]. If there is a suspicious finding, biopsy is warranted. However, if the imaging is negative with persistent clinical concern, skin punch biopsy is recommended. If the skin punch biopsy is benign and clinical suspicion persists, breast MRI is recommended for further evaluation.

Inflammatory breast cancer (IBC) is a rare subtype of breast cancer with a highly virulent course and a low 5-year survival rate of 25–50 % [54]. Patients typically present with rapid onset of breast erythema, edema, and peau d'orange [55]. Trimodality treatment including preoperative chemotherapy, mastectomy and radiation therapy has been shown to improve prognosis in patients who are able to complete the treatment regimen [55].

In patients with clinical suspicion of inflammatory breast cancer (IBC) and negative conventional imaging and negative skin punch biopsy, breast MRI may be helpful in diagnosing IBC [47]. In a comparison of PET/CT, MRI, mammography, and sonography in 80 patients with IBC, MRI was found to be the most accurate imaging technique in detecting a primary breast parenchymal lesion [56]. Certain MRI features may facilitate diagnosis of IBC. In a comparison of the MRIs of 48 patients with IBC and 52 patients with locally advanced breast cancer (LABC), IBC patients had multiple smaller focal masses than LABC patients, cutaneous and subcutaneous edema, thickening and pathologic enhancement of Cooper's ligaments, and skin thickening more often than LABC patients [57]. In a retrospective review of the MRI features of 80 women with IBC, MRI detected a primary breast lesion in 98 % of patients compared with 68 % with mammography [58]. Multiple small, confluent, heterogeneously enhancing masses and global skin thickening were key features of IBC on MRI.

In patients with suspected, but mammographically and sonographically occult IBC, MRI may be helpful in identifying a target for biopsy within the breast parenchyma to establish the diagnosis [55]. It may also be helpful in documenting the extent of disease in the incident breast and occult disease in the contralateral breast, as well as to provide a baseline to assess subsequent treatment response. It may also be a useful aide for surgical decision making in determining timing of mastectomy for IBC patients with a challenging clinical exam following preoperative therapy.

Skin changes of the nipple may also signify malignancy. In patients with skin changes including nipple excoriation and scaling or eczema and clinical suspicion of Paget's disease, the NCCN guidelines recommend mammogram and/or ultrasound as the initial imaging evaluation [47]. If there is a suspicious imaging finding, biopsy is warranted. However, if there are negative or probably benign imaging findings and persistent clinical concern, skin punch biopsy or nipple biopsy is recommended. If histology is benign and discordant with clinically suspicious findings, consideration should be given to breast MRI or surgical biopsy.

Paget's disease of the breast is a rare manifestation of breast cancer [59, 60]. Pathologically, the Paget cell originates from an intraductal carcinoma of the underlying duct system of the nipple or breast and extends into the nipple epidermis. It may be associated with an underlying in situ or invasive carcinoma and is often multicentric, diffuse, and extensive. Symptoms may include itching, burning, crusting, or erosion of the nipple. There is frequently a delay in diagnosis due to the infrequent occurrence of Paget's disease and its similar presentation to other dermatologic conditions. Treatment is the same as for other breast cancers.

In a surgical review of patients with nipple changes suspicious for Paget disease as the only physical finding, positive skin/nipple biopsy, and negative mammogram,

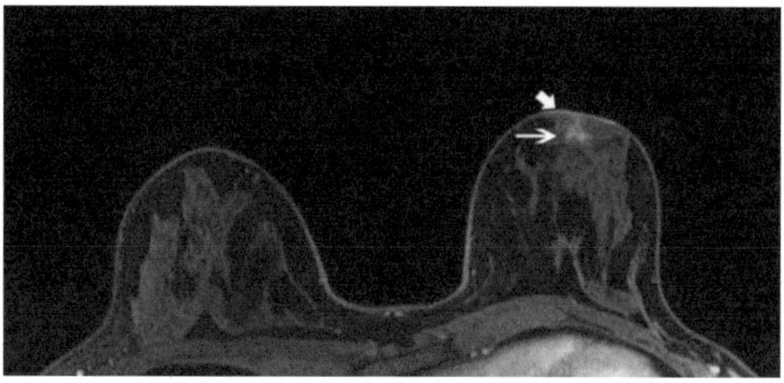

Fig. 7.6 Forty-two year old with left nipple inversion, erythema, and eczema-like appearance of the nipple-areolar complex. Mammogram (not shown) showed dense breast tissue and was otherwise negative. Retroareolar ultrasound (not shown) was unremarkable. Due to suspicious clinical findings, the patient was referred for a problem solving MRI. Axial dynamic post contrast fat suppressed MRI demonstrates 0.7 cm focal hetereogeneous non mass enhancement (*arrow*) in the left retroareolar region with flattening of the nipple-areolar complex and skin enhancement (*thick arrow*). MRI core biopsy revealed ductal carcinoma in situ, intermediate to high nuclear grade, with pagetoid spread, involving the nipple epidermis. This was consistent with Paget's disease of the nipple. The patient elected bilateral mastectomy

MRI detected otherwise occult malignancy in 4 (50 %) of 8 patients and accurately demonstrated extent of disease in 4 of 4 patients [61]. The authors concluded that in the setting of negative mammography, MRI can facilitate treatment planning for patients with Paget disease.

In summary, patients with skin changes suggestive of IBC or Paget's disease and negative conventional imaging may benefit from breast MRI as a problem solving tool, to identify malignancy and to guide biopsy (Fig. 7.6).

7.7 Conclusion

In our review of the current literature on problem solving MRI for imaging or clinical findings, there are relatively few indications for problem solving breast MRI. If there is a suspicious mammographic or sonographic finding, biopsy should be performed based upon that modality: MRI does not have sufficient negative predictive value to avoid biopsy of a suspicious mammographic or sonographic finding. Mammographic or sonographic BIRADS 3 lesions have such a high probability of benignity that adding breast MRI to the diagnostic imaging algorithm is unlikely to offer a favorable cost-benefit ratio. Breast MRI may rarely be indicated for equivocal or inconclusive findings at diagnostic mammographic and sonographic evaluation, and when biopsy cannot be performed. There may be diagnostic uncertainty if a lesion is present on some but not all diagnostic views, if there is uncertainty if a lesion is real or apparent changes are due to a technical factor: MRI may be helpful in these circumstances. MRI may be helpful for possible recurrence vs scar in patients with prior lumpectomy and radiation for breast cancer and difficult clinical examination.

For most clinical symptoms such as palpable findings or breast pain, for which conventional imaging is negative, MRI is not indicated. However, patients with skin changes suggestive of IBC or Paget's disease and negative conventional imaging may benefit from breast MRI as a problem solving tool, to identify malignancy and to guide biopsy. Further investigation of the role for breast MRI in suspicious nipple discharge is warranted. Although MRI does not demonstrate some benign and malignant causes of discharge, it demonstrates lesion extent better than ductography, and evaluates the whole breast and not one cannulated central ductal system.

As future research continues, the role of breast MRI as a problem solving tool will continue to evolve.

References

1. Kuhl C. The current status of breast MR imaging. Part I. Choice of technique, image interpretation, diagnostic accuracy, and transfer to clinical practice. Radiology. 2007;244(2):356–78.
2. Sung JS, Dershaw DD. Breast magnetic resonance imaging for screening high-risk women. Magn Reson Imaging Clin N Am. 2013;21(3):509–17.
3. Kuhl CK. Current status of breast MR imaging. Part 2. Clinical applications. Radiology. 2007;244(3):672–91.
4. Sickles EA, Miglioretti DL, Ballard-Barbash R, Geller BM, Leung JW, Rosenberg RD, et al. Performance benchmarks for diagnostic mammography. Radiology. [Research Support, N.I.H., Extramural Research Support, U.S. Gov't, P.H.S.].2005;235(3):775–90.
5. D'Orsi CJ, Sickles EA, Mendelson EB, Morris EA, et al. ACR BI-RADS® Atlas, Breast Imaging Reporting and Data System. Reston, VA, American College of Radiology; 2013.
6. DeMartini W, Lehman C. A review of current evidence-based clinical applications for breast magnetic resonance imaging. Top Magn Reson Imaging. [Meta-Analysis Review].2008;19(3):143–50.
7. Leung JW. MR imaging in the evaluation of equivocal clinical and imaging findings of the breast. Magn Reson Imaging Clin N Am. [Review].2010 May;18(2):295–308 , ix–x.
8. Olsen ML, Morton MJ, Stan DL, Pruthi S. Is there a role for magnetic resonance imaging in diagnosing palpable breast masses when mammogram and ultrasound are negative? J Womens Health (Larchmt). [Research Support, Non-U.S. Gov't].2012;21(11):1149–54.
9. Soo MS, Rosen EL, Baker JA, Vo TT, Boyd BA. Negative predictive value of sonography with mammography in patients with palpable breast lesions. AJR Am J Roentgenol. [Comparative Study].2001;177(5):1167–70.
10. Shetty MK, Shah YP, Sharman RS. Prospective evaluation of the value of combined mammographic and sonographic assessment in patients with palpable abnormalities of the breast. J Ultrasound Med. [Evaluation Studies]. 2003;22(3):263–268; quiz 9–70.
11. Moy L, Slanetz PJ, Moore R, Satija S, Yeh ED, McCarthy KA, et al. Specificity of mammography and US in the evaluation of a palpable abnormality: retrospective review. Radiology. 2002;225(1):176–81.
12. Bluemke DA, Gatsonis CA, Chen MH, DeAngelis GA, DeBruhl N, Harms S, et al. Magnetic resonance imaging of the breast prior to biopsy. JAMA. [Clinical Trial Multicenter Study Research Support, U.S. Gov't, P.H.S.].2004;292(22):2735–42.
13. Bazzocchi M, Zuiani C, Panizza P, Del Frate C, Soldano F, Isola M, et al. Contrast-enhanced breast MRI in patients with suspicious microcalcifications on mammography: results of a multicenter trial. AJR Am J Roentgenol. [Multicenter Study Research Support, Non-U.S. Gov't].2006;186(6):1723–32.

14. Cilotti A, Iacconi C, Marini C, Moretti M, Mazzotta D, Traino C, et al. Contrast-enhanced MR imaging in patients with BI-RADS 3-5 microcalcifications. Radiol Med. [Evaluation Studies].2007;112(2):272–86.
15. Yau EJ, Gutierrez RL, DeMartini WB, Eby PR, Peacock S, Lehman CD. The utility of breast MRI as a problem-solving tool. Breast J. [Evaluation Studies].2011;17(3):273–80.
16. Strobel K, Schrading S, Hansen NL, Barabasch A, Kuhl CK. Assessment of BI-RADS category 4 lesions detected with screening mammography and screening US: utility of MR imaging. Radiology. [Evaluation Studies].2015;274(2):343–51.
17. Uematsu T, Yuen S, Kasami M, Uchida Y. Dynamic contrast-enhanced MR imaging in screening detected microcalcification lesions of the breast: is there any value? Breast Cancer Res Treat. 2007;103(3):269–81.
18. Gokalp G, Topal U. MR imaging in probably benign lesions (BI-RADS category 3) of the breast. Eur J Radiol. 2006;57(3):436–44.
19. Dorrius MD, Pijnappel RM, Jansen-van der Weide MC, Oudkerk M. Breast magnetic resonance imaging as a problem-solving modality in mammographic BI-RADS 3 lesions. Cancer Imaging. [Review].2010;10(Spec no A):S54–8.
20. American College of Radiology Practice Parameter for the Performance of Contrast-Enhanced Magnetic Resonance Imaging (MRI) of the Breast. [updated 20141.2.16]; Available from: http://www.acr.org/.
21. Moy L, Elias K, Patel V, Lee J, Babb JS, Toth HK, et al. Is breast MRI helpful in the evaluation of inconclusive mammographic findings? AJR Am J Roentgenol. 2009;193(4):986–93.
22. Giess CS, Chikarmane SA, Sippo DA, Birdwell RL. Breast MR Imaging for Equivocal Mammographic Findings: Help or Hindrance? Radiographics. 2016;36(4):943–56. doi: 10.1148/rg.2016150205. Epub 2016 Jun 10.
23. Sardanelli F, Melani E, Ottonello C, Parodi RC, Imperiale A, Massa T, et al. Magnetic resonance imaging of the breast in characterizing positive or uncertain mammographic findings. Cancer Detect Prev. 1998;22(1):39–42.
24. Lee CH, Smith RC, Levine JA, Troiano RN, Tocino I. Clinical usefulness of MR imaging of the breast in the evaluation of the problematic mammogram. AJR Am J Roentgenol. 1999;173(5):1323–9.
25. Spick C, Szolar DH, Preidler KW, Tillich M, Reittner P, Baltzer PA. Breast MRI used as a problem-solving tool reliably excludes malignancy. Eur J Radiol. 2015;84(1):61–4.
26. Oztekin PS, Kosar PN. Magnetic resonance imaging of the breast as a problem-solving method: to be or not to be? Breast J. 2014;20(6):622–31.
27. Lee CH. Problem solving MR imaging of the breast. Radiol Clin North Am. [Review].2004; 42(5):919–34 , vii.
28. Houssami N, Abraham LA, Miglioretti DL, Sickles EA, Kerlikowske K, Buist DS, et al. Accuracy and outcomes of screening mammography in women with a personal history of early-stage breast cancer. JAMA. [Multicenter Study Research Support, N.I.H., Extramural Research Support, Non-U.S. Gov't].2011;305(8):790–9.
29. Heywang-Kobrunner SH, Schlegel A, Beck R, Wendt T, Kellner W, Lommatzsch B, et al. Contrast-enhanced MRI of the breast after limited surgery and radiation therapy. J Comput Assist Tomogr. 1993;17(6):891–900.
30. Viehweg P, Heinig A, Lampe D, Buchmann J, Heywang-Kobrunner SH. Retrospective analysis for evaluation of the value of contrast-enhanced MRI in patients treated with breast conservative therapy. MAGMA. [Clinical Trial].1998;7(3):141–52.
31. Gilles R, Guinebretiere JM, Shapeero LG, Lesnik A, Contesso G, Sarrazin D, et al. Assessment of breast cancer recurrence with contrast-enhanced subtraction MR imaging: preliminary results in 26 patients. Radiology. 1993;188(2):473–8.
32. Preda L, Villa G, Rizzo S, Bazzi L, Origgi D, Cassano E, et al. Magnetic resonance mammography in the evaluation of recurrence at the prior lumpectomy site after conservative surgery and radiotherapy. Breast Cancer Res. [Comparative Study].2006;8(5):R53.
33. Quinn EM, Coveney AP, Redmond HP. Use of magnetic resonance imaging in detection of breast cancer recurrence: a systematic review. Ann Surg Oncol. [Review].2012;19(9):3035–41.

34. Leis HP, Jr. Management of nipple discharge. World J Surg. [Review]. 1989;13(6):736–742.
35. Chen L, Zhou WB, Zhao Y, Liu XA, Ding Q, Zha XM, et al. Bloody nipple discharge is a predictor of breast cancer risk: a meta-analysis. Breast Cancer Res Treat. [Meta-Analysis Research Support, Non-U.S. Gov't Review].2012;132(1):9–14.
36. Kalu ON, Chow C, Wheeler A, Kong C, Wapnir I. The diagnostic value of nipple discharge cytology: breast imaging complements predictive value of nipple discharge cytology. J Surg Oncol. 2012;106(4):381–5.
37. Orel SG, Dougherty CS, Reynolds C, Czerniecki BJ, Siegelman ES, Schnall MD. MR imaging in patients with nipple discharge: initial experience. Radiology. 2000;216(1):248–54.
38. Nakahara H, Namba K, Watanabe R, Furusawa H, Matsu T, Akiyama F, et al. A comparison of MR imaging, galactography and ultrasonography in patients with nipple discharge. Breast Cancer. [Comparative Study].2003;10(4):320–9.
39. Morrogh M, Morris EA, Liberman L, Borgen PI, King TA. The predictive value of ductography and magnetic resonance imaging in the management of nipple discharge. Ann Surg Oncol. 2007;14(12):3369–77.
40. Schwab SA, Uder M, Schulz-Wendtland R, Bautz WA, Janka R, Wenkel E. Direct MR galactography: feasibility study. Radiology. [Comparative Study].2008;249(1):54–61.
41. Wenkel E, Janka R, Uder M, Doellinger M, Melzer K, Schulz-Wendtland R, et al. Does direct MR galactography have the potential to become an alternative diagnostic tool in patients with pathological nipple discharge? Clin Imaging. 2011;35(2):85–93.
42. Nicholson BT, Harvey JA, Patrie JT, Mugler 3rd JP. 3D-MR ductography and contrast-enhanced MR mammography in patients with suspicious nipple discharge; a feasibility study. Breast J. 2015;21(4):352–62.
43. Lorenzon M, Zuiani C, Linda A, Londero V, Girometti R, Bazzocchi M. Magnetic resonance imaging in patients with nipple discharge: should we recommend it? Eur Radiol. 2011; 21(5):899–907.
44. Sanders LM, Daigle M. The rightful role of MRI after negative conventional imaging in the management of bloody nipple discharge. Breast J. 2015;22(2):209–12.
45. Morrogh M, Park A, Elkin EB, King TA. Lessons learned from 416 cases of nipple discharge of the breast. Am J Surg. 2010;200(1):73–80.
46. Harvey JA, Mahoney MC, Newell MS, Bailey L, Barke LD, D'Orsi C, et al. ACR appropriateness criteria palpable breast masses. J Am Coll Radiol. 2013;10(10):742-9 e1–3.
47. Bevers TB, Anderson BO, Bonaccio E, Buys S, Daly MB, Dempsey PJ, et al. NCCN clinical practice guidelines in oncology: breast cancer screening and diagnosis. J Natl Compr Canc Netw. [Practice Guideline Review].2009;7(10):1060–96.
48. Dennis MA, Parker SH, Klaus AJ, Stavros AT, Kaske TI, Clark SB. Breast biopsy avoidance: the value of normal mammograms and normal sonograms in the setting of a palpable lump. Radiology. 2001;219(1):186–91.
49. Murphy IG, Dillon MF, Doherty AO, McDermott EW, Kelly G, O'Higgins N, et al. Analysis of patients with false negative mammography and symptomatic breast carcinoma. J Surg Oncol. [Comparative Study].2007;96(6):457–63.
50. Lehman CD, Lee AY, Lee CI. Imaging management of palpable breast abnormalities. AJR Am J Roentgenol. [Research Support, Non-U.S. Gov't Review].2014;203(5):1142–53.
51. Tumyan L, Hoyt AC, Bassett LW. Negative predictive value of sonography and mammography in patients with focal breast pain. Breast J. [Comparative Study].2005;11(5):333–7.
52. Lumachi F, Ermani M, Brandes AA, Boccagni P, Polistina F, Basso SM, et al. Breast complaints and risk of breast cancer. Population-based study of 2,879 self-selected women and long-term follow-up. Biomed Pharmacother. 2002;56(2):88–92.
53. Duijm LE, Guit GL, Hendriks JH, Zaat JO, Mali WP. Value of breast imaging in women with painful breasts: observational follow up study. BMJ. 1998;317(7171):1492–5.
54. Hance KW, Anderson WF, Devesa SS, Young HA, Levine PH. Trends in inflammatory breast carcinoma incidence and survival: the surveillance, epidemiology, and end results program at the National Cancer Institute. J Natl Cancer Inst. 2005;97(13):966–75.

55. Yeh ED, Jacene HA, Bellon JR, Nakhlis F, Birdwell RL, Georgian-Smith D, et al. What radiologists need to know about diagnosis and treatment of inflammatory breast cancer: a multidisciplinary approach. Radiographics. 2013;33(7):2003–17.
56. Yang WT, Le-Petross HT, Macapinlac H, Carkaci S, Gonzalez-Angulo AM, Dawood S, et al. Inflammatory breast cancer: PET/CT, MRI, mammography, and sonography findings. Breast Cancer Res Treat. [Review].2008;109(3):417–26.
57. Renz DM, Baltzer PA, Bottcher J, Thaher F, Gajda M, Camara O, et al. Inflammatory breast carcinoma in magnetic resonance imaging: a comparison with locally advanced breast cancer. Acad Radiol. [Comparative Study].2008;15(2):209–21.
58. Le-Petross HT, Cristofanilli M, Carkaci S, Krishnamurthy S, Jackson EF, Harrell RK, et al. MRI features of inflammatory breast cancer. AJR Am J Roentgenol. [Comparative Study].2011;197(4):W769–76.
59. Kister SJ, Haagensen CD. Paget's disease of the breast. Am J Surg. 1970;119(5):606–9.
60. Sakorafas GH, Blanchard K, Sarr MG, Farley DR. Paget's disease of the breast. Cancer Treat Rev. [Review]. 2001;27(1):9–18.
61. Morrogh M, Morris EA, Liberman L, Van Zee K, Cody 3rd HS, King TA. MRI identifies otherwise occult disease in select patients with Paget disease of the nipple. J Am Coll Surg. [Research Support, Non-U.S. Gov't].2008;206(2):316–21.

Chapter 8
Post-operative Findings/Recurrent Disease

Amy Melsaether and Yiming Gao

Abstract Breast cancer treatment has evolved since William Halsted, MD, an American surgeon, introduced the radical mastectomy in 1882 (Halsted, Ann Surg 20:497, 1894). The modified radical mastectomy gained popularity in the 1970s (www.cancer.org/cancer/cancerbasics/thehistoryofcancer/the-history-of-cancer-cancer-treatment-surgery. Accessed 11/23/2015) and in 1985. Fisher et al. established lumpectomy, or breast conservation therapy (BCT), and radiation as treatment for early stage breast cancers (Fisher et al., N Engl J Med 312(11):665–673, 1985). The National Institutes of Health soon endorsed and thus popularized this less invasive treatment (Consensus statement: treatment of early-stage breast cancer. National Institutes of Health Consensus Development Panel. J Natl Cancer Inst Monogr. 1992;11:1–5. Review). Today, while BCT and radiation remain the standard of care for stage I and II cancers, mastectomy and reconstruction procedures have been updated and rising ipsilateral and contralateral prophylactic mastectomy rates have been documented (Jones et al., Ann Surg Oncol 16(10):2691–2696, 2009; Tuttle et al., J Clin Oncol 25(33):5203–5209, 2007; McGuire et al., Ann Surg Oncol 16(10):2682–2690, 2009; Dragun et al., Am J Clin Oncol 36(4):375–380, 2013).

As women survive their breast cancers and continue screening with mammogram, ultrasound and often MRI, differentiating multi-modality post-operative and post-radiation changes from signs of malignancy is key both for the avoidance of unnecessary biopsies and for the early detection of subsequent cancers in this elevated risk population. In this chapter, we will cover normal post-lumpectomy and post-radiation findings on mammogram, ultrasound, and MRI and contrast these post-treatment changes with imaging features of recurrent cancers. We will also discuss mastectomy techniques, including the modified radical mastectomy and skin- and nipple-sparing mastectomies together with autologous and implant reconstructions, along with tips for avoiding common pitfalls.

A. Melsaether, MD (✉) • Y. Gao, MD
Department of Radiology, NYU School of Medicine, New York, NY, USA
e-mail: amy.melsaether@nyumc.org; yiming.gao@nyumc.org

S.L. Heller, L. Moy (eds.), *Breast Oncology: Techniques, Indications, and Interpretation*, DOI 10.1007/978-3-319-42563-4_8

Keywords Lumpectomy • Breast conservation therapy • Mastectomy • MRI • Mammogram • Ultrasound • Post-operative • Post surgical • Breast reconstruction • Fat necrosis • Seroma • Recurrence • Benign • Malignant • Flap reconstruction • Breast cancer treatment • Breast cancer surveillance

8.1 Breast Conservation Therapy (BCT)

8.1.1 Patient Selection

The standard of care for breast conservation therapy (BCT) is well established via multidisciplinary consensus of the American College of Surgeons, American College of Radiology, the College of American Pathologists, and the Society of Surgical Oncology [1]. This therapy typically consists of surgical excision followed by whole breast radiation. A woman with an early stage small unifocal tumor (<5 cm) in a breast large enough to allow adequate resection and satisfactory cosmesis is a good candidate for breast conservation. Contraindications of BCT (and hence indications for mastectomy) include multicentric or extensive disease in the breast, prior radiation involving the breast region, pregnancy (first and second trimesters), and collagen vascular disease (due to poor radiation tolerance). The goal of BCT is resection of tumor with tissue margins free of tumor. Although the strongest predictor of local disease recurrence is positive surgical margins [2], there has been little consensus on what constitutes an optimal margin. Despite the 2014 guideline of "no ink on tumor" by the Society of Surgical Oncology, the American Society of Breast Surgeons, and the American Society for Radiation Oncology [3], there is evidence that BCT using this criteria leaves behind more residual tumor than the traditional ≥2 mm negative tissue margin [4], and further studies with long term follow-up of local recurrence rates are needed.

8.1.2 Imaging Findings

Because there is significant overlap in imaging findings of benign post treatment changes and those of new/recurrent disease in the breast, it is essential to understand imaging findings in the context of chronology. The most prominent post surgical and post radiation changes typically diminish over a span of 2–3 years to reach a stable appearance of the post treatment breast (Fig. 8.1), at which time tumor recurrence also begins to surface again [5]. Because recurrence is rare in the first year or two after BCT, early post-surgical imaging followup is generally favored to provide baseline imaging and so to avoid unnecessary biopsies. The first post lumpectomy mammogram is acquired prior to radiation therapy if the treated disease contains

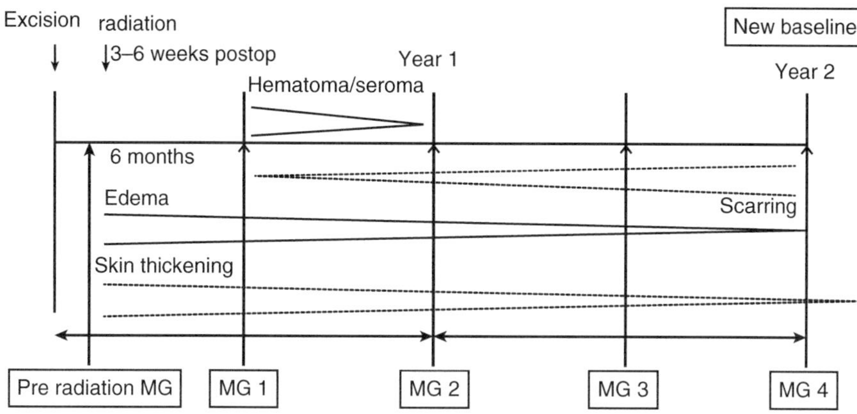

Fig. 8.1 Typical timeline of mammographic (MG) findings following Breast Conservation Therapy

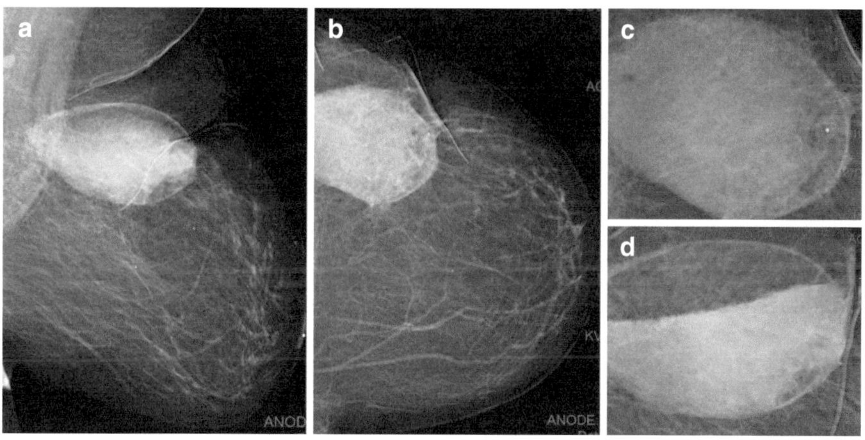

Fig. 8.2 Status post recent left lumpectomy with a circumscribed hyperdense oval mass in the surgical bed in the upper outer quadrant deep to the scar marker on MLO (**a**) and CC views (**b**). Delayed lateral view (**d**) demonstrates layering of internal fluid, which appears dense en face (**c**), consistent with a post surgical fluid collection

calcifications, in order to assess for residual disease [6]. Magnification views of the lumpectomy bed allow high resolution evaluation. Mammographic surveillance typically begins approximately 6 months after BCT.

Early findings of postoperative collections such as seroma and/or hematoma, breast edema and skin thickening, are most pronounced within the first 6 months (Fig. 8.1). Postoperative seromas/hematomas are relatively discrete hyperdense oval masses on mammogram, occasionally with internal dependent layering, confirming it as a fluid collection (Fig. 8.2). Ultrasound helps further characterize postoperative collections if findings on mammogram are unclear, typically showing a simple or complex fluid collection closely associated with the surgical incision

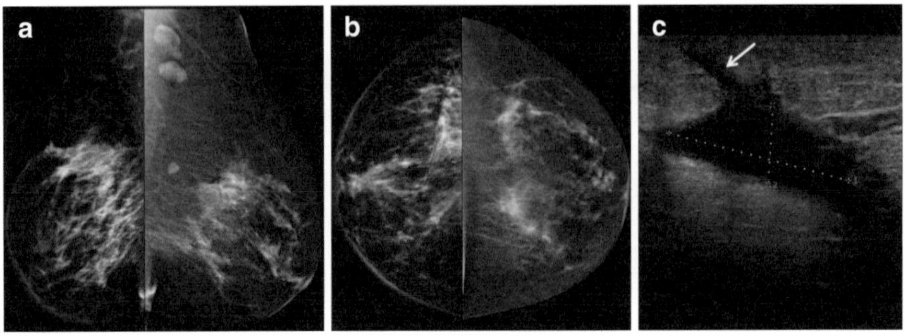

Fig. 8.3 Four months following right lumpectomy and radiation therapy for breast cancer. There is moderate skin thickening and breast edema (trabecular thickening) involving the right breast seen on MLO view (**a**) and CC view (**b**) as compared to the untreated normal appearing left breast. There is an anechoic postoperative seroma in the superior right breast in the surgical bed, extending to the skin at the site of surgical excision (*arrow*) (**c**)

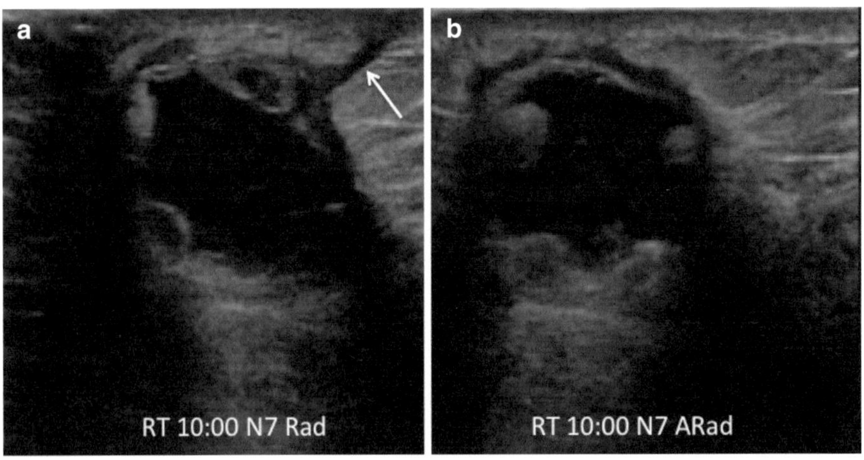

Fig. 8.4 Five months following right lumpectomy and radiation therapy, there is a thick walled complex fluid collection with suggestion of internal septations (**a**, **b**) in the surgical bed with peripheral nodular granulation tissue and scarring extending to skin (**a**) (*arrow*) at the level of the surgical incision

seen as a hypoechoic track extending to the skin (Figs. 8.3 and 8.4). On MRI, a seroma appears as a circumscribed fluid-filled structure with smooth rim enhancement (Fig. 8.5), and a hematoma appears as a nonenhancing mass of varying internal signal depending on chronicity. Although seromas can have benign nodular or irregular enhancing components due to granulation tissue or fat necrosis, these should be viewed with suspicion and residual/recurrent malignancy must be excluded (Fig. 8.6). Postoperative collections usually resolve by one year, but some can persist indefinitely. As a collection decreases in size, the diminishing surgical cavity evolves into a coalescing scar made of dense connective tissue and

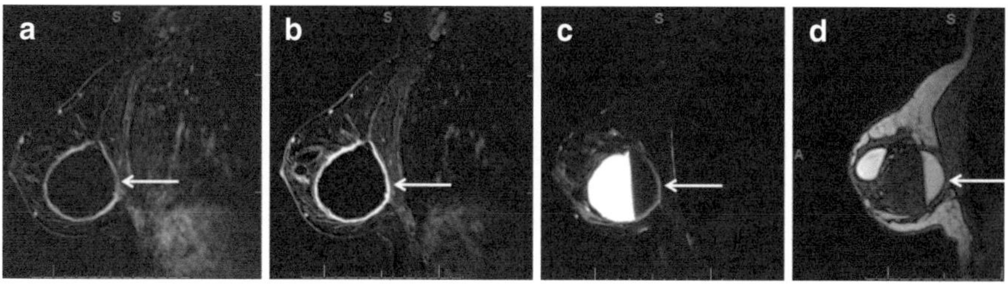

Fig. 8.5 Post surgical seroma with circumscribed margin and smooth thin rim persistent enhancement on T1 post contrast subtraction images at early (**a**) and late (**b**) phases. Internal fat-fluid level (**c**, **d**) is related to history of prior free fat injection in this patient

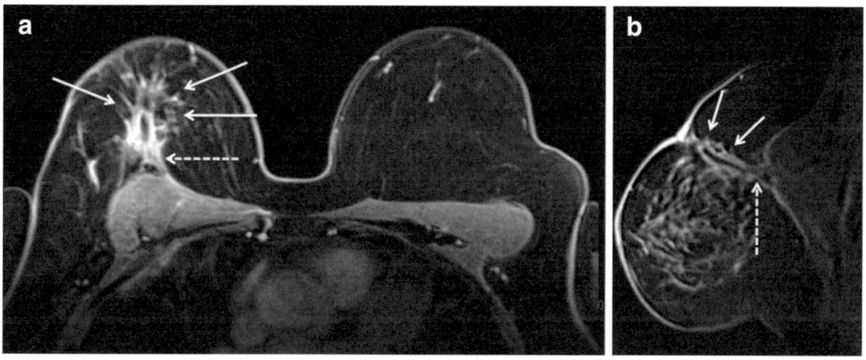

Fig. 8.6 Fifteen months status post right breast lumpectomy and radiation therapy. Axial (**a**) and sagittal (**b**) T1 post contrast images show a nearly completely resolved seroma surrounded by a thickened and nodular residual capsule (**a**) and new heterogeneous irregular spiculated peripheral enhancement (**b**) (*arrows*, *solid*). In addition, the posterior aspect of the irregular enhancement demonstrates washout kinetics on imaging and correlates with positive deep surgical margin at histologic analysis (**a**, **b**) (*arrows*, *dashed*). This underwent MR guided biopsy, confirming presence of residual DCIS

fibrosis. This is seen on mammogram as an area of architectural distortion with central equal/low density and peripheral radiating spiculations interspersed by fat. This classic appearance of fibrotic bands of a scar entrapping areas of fat necrosis is well depicted on digital breast tomosynthesis (Fig. 8.7a, b). In contrast, a cancer associated with spiculations due to adjacent desmoplastic reactions is more hyperdense and mass-like centrally on mammogram. Benign fat necrosis calcifications at lumpectomy scar typically develop 2–5 years post radiation, and early evolving benign calcifications may mimic malignancy. On ultrasound, scarring typically appears as hypoechoic spiculations extending to the skin (Fig. 8.7c). On MRI, post lumpectomy scar tissue may enhance for up to 18 months, but after this period enhancement is expected to subside [7] (Fig. 8.8). New or increased enhancement at the scar on MRI, particularly after 18 months, requires exclusion of recurrent disease. However, in our practice on our 3.0T magnet, we have seen enhancement at the lumpectomy site several years after surgery. In these cases, we verify that the

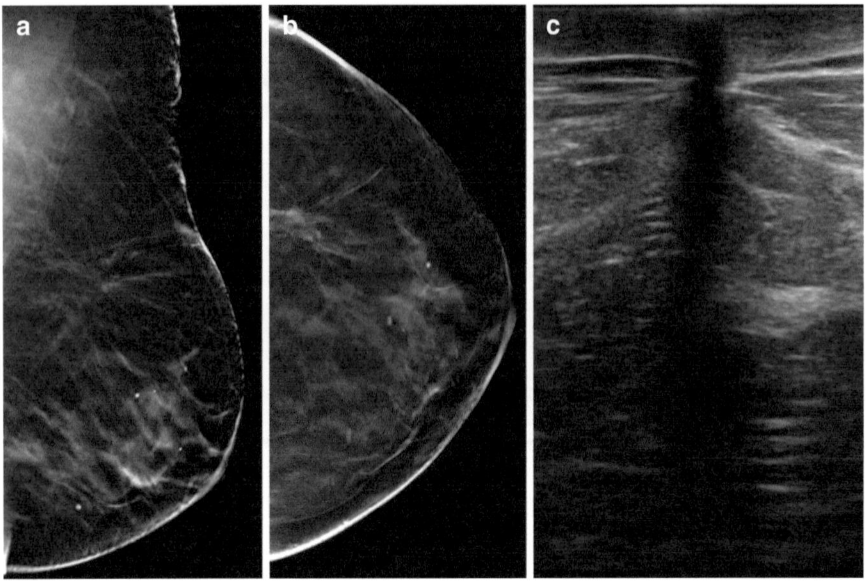

Fig. 8.7 Left lumpectomy scar seen on tomosynthesis images on MLO (**a**) and CC (**b**) views, showing central lucent fatty attenuation and peripheral spiculations of fibrotic bands interspersed with fat. A separate case of post lumpectomy scar seen on ultrasound as a hypoechoic band extending to the skin (**c**)

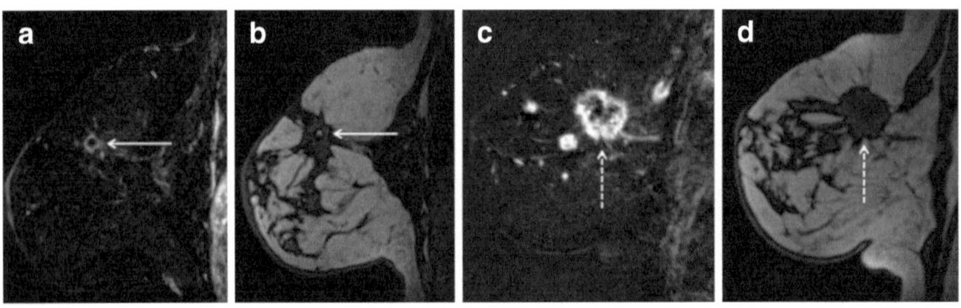

Fig. 8.8 Post lumpectomy breast on T1 post contrast subtraction (**a**) and T1 non fat saturated (**b**) sequences show an area of retracted scarring containing central area of fat with rim enhancement, consistent with fat necrosis. This is in stark comparison with T1 post contrast subtraction (**c**) and T1 non fat saturated (**d**) sequences showing the same breast with interval increased bulk and now mass like configuration of the scar, with tumor replacement of previously seen central fat, consistent with recurrent malignancy. In addition to the new irregular enhancing mass at the scar, there is additional adjacent satellite disease (**c**)

enhancement is not increasing as compared with prior exams. This enhancement may be explained by the relatively increased relaxation time for both fat and glandular tissue at 3T compared to that of gadolinium. The resulting relative difference in signal intensity between enhancing lesions and nonenhancing tissues is therefore increased at 3T, thus making enhancing lesions more conspicuous [8, 9].

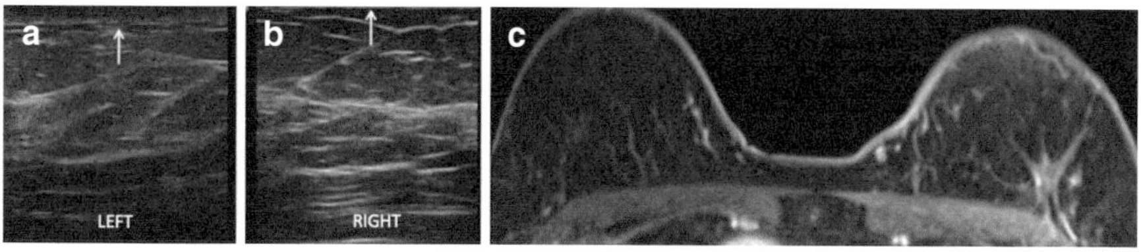

Fig. 8.9 Five months following left lumpectomy and radiation therapy for breast cancer. Asymmetric left breast skin thickening (*arrow*) (**a**) and tissue edema which manifests as diffusely increased stromal echogenicity (**a**) are seen as compared to the normal right breast (**b**). Similarly, left breast skin thickening is seen on MRI (**c**)

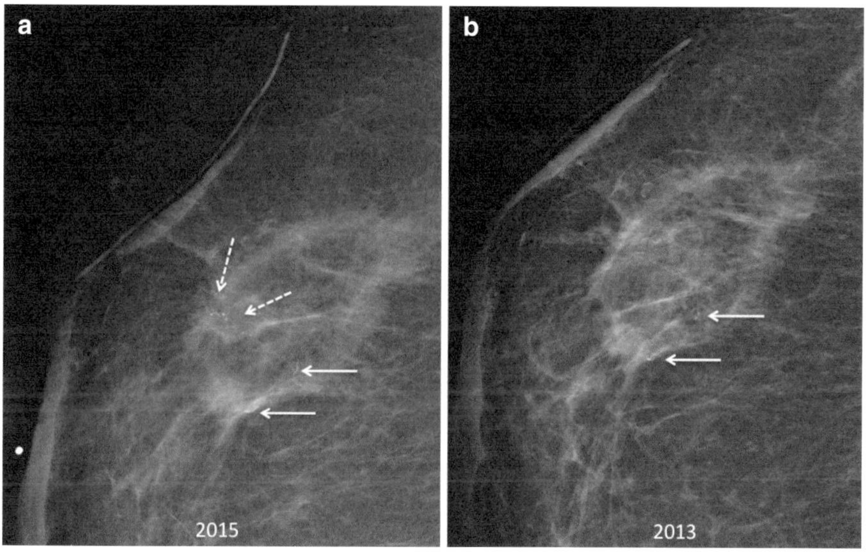

Fig. 8.10 New pleomorphic calcifications in the right lumpectomy bed two and half years following breast conservation therapy for invasive ductal carcinoma (**a**) (*arrows, dashed*) were biopsied yielding DCIS, consistent with recurrence. In contrast, the adjacent curvilinear slow evolving calcifications at the periphery of an area of fat necrosis are distinct in appearance (**a**, **b**) (*arrows, solid*). Nevertheless, there is significant overlap in appearance between early evolving calcifications of fat necrosis and malignant calcifications

Following whole breast radiation, skin thickening and breast edema share similar timelines of recovery to near normal/normal by approximately 2 years (Fig. 8.1). Skin thickening and breast edema (trabecular thickening) are best evaluated in comparison with the contralateral normal breast on mammogram (Fig. 8.3a, b), ultrasound, and MRI (Fig. 8.9). On MRI, post radiation "quiescence" in the treated breast may also be seen as asymmetrically decreased background parenchymal enhancement and fibrocystic changes (Fig. 8.10). Overall, new or increased findings usually warrant biopsy to exclude recurrent disease given expected pattern of evolution/resolution of most post surgical changes over time.

8.2 Tumor Recurrence and Imaging Surveillance

True recurrence occurs at the site of original tumor and signifies local treatment failure. Recurrence is rare before 2 years post treatment, but may occur as early as 2–5 years following BCT [6]. Patients who undergo lumpectomy without radiation, have positive surgical margins, multifocal disease, or ER-negative cancers are at further increased risk of recurrence [10]. Up to 50 % of recurrence is detected on mammogram, which can present as new suspicious calcifications in the lumpectomy bed (Fig. 8.10), developing asymmetry, new mass or architectual distortion. Ultrasound may help to identify a mass at or adjacent to the scar. MRI is useful in distinguishing between benign entities such as a scar or fat necrosis from recurrence when mammogram and ultrasound are indeterminate. Although protocols vary, most centers perform post treatment mammographic surveillance every 6 months following BCT for 2–5 years with subsequent annual mammograms. This is accompanied by annual clinical breast exam to detect imaging occult recurrence.

8.3 Mastectomy

Conventional indications for mastectomy were covered earlier in this chapter as were contraindications for BCT. In addition, some patients eligible for BCT choose mastectomy instead. Contralateral prophylactic mastectomy is increasingly requested in the setting of unilateral breast cancer and bilateral prophylactic mastectomy is accepted treatment for high risk patients, typically in the setting of BRCA mutations [11].

8.3.1 Techniques

Modified radical mastectomy (MRM) is, in the absence of pectoralis muscle invasion, the most extensive mastectomy performed today and includes complete removal of the breast tissue, skin envelope, nipple areolar complex and level I and II axillary nodes. This surgery is appropriate in locally advanced cancers including inflammatory breast cancers and is the surgery of choice when a woman is not planning reconstruction [12]. Newer techniques include the skin sparing mastectomy (SSM), which preserves the skin envelope and inframammary fold while removing the breast tissue and nipple areolar complex [13], and the nipple sparing mastectomy (NSM), which preserves the skin envelope and nipple areolar complex while removing the breast tissue. SSM facilitates breast reconstruction, provides a superior cosmetic outcome as compared with MRM, and can often be performed in lieu of MRM, provided there is approximately 5 mm between the tumor margin and the

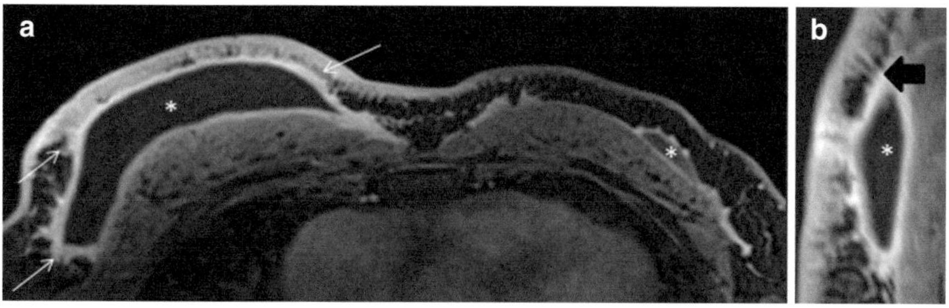

Fig. 8.11 A 50 year old man with a history of right breast invasive ductal cancer (IDC) underwent bilateral mastectomies 18 months prior and now presents with elevated cancer antigen 27.29. The post-contrast T1-weighted fat-suppressed axial image (**a**) shows bilateral seromas (*asterisks*), left greater than right. The thicker enhancing rim seroma (*thin arrows*, **a**) with spiculations (*thick arrow*) seen best on the post-contrast T1-weighted fat-suppressed sagittal image (**b**) appropriately prompted biopsy; results were benign post-operative changes

skin. NSM provides the best cosmetic outcome and is most often performed in the prophylactic setting. In the setting of cancer treatment, indications for NSM put forth by Voltura et al. include a tumor size <4.5 cm, distance from the areola of >2.5 cm and distance from the center of the nipple >4 cm [14].

8.3.2 Imaging Findings

The post-mastectomy or post-reconstructed breast is not usually imaged to screen for recurrent disease. However, MRI has been shown to be useful in evaluating the post-mastectomy or post-resonstruction breast for post-treatment changes versus recurrence. In addition, imaging of mastectomy or reconstruction may occur during MRI evaluation of the contralateral breast. In MRM without reconstruction, MR imaging findings are straightforward and include the absence of a breast with simply the pectoralis muscles, subcutaneous fat and overlying skin. As in any post-operative setting, edema, presenting as increased skin thickness and increased signal on T2 weighted images will be present initially and will subside over time. As in any post-operative setting, seromas and hematomas can form. Clean seromas can be distinguished by smooth, thin margins. However, seromas may have shaggier enhancing margins which can raise concern for tumor (Fig. 8.11). In this case, lesion enhancement kinetics and pathology reports can be useful. Progressive enhancement is more consistent with post-operative changes and scarring while washout enhancement is more concerning for malignancy. With reported clean margins, when imaging is within 6 months of the date of surgery, and when the enhancement pattern is persistent, a short-interval (6 month) follow-up study may be appropriate in lieu of biopsy. However, in cases without clean margins or in any case where enhancement demonstrates wash-out kinetics or has increased compared with a prior study, biopsy should be performed.

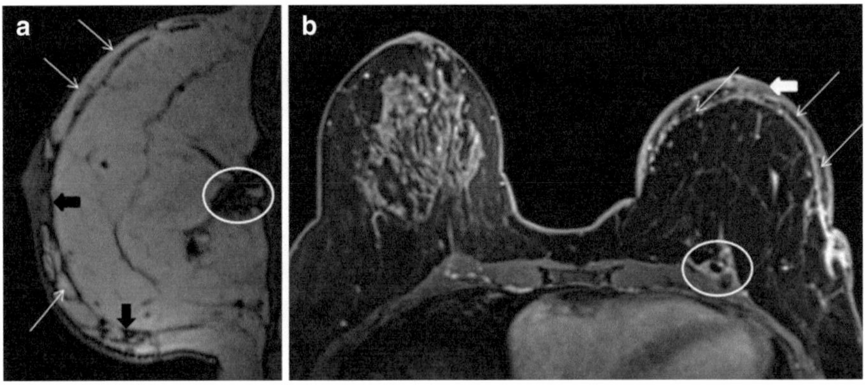

Fig. 8.12 A 58 year old woman with a history of left breast IDC underwent nipple sparing mastectomy and TRAM reconstruction. The line between the fat from the flap and the native subcutaneous fat (*thin arrows*) is well seen on both the T1-weighted non-fat-suppressed sagittal (**a**) and the T1-weighted post-contrast fat-suppressed axial (**b**) images. A small amount of residual breast tissue can be seen (*thick arrow*), most notably beneath the nipple. The vascular pedicle (*circled*) is also well seen on both images

In SMS and NSM, the imaging appearance will depend on the type of reconstruction. In all cases, however, there will be a thin rim of native subcutaneous fat beneath the conserved skin. In up to 60 % of cases, there will also be some amount of residual breast tissue [15] (Fig. 8.12). This finding is normal and not a failure of mastectomy. In NSM, competing techniques stress the importance of complete removal of all ductal tissue including the nipple core versus the importance of an approximately 5 mm residual layer of glandular tissue to preserve perfusion and protect against nipple necrosis [16]. In the former case, there will be very little or no residual ductal tissue and in the latter case, there will be some residual ductal tissue under the native nipple areolar complex (Fig. 8.12). In therapeuric NSM, intraoperative radiation can be used to decrease recurrence rates in spite of residual tissue [17].

8.4 Reconstruction Techniques

Breast reconstruction can be performed with autologous pedicled or free flaps or with synthetic implants. Nipple reconstruction further improves cosmetic outcomes.

8.4.1 Pedicled Flaps

The pedicled transverse rectus abdominus myocutnaeous (TRAM) flap is a well-established technique where an island of skin, fat and muscle from the abdomen is cut and tunneled underneath the skin to the contralateral mastectomy site, where this

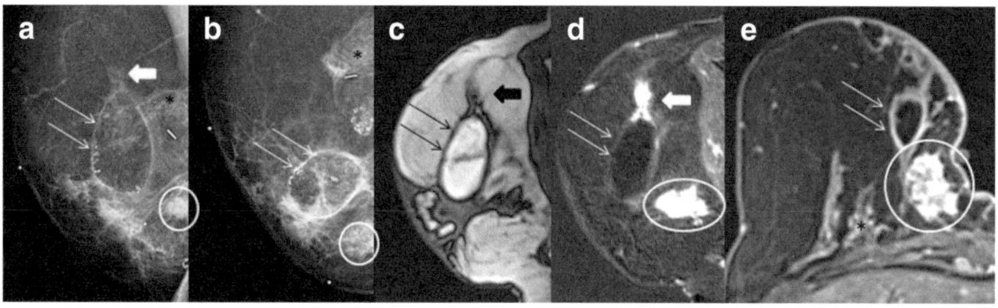

Fig. 8.13 A 68 year old woman with a history of right IDC, status post mastectomy and TRAM reconstruction had a history of palpable fat necrosis and presented with a new palpable mass. The fat necrosis is well seen as a lucent centered mass (*long arrows*) with peripheral calcifications on MLO and CC mammographic views (**a**, **b**) and follows fat signal on T1 (**c**) and sagittal and axial fat-suppressed T1 weighted images (**d**, **e**). Suspicious enhancement superior to the fat necrosis (*thick arrows*) appears consistent with fat on the unenhanced, non-fat-suppressed T1 sequence (**c**) and MLO mammogram (**a**); this was biopsied and was found to be benign fat necrosis. The new palpable mass, (*circled*) is seen as a high density mass in the inferomedial right breast on mammogram (**a**, **b**), and as an irregular, solid heterogeneously enhancing mass on MRI. Biopsy of this mass demonstrated recurrent IDC. Incidentally, the TRAM pedicle (*asterisk*) with atrophied muscle is well seen on mammogram (**a**, **b**) and MRI (**e**). A special thank you to Sara Shaylor, MD for these images

tissue is used to for a new breast mound. The now transversely oriented skin island can fill in the nipple defect in a SSM, and the superior epigastric vascular supply remains intact [18]. Pedicled latissimus dorsi flaps can also be used [19].

Imaging findings include a deep and inferior vascular pedicle, adjacent muscle, typically with fatty infiltration related to disuse and denervation atrophy, and a subcutaneous line where the residual subcutaneous fat meets the transferred autologous fat (Fig. 8.12). Fat necrosis is very common in TRAM reconstructions, occurring in nearly 60 % of patients within 2 months of surgery [20]. Patients often present with a palpable mass, which can be imaged mammographically to distinguish between fat necrosis and recurrence (Fig. 8.13a, b). Fat necrosis will often show a lucent center and concave margins, while recurrence will have convex margins. On MRI, fat necrosis can appear suspicious, with irregular peripheral enhancement. Often a careful search for central fat on T1-weighted images without fat saturation and T2-weighted images with fat saturation can confirm fat necrosis, while solid enhancing masses are worrisome for malignancy (Fig. 8.13c–e). Here too, concave margins can suggest benign necrosis while a bulging, convex margin suggests recurrence (Fig. 8.8). Post-operative edema, skin thickening, seromas and hematomas are also common.

8.4.2 *Free Flaps*

Free flaps, mostly named for their donor artery, include the free TRAM, the deep and superficial inferior epigastric perforator (artery) (DIEP and SIEP or SIE(A)) flaps, the superior and inferior gluteal artery perforator (SGAP and IGAP) flaps and the transverse upper gracilis (TUG) flap [21]. Free flap reconstructions require microsurgery between the donor vessel and, most often, the internal mammary artery, and are more difficult to perform than pedicled reconstructions. However, free flaps have several advantages over the conventional pedicled TRAM flap including preservation of abdominal wall strength, more options for tissue harvesting, and importantly, improved blood flow. **Imaging findings** in free flap reconstructions are similar to those in pedicled reconstructions, except the vascular pedicle is higher, attached to the internal mammary artery at the level of the anterior second through fourth ribs. Adjacent muscle can be seen in non-muscle sparing flaps including the TUG and, variably, the free TRAM. Free flaps can also be complicated by fat necrosis in the first 6 months [20], although at much lower rates (near 20 %) as compared with the pedicled TRAM.

8.4.3 Implant Reconstruction

Implant reconstruction is the most common breast reconstruction technique and can be used alone or in conjunction with autologous reconstruction (Fig. 8.14). In 2014, it was estimated that over 102,000 breast reconstructions were performed in the United States [22], 70 % of which were implant based [23]. A two-step expander/silicone implant reconstruction is the most often used technique, which allows for shape preservation and revascularization following mastectomy, although with the development of the acellular dermal matrix (ADM), single step reconstruction with

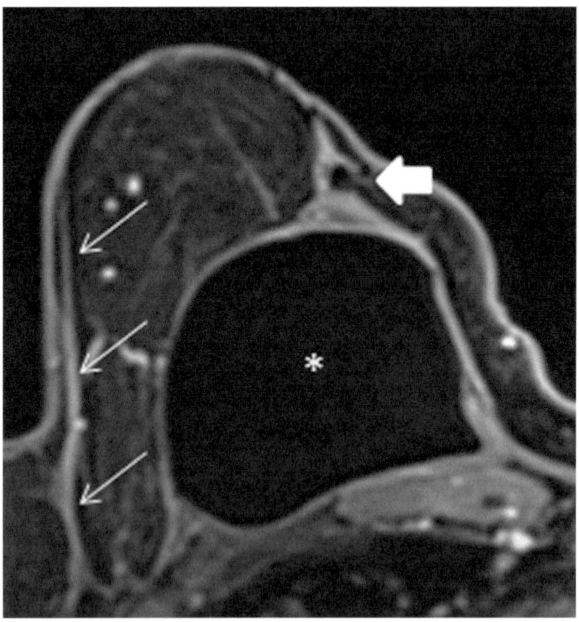

Fig. 8.14 A 62 year old woman with a history of right IDC, status post mastectomy and TRAM reconstruction underwent subsequent silicone implant placement to achieve greater symmetry with the contralateral breast. The vascular pedicle (*thick arrow*) and line between the TRAM and native subcutaneous fat (*thin arrows*) are seen in addition to the subpectoral silicone implant (*asterisk*)

immediate implant placement is becoming more common [24]. While both silicone and saline implants can be used for augmentation, silicone implants are more commonly used and continue to be refined. The most recent adaptation includes higher density and higher viscosity "cohesive" silicone gel which allows implants to maintain their shape even when cut [25]. About 10 % of saline implants rupture by 10 years after implantation. These ruptures most commonly present clinically as a change in breast size as the saline flows freely and is resorbed; imaging is therefore not necessary [26]. About 9–12 % of silicone implants rupture 8 years after implantation [27]. Unlike saline implant rupture, silicone implant rupture is commonly asymptomatic. The FDA recommends MRI screening for silicone implant rupture 3 years after implantation and every 2 years thereafter. Cohesive gel implants are relatively new and rupture data is limited but encouraging. Rupture rate appears to be about 1 % at 6 years after implantation [28].

8.4.4 Imaging Findings

Most tissue expanders are not MRI compatible and MRI should generally be deferred until expanders have been replaced with implants. Silicone implants will follow silicone signal on silicone sensitive and on silicone suppressed MRI sequences. Enhancement around an implant is not typical and should be viewed with suspicion (Fig. 8.15). Radial folds and a small amount of reactive fluid surrounding the implant are normal findings. Contour deformity with an implant bulge,

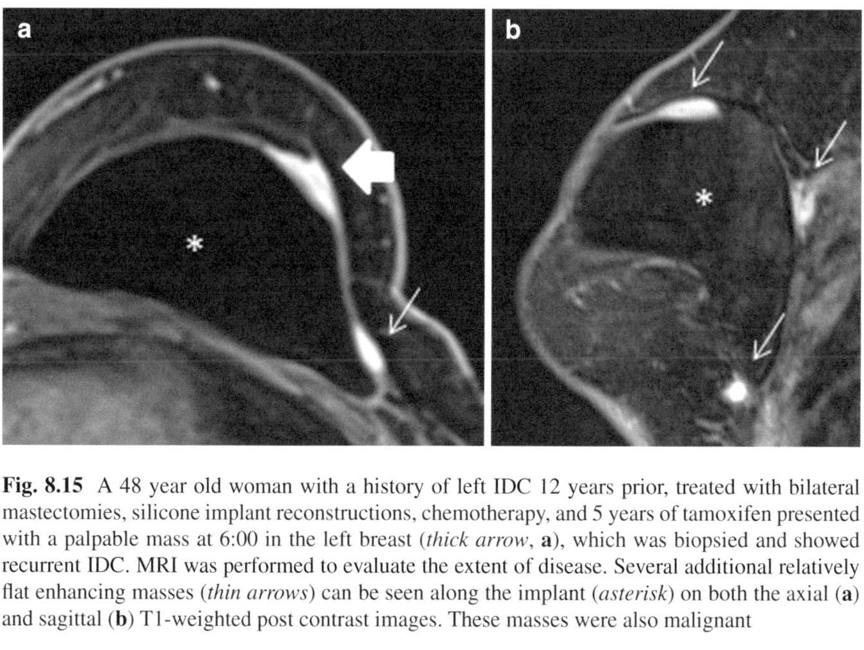

Fig. 8.15 A 48 year old woman with a history of left IDC 12 years prior, treated with bilateral mastectomies, silicone implant reconstructions, chemotherapy, and 5 years of tamoxifen presented with a palpable mass at 6:00 in the left breast (*thick arrow*, **a**), which was biopsied and showed recurrent IDC. MRI was performed to evaluate the extent of disease. Several additional relatively flat enhancing masses (*thin arrows*) can be seen along the implant (*asterisk*) on both the axial (**a**) and sagittal (**b**) T1-weighted post contrast images. These masses were also malignant

an irregular margin, mixed signal intensity of the implant margin and keyhole and teardrop signs all suggest possible rupture while subcapsular lines and the linguine sign are compatible with definitive rupture [29]. Siliconomas generally suggest extracapsular rupture, but can also be the result of prior rupture and implant replacement; thus, a thorough clinical and surgical history is necessary. A detailed description of implants and ruptures can be found in the dedicated chapter in this same volume.

8.4.5 Nipple Reconstruction

Recreation of the nipple areolar complex (NAC), which can be performed about 3–4 months after reconstruction, provides a more natural appearing breast. To recreate the NAC, several options are available including grafts, local flaps, and flaps with augmentation [30]. Most commonly seen in our practice is a local flap consisting of a tri-lobed or star-shaped subdermal incision. The flap "arms" are then reconstructed into a nipple shape and subcutaneous fat is often added to augment the reconstructed nipple size. Tattooing for color matching is typically performed 6–12 weeks after surgery.

Mammographic imaging of a reconstructed NAC may show typical skin calcifications along the incision site. Theoretically, the punctate hyperdense foci seen in the lymph nodes of women with upper extremity tattoos [31] could be seen in this setting as well. Finally, on MRI a native nipple will typically show a thin rim of hyperintense signal on contrast enhanced T1-weighted imaging, while the reconstructed nipple will enhance similarly to the adjacent skin.

References

1. Morrow M, Strom EA, Bassett LW, et al. Standard for breast conservation therapy in the management of invasive breast carcinoma. CA Cancer J Clin. 2002;52:277–300.
2. Tatter PI, Kaplan J, Bleiweiss I, et al. Lumpectomy margins, reexcision, and local recurrence of breast cancer. Am J Surg. 2000;179:81–5.
3. Moran MS, Schnitt SJ, Giuliano AE, et al. Society of Surgical Oncology-American Society for Radiation Oncology consensus guideline on margins for breast-conserving surgery with whole-breast irradiation in stages I and II invasive breast cancer. Int J Radiat Oncol Biol Phys. 2014;88(3):553–64.
4. Merrill AL, Coopey SB, Tang R, et al. Implications of new lumpectomy margin guidelines for breast conservation surgery: changes in reexcision rates and predicted rates of residual tumor. Ann Surg Oncol. 2015;23(3):729–34 [Epub ahead of print].
5. Mendelson EB. Evaluation of the postoperative breast. Radiol Clin North Am. 1992; 30:107–38.
6. Dershaw DD. Mammography in patients with breast cancer treated with breast conservation (lumpectomy with or without radiation). AJR. 1995;164:309–16.

7. Gutierrez R, Horst KC, Dirbas FM, Ikeda DM. Breast imaging following breast conservation therapy. Breast surgical techniques and interdisciplinary management. F.M. Dirbas and C.E.H. Scott-Conner (eds.) Springer 2011 Edition. DOI 10.1007/978-1-4419-6076-4_81
8. Rahbar H, Partridge SC, DeMartini WB, Thursten B, Lehman CD. Clinical and technical considerations for high quality breast MRI at 3 Tesla. J Magn Reson Imaging. 2013;37(4):778–90. doi:10.1002/jmri.23834.
9. Bedair R, Graves MJ, Patterson AJ, McLean MA, Manavaki R, Wallace T, Reid S, Mendichovszky I, Griffiths J, Gilbert FJ. Effect of radiofrequency transmit field correction on quantitative dynamic contrast-enhanced MR imaging of the breast at 3.0 T. Radiology. 2015;279(2):368–77 , 150920.
10. Anderson SJ, Wapnir I, Dignam JJ, et al. Prognosis after ipsilateral breast tumor recurrence and locoregional recurrence in patients treated by breast-conservation therapy in five National Surgical Adjuvant Breast and Bowel Project protocols of node-negative breast cancer. J Clin Oncol. 2009;27(15):2466–73.
11. Ingham SL, Sperrin M, Baildam A, Ross GL, Clayton R, Lalloo F, et al. Risk-reducing surgery increases survival in BRCA1/2 mutation carriers unaffected at time of family referral. Breast Cancer Res Treat. 2013;142:611–8.
12. Loukas M, Tubbs RS, Mirzayan N, Shirak M, Steinberg A, Shoja MM. The history of mastectomy. Am Surg. 2011;77(5):566–71.
13. Toth BA, Lappert P. Modified skin incisions for mastectomy: the need for plastic surgical input in preoperative planning. Plast Reconstr Surg. 1991;87(6):1048–53.
14. Voltura AM, Tsangaris TN, Rosson GD, Jacobs LK, Flores JI, Singh NK, Argani P, Balch CM. Nipple-sparing mastectomy: critical assessment of 51 procedures and implications for selection criteria. Ann Surg Oncol. 2008;15(12):3396–401.
15. Torresan RZ, dos Santos CC, Okamura H, Alvarenga M. Evaluation of residual glandular tissue after skin-sparing mastectomies. Ann Surg Oncol. 2005;12(12):1037–44.
16. Chung AP, Sacchini V. Nipple-sparing mastectomy: where are we now? Surg Oncol. 2008 Dec;17(4):261–6.
17. Benediktsson KP, Perbeck L. Survival in breast cancer after nipple-sparing subcutaneous mastectomy and immediate reconstruction with implants: a prospective trial with 13 years median follow-up in 216 patients. Eur J Surg Oncol. 2008;34:143–8.
18. Jatoi I, Kaufmann M, Petit JY. Atlas of breast surgery. Heidelberg: Springer; 2006.
19. Sternberg EG, Perdikis G, McLaughlin SA, Terkonda SP, Waldorf JC. Latissimus dorsi flap remains an excellent choice for breast reconstruction. Ann Plast Surg. 2006;56(1):31–5.
20. Garvey PB, Buchel EW, Pockaj BA, et al. DIEP and pedicled TRAM flaps: a comparison of outcomes. Plast Reconstr Surg. 2006;117(6):1711–9 ; discussion 1720–1721.
21. Tachi M, Yamada A. Choice of flaps for breast reconstruction. Int J Clin Oncol. 2005; 10(5):289–97.
22. Surgeons ASoP. 2014 Reconstructive Plastic Surgery Statistics 2014.
23. Albornoz CR, Bach PB, Mehrara BJ, et al. A paradigm shift in U.S. Breast reconstruction: increasing implant rates. Plast Reconstr Surg. 2013;131(1):15–23.
24. Serletti JM, Fosnot J, Nelson JA, Disa JJ, Bucky LP. Breast reconstruction after breast cancer. Plast Reconstr Surg. 2011;127(6):124e–35e; Colwell AS. Current strategies with 1-stage prosthetic breast reconstruction. Gland Surg. 2015;4(2):111–5.
25. Stevens WG, Hirsch EM, Tenenbaum MJ, Acevedo M. A prospective study of 708 form-stable silicone gel breast implants. Aesthet Surg J. 2010;30(5):693–701.
26. Walker PS, Walls B, DK M. Silicone implants Natrelle saline-filled breast implants: a prospective 10-year study. Aesthet Surg J. 2009;29(1):19–25.
27. Hölmich LR, Friis S, Fryzek JP, et al. Incidence of silicone breast implant rupture. Arch Surg. 2003;138(7):801–6.
28. Cunningham B, McCue J. Safety and effectiveness of Mentor's MemoryGel implants at 6 years. Aesthetic Plast Surg. 2009;33(3):440–4.

29. Juanpere S, Perez E, Huc O, et al. Imaging of breast implants—a pictorial review. Insights Imaging. 2011;2(6):653–70.
30. Nimboriboonporn A, Chuthapisith S. Nipple-areola complex reconstruction. Gland Surg. 2014;3(1):35–42.
31. Honegger MM, Hesseltine SM, Gross JD, Singer C, Cohen JM. Tattoo pigment mimicking axillary lymph node calcifications on mammography. AJR Am J Roentgenol. 2004;183(3):831–2.

Part III
MRI Findings, Interpretation, and Management

Chapter 9
In Situ Disease on Breast MRI

Heather I. Greenwood and Bonnie N. Joe

Abstract Ductal Carcinoma in Situ is a non-invasive form of breast cancer, in which malignant ductal epithelial cells proliferate, but do not invade through the basement membrane. It is a heterogeneous disease, and is a non-obligate precursor to invasive carcinoma. With the advent of screening mammography the incidence of DCIS has greatly increased. MRI is the most sensitive examination for detecting DCIS. The most common presenting morphology of DCIS is nonmass enhancement, with a clumped internal enhancement pattern and with a segmental distribution pattern. There is great variety in the kinetic patterns of DCIS, and therefore assessment must be based on morphology. Additional tools, such as diffusion weighted imaging have been shown to be promising in helping detect clinically relevant DCIS.

Keywords Ductal Carcinoma in Situ (DCIS) • MRI • Nonmass enhancement • Clumped internal enhancement • Clustered ring internal enhancement • Segmental distribution • Diffusion Weighted Imaging (DWI) • Overdiagnosis • Overtreatment • Oncotype DX 12-gene assay (DCIS Score)

9.1 Background

Ductal carcinoma in situ (DCIS) is a noninvasive breast cancer, referred to as stage 0 breast cancer. At pathology DCIS shows the proliferation of malignant ductal epithelial cells that line a terminal ductal lobular unit without evidence of invasion

H.I. Greenwood, MD (✉) • B.N. Joe, MD, PhD
Department of Radiology and Biomedical Imaging, University of California, San Francisco Medical Center at Mt. Zion, San Francisco, CA, USA
e-mail: heather.greenwood@ucsf.edu

S.L. Heller, L. Moy (eds.), *Breast Oncology: Techniques, Indications, and Interpretation*, DOI 10.1007/978-3-319-42563-4_9

through the basement membrane. DCIS represents a broad spectrum of disease, and is a non-obligate precursor to invasive breast cancer [1–3]. Some lesions may remain clinically quiescent, while others are precursors to invasive breast cancer.

DCIS is rarely symptomatic. With the advent of screening mammography, there has been a significant increase in the incidence of DCIS from 18.7 per 100,000 in 1973–1975 to 32.5 per 100,000 in 2005 [4], a 17-fold increase. DCIS now accounts for up to 25 % of screen detected breast cancers [5].

The term DCIS includes a markedly heterogeneous group of lesions which differ in genetic and molecular abnormalities, histopathologic features, and biologic markers [6]. DCIS is classified according to its tumor grade (high, intermediate, low) architectural pattern (solid, cribiform, papillary, micropapillary, comedo-type), and the presence or absence of necrosis.

Despite the fact that not all cases of DCIS progress to IDC, women who have been diagnosed with DCIS report similar psychologic morbidity as women with invasive cancer [7, 8]. With this similar psychologic morbidity as well as the great heterogeneity of DCIS, there is currently a significant controversy regarding the clinical significance of DCIS, as well as the possible overdiagnosis and overtreatment of DCIS.

The definition of overdiagnosis is "the detection of cancers that would never have been found were if not for the screening test" [9]. Overdiagnosis is considered a harm of screening mammography, and may be considered the most adverse outcome of screening mammography. Autopsy series of women not known to have breast cancer in their lifetime show a prevalence of DCIS of about 10–15 % [10–12].

It is not possible to recognize which cases of breast cancer are cases of overdiagnosis at the individual level; the number may only be estimated at a population level based on data from years of screening mammography. Puliti et al. conducted a literature review of observational studies providing estimates of breast cancer overdiagnosis in a European population based mammographic screening program. The analysis of the papers in the review and of the biases that may affect the estimates found that the most likely estimate of overdiagnosis, "expressed as a percentage of the expected incidence in the absence of screening", was low, and ranged from 1 to 10 %. The authors found the much higher estimates of overdiagnosis in the literature they reviewed to be related to "the lack of adjustment for breast cancer risk and/or lead time bias" [13].

An additional factor in over diagnosis may be secondary to high inter-observer pathologist variability and discrepancies in the classification of DCIS [14–20]. Several of the discrepancies in this classification come from the criteria used to distinguish between atypical ductal hyperplasia (ADH) and DCIS [17]. The architectural appearance and extent of disease process are not simultaneously present in ADH: the diagnosis of ADH is therefore made when some features of DCIS are present, however others are absent [21, 22]. Rosai et al. reported an "unacceptably high" interobserver variation between experienced pathologists in the context of ADH versus DCIS categorization [19]. Thus the issue of over diagnosis, is one shared by both radiologists and pathologists.

Despite the heterogeneous nature of DCIS, it has been shown that almost all invasive cancers arise from DCIS [23]. Long term (30 year) follow-up of low grade DCIS treated only with biopsy without definitive excision or radiation therapy demonstrates a 30–60 % incidence of IDC, usually at or near the site of DCIS [24]. Half of recurrent cases of DCIS lesions manifest as invasive cancer, and 20 % of DCIS cases result in distant metastatic disease in 10 years [25]. It is therefore essential to have an accurate test for the diagnosis and detection of DCIS.

The goal of treating DCIS is to prevent the development of invasive cancer and to decrease the rate of local recurrence. Traditionally DCIS has been treated in most women with breast conservation therapy (lumpectomy) either with or without radiation therapy. Several randomized controlled trials have shown that adding radiation treatment following lumpectomy decreases the risk of local recurrence and invasive local recurrence by 50 % [26–31]. However, some patients at low risk of recurrence may not require radiation therapy.

A challenge in the treatment of DCIS is that clinical factors and pathologic features of DCIS have not been shown to consistently help clinicians determine patients at low risk. The Oncotype DX 12-gene assay (DCIS Score) is a multigene expression assay that generates individualized estimates of the 10-year risk of any local recurrence (LR). The score is generated from an algorithm that includes 12/21 genes in the Oncotype DX invasive assay. The Oncotype DX Score has been shown to predict local recurrence in patients who have undergone breast conservation therapy alone [32]. Therefore, the Oncotype DX score in combination with other well-established risk factors has the potential to be a useful tool in decreasing the overtreatment of DCIS.

9.2 Sensitivity of Imaging Modalities

An accurate assessment of the extent of DCIS is required for successful breast conservation therapy, as patients with positive margins after surgery and patients with residual synchronous foci of DCIS have an increased risk of recurrence. Several studies have shown that MRI is the most sensitive imaging examination for the detection of DCIS. The overall sensitivity of MRI for DCIS has been shown to be approximately 92 %, versus 56 % for mammography [33]. MRI detection is related to contrast uptake. Contrast uptake, or enhancement, is secondary to tumor vascularity, vessel density and permeability. Therefore, MRI, unlike mammography may detect not just calcified DCIS, but also noncalcified DCIS.

Over the past several years, studies have demonstrated the increasing sensitivity of MRI for detecting DCIS. Early studies looking at the sensitivity of MRI for DCIS were performed at a higher temporal resolution and lower spatial resolution, focused on mass lesions, and were also performed in patients with a new diagnosis of breast cancer, generally diagnosed by either mammogram or ultrasound [34]. More recent studies have used higher spatial resolution MRI technique, focused on nonmass enhancement distinct from background parenchymal enhancement (BPE), and evaluated a high risk screening population. These more recent studies have shown a greatly increased sensitivity of MRI for detecting DCIS [33, 34].

Not only is MRI the most sensitive examination for the detection of DCIS but it's sensitivity increases with increasing histologic grade. MRI has been shown to have a sensitivity of 80 % for low grade DCIS, 91 % for intermediate grade, and 98 % for high grade DCIS [33]. Thus MRI is the most sensitive at detecting the type of DCIS that is most likely to progress to invasive carcinoma and to recur.

In addition, contrast enhancement is a biomarker of protease and angiogenic activity. There is increasing vascularity with increasing grades of DCIS. Protease activity is required to penetrate into the basement membrane and beyond it [35]. These factors suggest that DCIS detected on MRI may be more clinically relevant. Therefore, MRI may prove a useful tool in the evaluation of DCIS and may help to allay criticism of mammographic overdetection.

9.3 MRI Features of DCIS

9.3.1 Morphology

Given that MRI has been shown to be the most sensitive imaging modality for the detection of DCIS, it is important to recognize the various MR imaging presentations of DCIS. The most common presenting morphology of DCIS is nonmass enhancement, seen in 60–81 % of cases [36–38]. Nonmass enhancement (NME) is defined as enhancement of an area that is not a mass. The term NME has replaced nonmass like enhancement in the BI-RADS lexicon [39]. Nonmass enhancement is further defined by its internal enhancement pattern as well as its distribution. The most common internal enhancement pattern seen when DCIS presents as NME is a clumped pattern, defined as cobblestone-like enhancement with occasional confluent areas. This internal enhancement pattern is seen in approximately 41–64 % of cases presenting as NME (Fig. 9.1). Less frequently when DCIS presents as NME, it may present with a heterogeneous (16–29 % of cases) or homogenous (0–16 % of cases) internal enhancement pattern [36–38].

In the second edition of BI-RADS for MR, the internal enhancement pattern "clustered ring" has been added. This is defined as small rings of enhancement, which are clustered together (Figs. 9.2 and 9.3) [39]. A study by Tozaki et al. showed that this finding was seen in 63 % of cases of malignancy (including both invasive and non-invasive), versus only 4 % of benign cases. The specificity for malignancy of the finding of clustered ring enhancement was 96 % [40].

When DCIS presents as NME, the most common distribution pattern is a segmental distribution, seen in approximately 14–77 % of cases [36–38, 41]. This is defined as a triangular region of enhancement, apex pointing to the nipple, suggesting a duct or its branches (Fig. 9.4) [39]. It may also present less commonly in a

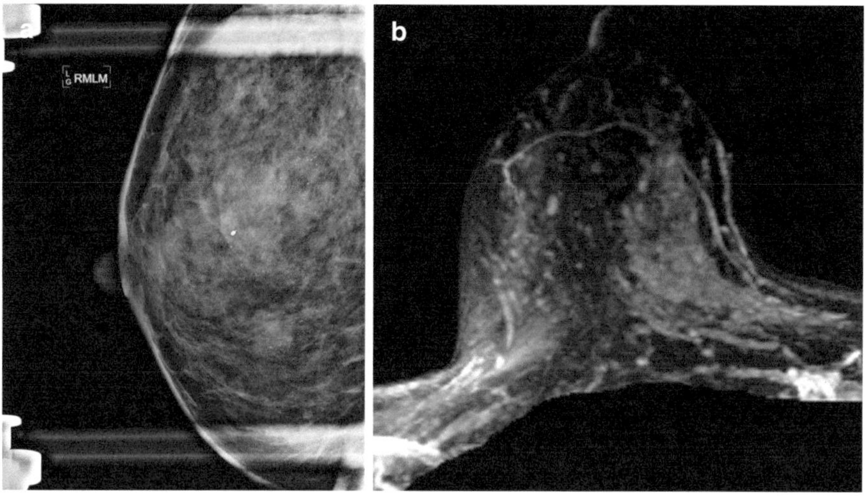

Fig. 9.1 High nuclear grade DCIS in a 47 year old found on screening mammography. (**a**) CC spot magnification view demonstrates segmental pleomorphic calcifications (**b**) MRI performed for extent of disease, maximum intensity projection (MIP) images demonstrates regional nonmass enhancement with a clumped internal enhancement pattern in the inner right breast

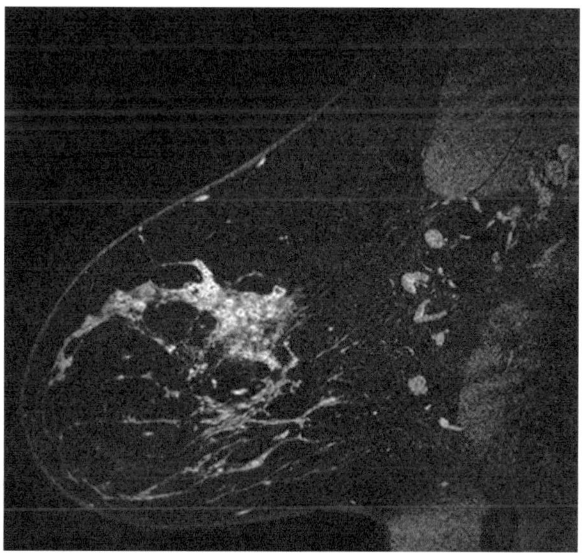

Fig. 9.2 Sagittal post-contrast subtracted image demonstrates segmental NME with a clustered ring internal enhancement pattern, compatible with biopsy proven DCIS in a 38 year old

linear, focal, regional, or diffuse enhancement pattern [36–38, 41]. The MR BI-RADS 2nd edition has removed the distribution ductal from the lexicon [39].

DCIS may also present as a mass morphology on MRI. A mass is defined as a 3D space occupying structure with convex outward contour, which may or may not displace or otherwise affect the surrounding normal breast tissue [39]. This morphology

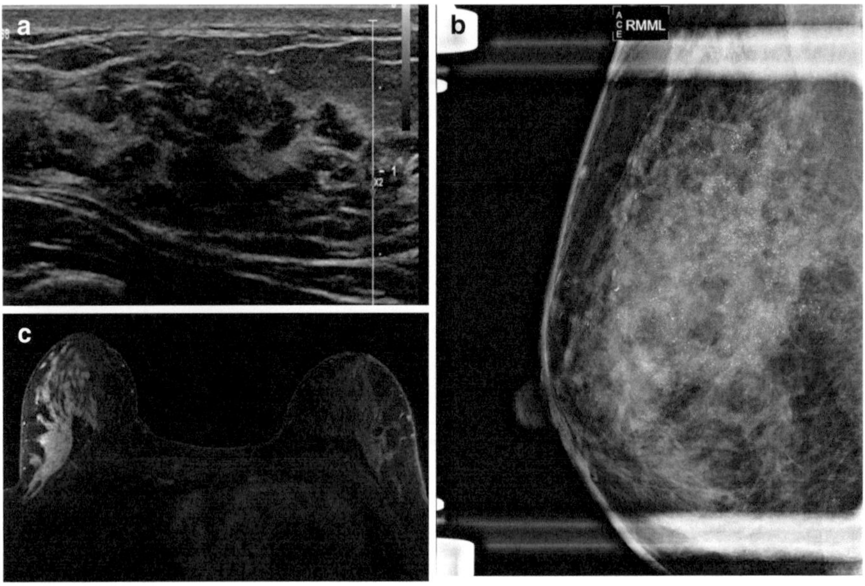

Fig. 9.3 28-year-old female with a palpable lump in the right breast. Given the patient's age she had an ultrasound examination to start. (**a**) Ultrasound images show an irregular mass containing multiple echogenic foci (**b**) Subsequently performed CC mammogram demonstrates fine pleomorphic calcifications. (**c**) MRI performed for extent of disease demonstrates regional NME with a clustered ring internal enhancement pattern, consistent with biopsy proven DCIS

has been seen in approximately 14–41 % of cases of DCIS on MRI [36–38]. Masses are further defined by shape, margin, and internal enhancement patterns. When DCIS presents as a mass on MRI it most commonly is an irregular mass, seen in 14–83 % of cases (Fig. 9.5). Less frequently it may present as an oval or round mass [36, 37, 42]. Of note, the 2nd edition of the MR BI-RADS lexicon has removed the shape lobular for mass lesions to be consistent with the mammogram and ultrasound sections. Masses with up to 3 lobulations now simply are described as "oval" [39]. The literature describes various mass margins when DCIS presents as a mass on MRI, including irregular (14–92 % of cases) and spiculated (0–92 % of cases) (Fig. 9.5). Infrequently DCIS presenting as a mass may have smooth margins (4–8 % cases) [36, 37, 42]. DCIS manifesting as a mass on MRI, may have various internal enhancement patterns. The most common pattern is heterogeneous (9–67 %), followed by homogenous (9–25 %), and less commonly rim enhancement (0–8 %) (Fig. 9.6) [36, 37]. To our knowledge, there has not been a report of non-enhancing dark internal septa in reports of DCIS seen as a mass on MRI. Of note, the terms central enhancement and enhancing septations have been removed from the new BI-RADS lexicon [39].

The least common morphologic appearance of DCIS is a focus [36–38]. A focus is defined as a lesion <5 mm, which is too small to further characterize (Fig. 9.7) [39]. The new BI-RADS edition has removed the term foci from the lexicon [39].

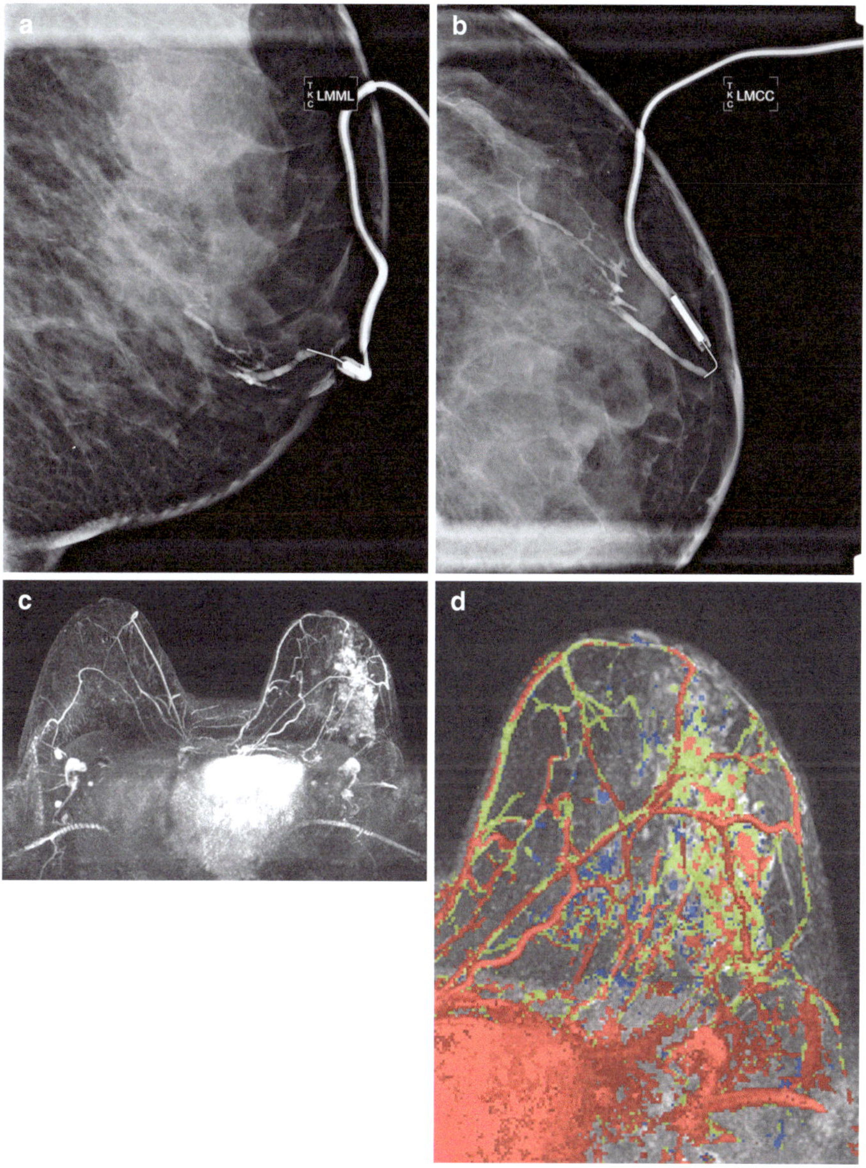

Fig. 9.4 34 year old with left bloody nipple discharge, normal mammogram and ultrasound. (**a**) LM and (**b**) CC views from a ductogram show an intraductal-filling defect in a slightly lower, slightly outer duct. Left duct surgical excision revealed IDC and DCIS on pathology. (**c**) MRI post-contrast subtracted MIP demonstrated extensive clumped NME with a segmental distribution (**d**) Kinetic image demonstrates mixed, predominantly Type 2 and Type 3 delayed kinetics. MR guided biopsy revealed DCIS and IDC. Kinetic key: Type 1 = *blue*, Type 2 = *green*, Type 3 = *red*

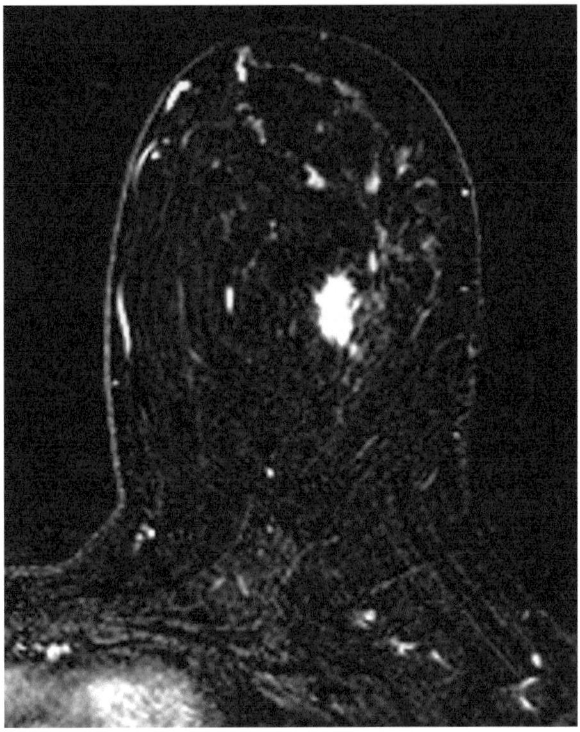

Fig. 9.5 Micropapillary DCIS in a 38-year-old woman with a palpable lump in the left breast. Post-contrast subtracted MR image shows an irregular mass, with spiculated margins, consistent with biopsy proven micropapillary DCIS

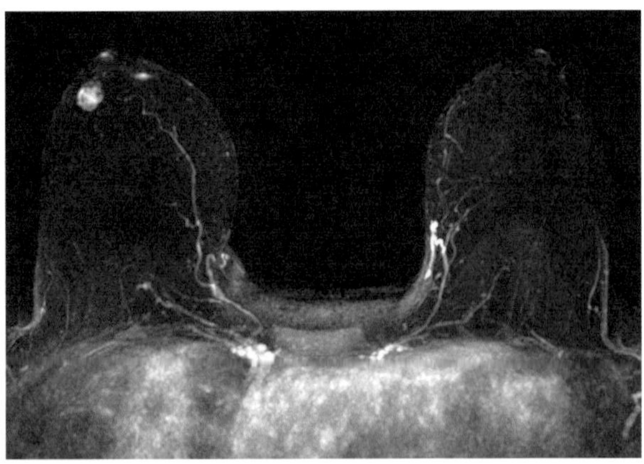

Fig. 9.6 High grade DCIS in a 38 year old female with new diagnosis of DCIS. Post-contrast MIP image demonstrates an oval mass with irregular margins and a heterogeneous internal enhancement pattern in the slightly outer right breast

Rosen et al. found that pure DCIS manifests as a focus in 12.5 % of cases while 3.0 % of invasive carcinomas manifest as a focus [38]. Van Goethem et al. found that a focus was seen in 20 % of DCIS cases versus 2.8 % invasive cancers [44]. Factors suggesting that a focus is malignant on MRI include: no T2 hyperintensity, lack of fatty hilum, washout kinetics, new or enlarging in size. Signs of benignity of

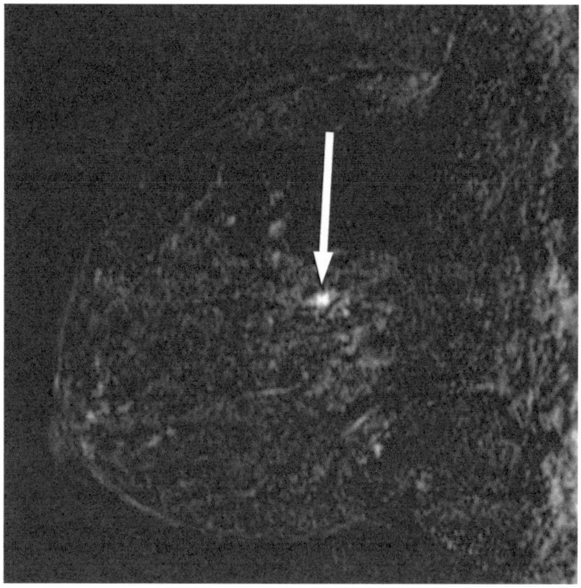

Fig. 9.7 Intermediate-grade DCIS in a 44 year old woman with negative mammographic findings who underwent screening MR imaging because of a strong family history of premenopausal breast cancer. Sagittal postcontrast subtraction image demonstrates a 4 mm focus that demonstrated type 3 (washout) kinetics (Reprinted with permission from Greenwood et al. [43], with permission from Radiology Society of North America (RSNA®))

a focus include: T2 hyperintensity, presence of a fatty hilum, persistent kinetics, and stability [39].

Jansen et al. found that there was no statistically significant difference between MR morphology in low, intermediate, and high nuclear grade DCIS lesions [36]. Additional studies by Chan et al., and Rahbar et al., also found no significant difference in MR morphology between high grade and non-high grade DCIS [37, 45]. At this point, no study to our knowledge has shown that MR morphology is able to predict nuclear grade of DCIS.

9.3.2 *Kinetics*

The kinetic pattern of DCIS varies widely. The initial enhancement phase is defined as occurring within the first 2 minutes after contrast injection or until peak enhancement is reached [39]. In the initial phase, the most common kinetic pattern for DCIS is a fast uptake, seen in 49–68 % of cases, less commonly an intermediate (<20 % of cases) or slow pattern (<20 % of cases) [36, 38, 46]. Of note, in the new BI-RADS 5th edition the term fast has replaced rapid [39]. The delayed enhancement phase is defined as following 2 minutes after contrast injection or after peak enhancement is reached and is used to described the shape of the curve [39]. There is a wide variety of delayed phase kinetic patterns seen in DCIS. The most common pattern is a plateau (type 2), seen in 20–52 % of cases (Fig. 9.8) followed by a washout pattern (type 3), in 28–44 % of cases, and persistent enhancement pattern is seen in 20–30 % of cases [36, 38, 46]. Given the significant variation in the kinetic patterns of DCIS,

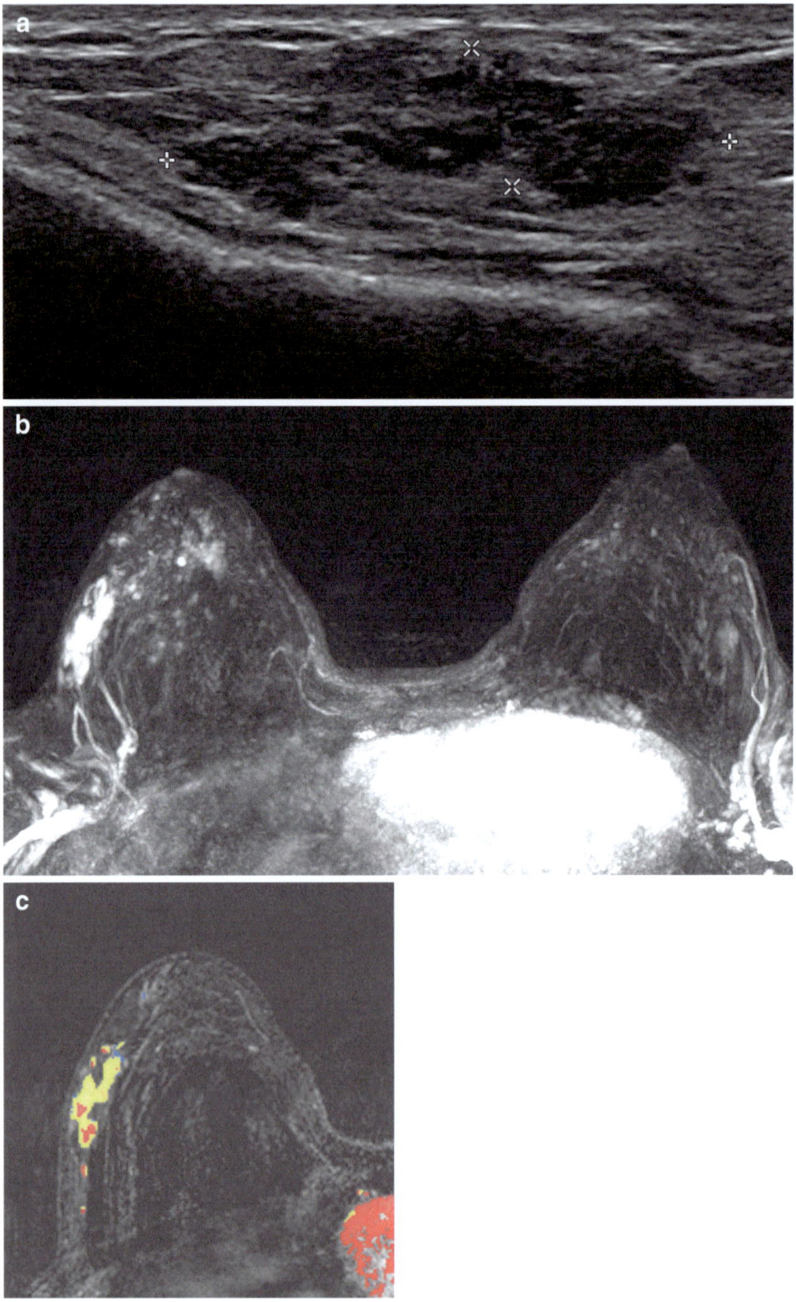

Fig. 9.8 High grade DCIS in a 56-year-old woman with a palpable lump (**a**) Ultrasound image demonstrates a hypoechoic mass with indistinct margins and echogenic foci, corresponding to calcifications on mammography. (**b**) MRI performed for extent of disease demonstrates corresponding segmental clumped NME (**c**) with predominantly Type 2 (plateau) delayed kinetic pattern, compatible with biopsy proven high grade DCIS (Kinetic key: *Blue* = type 1, *yellow* = type 2, *red* = type 3)

it is very important to base the assessment for DCIS on MRI primarily on morphology rather than kinetics.

Additional studies have looked at whether kinetic patterns may predict grade of DCIS. Jansen et al. found no significant difference in kinetic patterns, both initial and delayed, and grade of DCIS [36]. A study in 2012 by Rahbar et al. found no significant association between nuclear grade and delayed phase of enhancement. They did find a non-significant trend ($p = .05$) towards higher peak initial enhancement in high-grade DCIS lesions, compared to non-high grade, at 1.5 T [47]. However, a subsequent study by Rahbar et al. in 2015, found no statistically significant difference in kinetic patterns, initial and delayed, of various grades of DCIS when done at 3 T MR imaging [45].

9.3.3 1.5 T Versus 3 T

There has been increasing use of 3 T MRI for clinical dynamic contrast enhanced breast imaging over the last decade. As it has become apparent that high spatial resolution allows for more accurate detection of DCIS, it follows that 3 T MRI may have increased sensitivity for DCIS, as a benefit of 3 T imaging is higher signal to noise ratio, which allows for higher spatial resolution [48]. Rahbar et al. did a prospective study in patients newly diagnosed with pure DCIS. Each patient underwent a pre-operative breast MRI at both 1.5 T and 3 T imaging. They found that maximum DCIS lesion size on 3 T had a higher correlation with maximum size found on pathology than did 1.5 T [49]. 3 T may therefore be clinically helpful in pre-operative planning for DCIS lesions and further research in this area may be of clinical significance.

9.4 Diffusion Weighted Imaging

As discussed earlier, DCIS has a variable morphologic and kinetic presentation at MRI, which may present diagnostic challenges. No statistically significant difference in morphology has been shown to predict high grade versus non-high grade DCIS [36, 37, 45]. As the concerns for overdiagnosis and overtreatment grow, this becomes a challenge. In addition, another challenge is that breast MRI requires gadolinium administration with may limit accessibility. Diffusion weighted imaging (DWI) is a valuable MRI technique that may better be able to predict grade of DCIS and in addition it does not require any intravenous contrast. DWI quantifies the random motion of water in biologic tissue. The apparent diffusion coefficient (ADC) is the most common quantification of this water transport. Cancers are often more cellular than normal tissue, therefore restrict the diffusion of free water, and this forms the basis of DWI in oncology [50]. In breast cancer, a restricted ADC is widely accepted as a marker of cellularity [51–57].

Rahbar et al. looked at 74 pure DCIS lesions and found that quantitatively these lesions demonstrated higher DWI and lower ADC than normal tissue in the same patient, with a statistical significant difference [58]. In a subsequent study Rahbar et al. studied whether 3 T MRI was able to identify low risk DCIS. This study looked at the features of 36 DCIS lesions on MRI, 8 classified as low risk and 28 high risk. Again no statistically significant differences were found for morphologic features and kinetics between low risk and high risk DCIS. However, low risk DCIS lesions showed different DWI features, such as higher contrast to noise ratio and lower normalized ADCs than high-risk DCIS lesions [45].

Iima et al. studied 22 patients with pure DCIS and found that the ADC of high and intermediate grade DCIS were significantly lower than those of low-grade DCIS, and there was a significant negative trend between mean ADC and tumor grade. These preliminary results suggest that possibly DWI may be able to identify patients with low grade DCIS, which if confirmed could decrease patient anxiety and decrease invasive approaches [59].

An additional study by Rahbar et al., suggests that the combination of findings on DCE MRI and DWI may be able to predict low grade from high grade DCIS, with up to 81% accuracy. Larger size lesions corresponded with higher grade DCIS. A higher contrast to noise ratio (CNR), between each lesion and normal tissue on DWI (b = 600 s/mm^2) was seen in non-high grade DCIS which was thought to be related to greater T2-shine through, as no significant difference in ADC values between high grade and non-high grade lesions [45]. This lack of difference between ADC values and grade of DCIS is different than the results of Iima et al., as ADC values are technique-dependent, and further research is required in this area.

9.5 MRI Features Suggestive of Occult Invasion

Microinvasive DCIS is a subtype of disease which shows 1 mm or less of extension of cancer cells through the basement membrane. Hahn et al. found that microinvasive DCIS showed more suspicious MR imaging characteristics than pure DCIS. These findings included spiculated mass-type lesion, segmental distribution, and clustered ring enhancement of nonmass enhancement, and strong initial enhancement kinetics with washout kinetics [60].

The early identification of an invasive cancer along with DCIS, which is different than microvinasive cancer, is important because it results in changes to surgical management, including a sentinel node biopsy [61]. Wisner et al. looked at whether certain MRI BI-RADS criteria or radiologist perception correlated with invasive cancer after initial diagnosis of DCIS on core-biopsy. 13/51 patients with core-biopsy proven DCIS had invasion at excision. There was a significant positive correlation between the presence of a mass and invasion while nonmass enhancement had a significant negative correlation with invasion [62]. Goto et al. found that that certain MR findings of breast lesions, particularly in NME lesions, including large size of lesion and relatively higher signal intensity on fat-saturated-T2 W images, were suggestive of invasion in biopsy proven DCIS [63]. However, Nori et al. did not find MRI morphologic features to be significantly associated with prediction of

DCIS plus invasive cancer when looking at cases of DCIS diagnosed on percutaneous biopsy [64]. This is an area where future research attention may be helpful.

9.6 Summary

With the advent of screening mammography the incidence of DCIS has increased significantly. MRI has been shown to be the most sensitive examination in the detection of DCIS. Not only is MR the most sensitive imaging modality but it is likely the one to detect the most clinically relevant cases of DCIS, and it is therefore essential to recognize the various presentations of DCIS on MR imaging. The most common morphology of DCIS is nonmass enhancement, and the most common distribution for the NME is in a segmental pattern. The most common kinetic pattern of DCIS is a fast initial uptake, however there is great variation in the delayed phase. It is thus, essential to evaluate lesions based on the morphologic pattern.

Given the broad spectrum of disease that DCIS represents, and the significant current controversies regarding both overdiagnosis and overtreatment of DCIS, additional research evaluating MR and its various techniques, including DWI, may be extremely useful in helping increase the detection of clinically relevant cases of DCIS and improving prediction of nonprogressive DCIS.

References

1. Mossa-Basha M, Fundaro GM, Shah BA, Ali S, Pantelic MV. Ductal carcinoma in situ of the breast: MR imaging findings with histopathologic correlation 1. Radiographics. 2010;30: 1673–87.
2. Ozzello L. Ultrastructure of intra-epithelial carcinomas of the breast. Cancer. 1971;28: 1508–15.
3. Recht A, Rutgers E, Fentiman I, Kurtz J, Mansel R, Sloane J. The fourth EORTC DCIS consensus meeting (Château Marquette, Heemskerk, The Netherlands, 23–24 January 1998)—Conference report. Eur J Cancer. 1998;34:1664–9.
4. Virnig BA, Wang S-Y, Shamilyan T, Kane RL, Tuttle TM. Ductal carcinoma in situ: risk factors and impact of screening. JNCI Monographs. 2010;2010:113–6.
5. Lynge E, Ponti A, James T, Májek O, Euler-Chelpin MV, Anttila A, et al. Variation in detection of ductal carcinoma in situ during screening mammography: a survey within the International Cancer Screening Network. Eur J Cancer. 2014;50:185–92.
6. Colin C, Devouassoux-Shisheboran M, Sardanelli F. Is breast cancer overdiagnosis also nested in pathologic misclassification? Radiology. 2014;273:652–5.
7. Rakovitch E, Franssen E, Kim J, Ackerman I, Pignol J-P, Paszat L, et al. A comparison of risk perception and psychological morbidity in women with ductal carcinoma in situ and early invasive breast cancer. Breast Cancer Res Treat. 2003;77:285–93.
8. De Morgan S, Redman S, White KJ, Cakir B, Boyages J. 'Well, have I got cancer or haven't I?' The psycho-social issues for women diagnosed with ductal carcinoma in situ. Health Expect. 2002;5:310–8.
9. Gotzsche PC. Breast cancer screening. International Agency for Research on Cancer (IARC) handbooks of cancer prevention. Vol. 7 Radiographics, October special issue 2013.

10. Erbas B, Provenzano E, Armes J, Gertig D. The natural history of ductal carcinoma in situ of the breast: a review. Breast Cancer Res Treat. 2005;97:135–44.
11. Nielsen M, Thomsen J, Primdahl S, Dyreborg U, Andersen J. Breast cancer and atypia among young and middle-aged women: a study of 110 medicolegal autopsies. Br J Cancer. 1987;56: 814–9.
12. Welch HG. Using autopsy series to estimate the disease "Reservoir" for ductal carcinoma in situ of the breast: how much more breast cancer can we find? Ann Intern Med. 1997;127: 1023–8.
13. Puliti D, Duffy SW, Miccinesi G, Koning HD, Lynge E, Zappa M, et al. Overdiagnosis in mammographic screening for breast cancer in Europe: a literature review. J Med Screen. 2012;19:42–56.
14. Costarelli L, Campagna D, Mauri M, Fortunato L. Intraductal proliferative lesions of the breast—terminology and biology matter: premalignant lesions or preinvasive cancer? Int J Surg Oncol. 2012. doi:10.1155/2012/501904.
15. Douglas-Jones A, Gupta S, Attanoos R, Morgan J, Mansel R. A critical appraisal of six modern classifications of ductal carcinoma in situ of the breast (DCIS): correlation with grade of associated invasive carcinoma. Histopathology. 1996;29:397–409.
16. Elston C, Sloane J, Amendoeira I, Apostolikas N, Bellocq J, Bianchi S, et al. Causes of inconsistency in diagnosing and classifying intraductal proliferations of the breast. Eur J Cancer. 2000;36:1769–72.
17. Ghofrani M, Tapia B, Tavassoli FA. Discrepancies in the diagnosis of intraductal proliferative lesions of the breast and its management implications: results of a multinational survey. Virchows Arch. 2006;449:609–16.
18. Jain RK, Mehta R, Dimitrov R, Larsson LG, Musto PM, Hodges KB, et al. Atypical ductal hyperplasia: interobserver and intraobserver variability. Mod Pathol. 2011;24:917–23.
19. Rosai J. Borderline epithelial lesions of the breast. Am J Surg Pathol. 1991;15:209–21.
20. Sloane JP, Amendoeira I, Apostolikas N, Bellocq J, Bianchi S, Boecker W, et al. Consistency achieved by 23 european pathologists in categorizing ductal carcinoma in situ of the breast using five classifications. Eur J Cancer. 2220(36):1769–72.
21. Page DL, Rogers LW. Combined histologic and cytologic criteria for the diagnosis of mammary atypical ductal hyperplasia. European Commission Working Group on Breast. Hum Pathol. 1992;23:1095–7.
22. Tavassoli FA, Norris HJ. A comparison of the results of long-term follow-up for atypical intraductal hyperplasia and intraductal hyperplasia of the breast. Cancer. 1990;65:518–29.
23. Burstein HJ, Polyak K, Wong JS, Lester SC, Kaelin CM. Ductal carcinoma in situ of the breast. N Engl J Med. 2004;350:1430–41.
24. Cady B. How to prevent invasive breast cancer: Detect and excise duct carcinoma in situ. J Surg Oncol. 1998;69:60–2.
25. Bjiker N, Peterse JL, Julien JP, Fentiman IS, Duval C, Di Palma S, et al. Risk factors for recurrence and metastasis after breast-conserving therapy for ductal carcinoma-in-situ: analysis of Eurpoean Organization for Research and Treatment of Cancer Trial 10853. J Clin Oncol. 2001;19:2263–71.
26. Bijker N, Meijen P, Peterse JL, Bogaerts J, Van Hoorebeeck I, Julien JP, et al. Breast-conserving treatment with or without radiotherapy for ductal carcinoma in situ (DCIS): ten-year results of European Organisation for Research and Treatment of Cancer (EORTC) randomized phase III trial 10853. Eur J Cancer Suppl. 2006;4:108.
27. Correa C, McGale P, Taylor C, Want Y, Clarke M, Davies C, et al. Overview of the randomized trials of radiotherapy in ductal carcinoma in situ of the breast. JNCI Monographs. 2010; 2010:162–77.
28. Cuzick J, Sestak I, Pinder SE, Ellis IO, Forsyth S, Bundred NJ, et al. Effect of tamoxifen and radiotherapy in women with locally excised ductal carcinoma in situ: long-term results from the UK/ANZ DCIS trial. Lancet Oncol. 2011;12:21–9.
29. Fisher B, Land S, Mamounas E, Dignam J, Fisher ER, Wolmark N. Prevention of invasive breast cancer in women with ductal carcinoma in situ: An update of the national surgical adjuvant breast and bowel project experience. Semin Oncol. 2001;28:400–18.

30. Solin LJ. The impact of adding radiation treatment after breast conservation surgery for ductal carcinoma in situ of the breast. JNCI Monographs. 2010;2010:187–92.
31. Wapnir IL, Dignam JJ, Fisher B, Mamounas EP, Anderson SJ, Julian TB, et al. Long-term outcomes of invasive ipsilateral breast tumor recurrences after lumpectomy in NSABP B-17 and B-24 randomized clinical trials for DCIS. JNCI J Natl Cancer Inst. 2011;103:478–88.
32. Solin LJ, Gray R, Baehner FL, Butler SM, Hughes LL, Yoshizawa C, et al. A multigene expression assay to predict local recurrence risk for ductal carcinoma in situ of the breast. JNCI J Natl Cancer Inst. 2013;105:701–10.
33. Kuhl CK, Schrading S, Bieling HB, Wardelmann E, Leutner CC, Koenig R, et al. MRI for diagnosis of pure ductal carcinoma in situ: a prospective observational study. Lancet. 2007;370:485–92.
34. Lehman CD. Magnetic resonance imaging in the evaluation of ductal carcinoma in situ. JNCI Monographs. 2010;2010:150–1.
35. Jansen SA, Paunesku T, Fan X, Woloschak GE, Vogt S, Conzen SD, et al. Ductal carcinoma in situ: X-ray fluorescence microscopy and dynamic contrast-enhanced MR imaging reveals gadolinium uptake within neoplastic mammary ducts in a murine model 1. Radiology. 2009;253:399–406.
36. Jansen SA, Newstead GM, Abe H, Shimauchi A, Schmidt RA, Karczmar GS. Pure ductal carcinoma in situ: kinetic and morphologic MR characteristics compared with mammographic appearance and nuclear grade 1. Radiology. 2007;245:684–91.
37. Chan S, Chen J-H, Agrawal G, Lin M, Mehta RS, Carpenter PM, et al. Characterization of pure ductal carcinoma in situ on dynamic contrast-enhanced MR imaging: do nonhigh grade and high grade show different imaging features? J Oncol. 2010;2010:1–9.
38. Rosen EL, Smith-Foley SA, Demartini WB, Eby PR, Peacock S, Lehman CD. BI-RADS MRI enhancement characteristics of ductal carcinoma in situ. Breast J. 2007;13:545–50.
39. Morris EA, Comstock CE, Lee CH, et al. ACR BI-RADS® magnetic resonance imaging. In: ACR BI-RADS® Atlas, Breast Imaging Reporting and Data System. Reston: American College of Radiology; 2013.
40. Tozaki M, Igarashi T, Fukuda K. Breast MRI using the VIBE sequence: clustered ring enhancement in the differential diagnosis of lesions showing non-masslike enhancement. Am J Roentgenol. 2006;187:313–21.
41. Yamada T, Mori N, Watanabe M, Kimijima I, Okumoto T, Seiji K, et al. Radiologic-pathologic correlation of ductal carcinoma in situ 1. Radiographics. 2010;30:1183–98.
42. Menell JH, Morris EA, Dershaw DD, Abramson AF, Brogi E, Liberman L. Determination of the presence and extent of pure ductal carcinoma in situ by mammography and magnetic resonance imaging. Breast J. 2005;11:382–90.
43. Greenwood HI, Heller SL, Kim S, Sigmund EE, Shaylor SD, Moy L. Ductal carcinoma in situ of the breasts: review of MR imaging features. Radiographics. 2013;33:1569–88.
44. Van Goethem M, Schelfout K, Kersschot E, Colpaert C, Weyler J, Verslegers I, et al. Comparison of MRI features of different grades of DCIS and invasive carcinoma of the breast. Clin Imaging. 2006;30:225–32.
45. Rahbar H, Parsian S, Lam DL, Dontchos BN, Andeen NK, Rendi MH, et al. Can MRI biomarkers at 3 T identify low-risk ductal carcinoma in situ? Clin Imaging. 2015;40:125–9. doi:10.1016/j.clinimag.2015.07.026.
46. Vag T, Baltzer PAT, Dietzel M, Benndorf M, Gajda M, Camara O, et al. Kinetic characteristics of ductal carcinoma in situ (DCIS) in dynamic breast MRI using computer-assisted analysis. Acta Radiol. 2010;51:955–61.
47. Rahbar H, Partridge SC, Demartini WB, Gutierrez RL, Allison KH, Peacock S, et al. In vivo assessment of ductal carcinoma in situ grade: a model incorporating dynamic contrast-enhanced and diffusion-weighted breast MR imaging parameters. Radiology. 2012;263:374–82.
48. Soher BJ, Dale BM, Merkle EM. A review of MR physics: 3 T versus 1.5 T. Magn Reson Imaging Clin N Am. 2007;15:277–90.
49. Rahbar H, Demartini WB, Lee AY, Partridge SC, Peacock S, Lehman CD. Accuracy of 3 T versus 1.5 T breast MRI for pre-operative assessment of extent of disease in newly diagnosed DCIS. Eur J Radiol. 2015;84:611–6.

50. Koh D-M, Padhani AR. Diffusion-weighted MRI: a new functional clinical technique for tumour imaging. Br J Radiol BJR. 2006;79:633–5.
51. Chen X, Li W-L, Zhang Y-L, Wu Q, Guo Y-M, Bai Z-L. Meta-analysis of quantitative diffusion-weighted MR imaging in the differential diagnosis of breast lesions. BMC Cancer 2010; doi:10.1186/1471-2407-10-693/.
52. Fornasa F, Pinali L, Gasparini A, Toniolli E, Montemezzi S. Diffusion-weighted magnetic resonance imaging in focal breast lesions: analysis of 78 cases with pathological correlation. Radiol med La radiologia medica. 2010;116:264–75.
53. Kul S, Cansu A, Alhan E, Dinc H, Gunes G, Reis A. Contribution of diffusion-weighted imaging to dynamic contrast-enhanced MRI in the characterization of breast tumors. Am J Roentgenol. 2011;196:210–7.
54. Partridge SC, Demartini WB, Kurland BF, Eby PR, White SW, Lehman CD. Quantitative diffusion-weighted imaging as an adjunct to conventional breast MRI for improved positive predictive value. Am J Roentgenol. 2009;193:1716–22.
55. Partridge SC, Demartini WB, Kurland BF, Eby PR, White SW, Lehman CD. Differential diagnosis of mammographically and clinically occult breast lesions on diffusion-weighted MRI. J Magn Reson Imaging. 2010;31:562–70.
56. Sinha S, Lucas-Quesada FA, Sinha U, Debruhl N, Bassett LW. In vivo diffusion-weighted MRI of the breast: potential for lesion characterization. J Magn Reson. 2002;15:693–704.
57. Yabuuchi H, Matsuo Y, Kamitani T, Setoguchi T, Okafuji T, Soeda H, et al. Non-mass-like enhancement on contrast-enhanced breast MR imaging: Lesion characterization using combination of dynamic contrast-enhanced and diffusion-weighted MR images. Eur J Radiol. 2010;75:126–32. doi:10.1016/j.ejrad.2009.09.013.
58. Rahbar H, Partridge SC, Eby PR, Demartini WB, Gutierrez RL, Peacock S, et al. Characterization of ductal carcinoma in situ on diffusion weighted breast MRI. Eur Radiol. 2011;21:2011–9.
59. Iima M, Bihan DL, Okumura R, Okada T, Fujimoto K, Kanao S, et al. Apparent diffusion coefficient as an MR imaging biomarker of low-risk ductal carcinoma in situ: a pilot study. Radiology. 2011;260:364–72.
60. Hahn SY, Han B-K, Ko EY, Shin JH, Hwang J-Y, Nam M. MR features to suggest microinvasive ductal carcinoma of the breast: can it be differentiated from pure DCIS? Acta Radiol. 2013;54:742–8.
61. Intra M, Rotmensz N, Veronesi P, Colleoni M, Iodice S, Paganelli G, et al. Sentinel node biopsy is not a standard procedure in ductal carcinoma in situ of the breast. Ann Surg. 2008; 247:315–9.
62. Wisner DJ, Hwang ES, Chang CB, Tso HH, Joe BN, Lessing JN, et al. Features of occult invasion in biopsy-proven DCIS at breast MRI. Breast J. 2013;19:650–8.
63. Goto M, Yuen S, Akazawa K, Nishida K, Konishi E, Kajihara M, et al. The role of breast MR imaging in pre-operative determination of invasive disease for ductal carcinoma in situ diagnosed by needle biopsy. Eur Radiol. 2011;22:1255–64.
64. Nori J, Meattini I, Giannotti E, Abdulcadir D, Mariscotti G, Calabrese M, et al. Role of preoperative breast MRI in ductal carcinoma in situ for prediction of the presence and assessment of the extent of occult invasive component. Breast J. 2014;20:243–8.

Chapter 10
MRI Appearance of Invasive Breast Cancer

Lea Gilliland and Maria Piraner

Abstract This chapter reviews invasive cancers using both the molecular classification of subtypes of breast cancer and the traditional pathologic classification of breast cancers. MRI is a frequently used modality for evaluating breast cancer. Tumors demonstrate varying morphologic and enhancement characteristics depending on tumor type. Knowledge of the MRI appearance of various tumors is helpful for expanding the differential diagnosis.

Keywords Luminal A/Luminal B breast cancer • Her2 enriched breast cancer • Triple negative breast cancer • Invasive ductal carcinoma • Invasive lobular carcinoma • Papillary carcinoma • Micropapillary carcinoma • Mucinous carcinoma • Medullary carcinoma • Tubular cancer • Metaplastic carcinoma • Adenoid cystic carcinoma • Phyllodes tumor

10.1 Introduction

Dynamic contrast enhanced Breast MRI emerged in the 1990s as a novel technique to detect breast cancer. Its high sensitivity is based on tumor angiogenesis and neovascularity [1]. A 2008 meta-analysis of 44 studies demonstrated that MRI has a sensitivity of 90 % and a specificity of 72 % [2]. A 2007 prospective study of 171 patients in a high risk population reported that MRI detected 100 % of the cancers while mammography identified 33 % of cancers and ultrasound demonstrated 17 % [3]. Whereas mammography uses x-rays and ultrasound uses sound waves, MRI employs a powerful magnetic field, radiofrequency pulses, and high soft tissue contrast to capture tumor morphology.

L. Gilliland, MD (✉)
Department of Radiology, Emory University Hospital, Atlanta, GA, USA
e-mail: lcgilli@emory.edu

M. Piraner, MD
Department of Radiology and Imaging Sciences, Emory University Hospital, Atlanta, GA, USA

S.L. Heller, L. Moy (eds.), *Breast Oncology: Techniques, Indications, and Interpretation*, DOI 10.1007/978-3-319-42563-4_10

10.2 Categorization of Invasive Breast Disease

Invasive breast cancers may be categorized in a variety of ways. This chapter will review the molecular and histopathologic classification of types of invasive breast tumors and discuss morphologic and kinetic appearance of invasive breast disease on MRI. Although this chapter will focus predominantly on the MRI phenotypic appearance of invasive cancers, it is important to recognize that more recently, molecular classifications have been identified.

10.3 Molecular Classification

To determine the molecular signature of breast cancer, messenger RNA is isolated and tested against complementary DNA microarrays to determine which genes a cancer expresses, and which genes it lacks [4]. It has been noted that breast cancers can be divided into two large categories, depending on the pattern of gene expression. When tumor cells have characteristics similar to the epithelial cells lining the milk ducts, expressing cytokeratin 8/18 and genes associated with the estrogen receptor (ER), the cancers are labeled luminal cancers [4]. Alternatively, when cancer cells display characteristics similar to the myoepithelial cells (also known as basal cells) that line the inner surface of the basement membranes, expressing cytokeratin 5/6 and laminin, the cancers are grouped into the basal category [4]. These two large categories of luminal breast cancers and basal breast cancers are defined and classified on the basis of the presence or absence of ERs [4] which defines the morphology and behavior of a tumor. Luminal tumors also are characterized by an absence of overexpression of the gene ERBB2 (also known as the HER2/neu gene), a proto-oncogene that stimulates cellular growth [4].

Other markers of cell proliferation and invasiveness have been analyzed over the past decade and four subgroups of breast cancer have been adopted. These are luminal A, luminal B, HER2-enriched, and basal-like cancers. Luminal A breast cancers express both estrogen (ER) and progesterone (PR) receptors and are generally low grade. HER2/neu is not amplified and there is a low Ki-67 proliferative index. This is the most common type of breast cancer, representing 50 % of all breast cancers. 5-year survival is greater than 80 % [4]. Luminal B cancers also express ER and PR but have higher Ki-67 levels and, thus, greater proliferative activity. Luminal B cancers generally do not overexpress HER2/neu, but 30 % will be Her2-enriched [4]. Five-year survival is 40 %. HER2-enriched tumors have extra copies of the HER-2 gene and over produce a growth enhancing protein ERBB2. This results in increased cellular aggressiveness and fast growth. Sixty-six percent of HER2- enriched cancers overexpress HER2/neu and the remaining tumors express overexpress genes in the *ras* pathway [4] 30–40 % HER2- enriched cancers are ER and PR positive. Basal like subtypes lack ER, PR, and HER2/neu markers and overexpress oncogenes that favor cell proliferation and carcinogenesis such as p53. Eighty percent of triple negative breast cancers are basal-like. Basal-like cancer is more common in younger BRCA1 carriers and in young African American women [4]. Specific imaging findings can be seen in Luminal A, Luminal B, Her2-enriched, and basal type cancers.

10.3.1 Luminal A/Luminal B

Luminal A and Luminal B are grouped as ER+ HER2- cancers for imaging purposes. Mammographically, these cancers often present as masses; calcifications are seen in 41 % of these cancers. Ultrasound often demonstrates irregular masses with angular or microlobulated margins [4]. 117 ER-positive HER2- negative breast cancers were studied by Uematsu and colleagues and MRI findings were reported as 67 % mass enhancement and 33 % nonmass enhancement (NME). Masses were irregular (32 %) and oval in shape (38 %) with irregular margins (86 %) (Fig. 10.1). Heterogeneous internal enhancement was seen 97 % of the time with kinetics being plateau or washout in 79 % of cases. Lesions were iso- to hypointense on T2-weighted images 85 % of the time [5].

10.3.2 Her2 Enriched

Although Her 2 positive tumors are not a perfect correlate for the HER2 enriched subtype, 60 % of HER-2 positive tumors are HER-2 enriched tumors. MRI features of HER2-positive tumors have been documented. HER-2 positive tumors have been reported to present as masses with microcalcifications [4]. Calcifications have been noted in as many as 78 % of HER2-positive tumors [4]. HER-2 cancers are often associated with DCIS, more than other breast cancer subtypes. Youk and colleagues reported MR characteristics of 94 HER2-positive cancers: mass enhancement was noted in 90 %; 47 % of masses were round or oval and 41 % were lobulated. Margins were spiculated (51 %) and irregular (48 %). Heterogeneous enhancement was most commonly seen (79 %) and washout was the most common kinetic pattern (90 %) Her-2-positive cancers demonstrate non-mass enhancement more often than the other subtypes [4] (Fig. 10.2).

10.3.3 Triple Negative/Basal

MRI characteristics reflect histology in triple negative cancers/basal-like breast cancers [5–6]. Triple negative breast cancer (TNBC) refers to invasive cancers that lack estrogen receptors (ER negative), progesterone receptors (PR negative), and are human epidermal growth factor receptor negative (HER2 negative). The majority of TNBCs are basal like. TNBCs are associated with the BRCA1 mutation and early metastatic

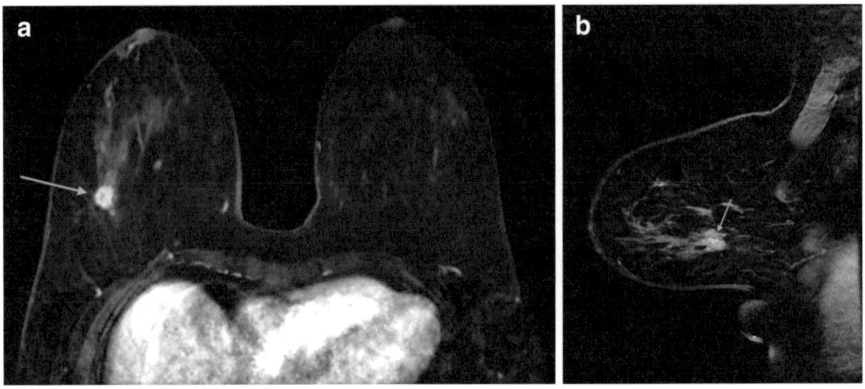

Fig. 10.1 Axial and sagittal T1 post contrast images demonstrate an irregularly shaped and irregularly marginated mass with heterogeneous enhancement (*arrows*). Biopsy demonstrated ER/PR + HER-2- IDC

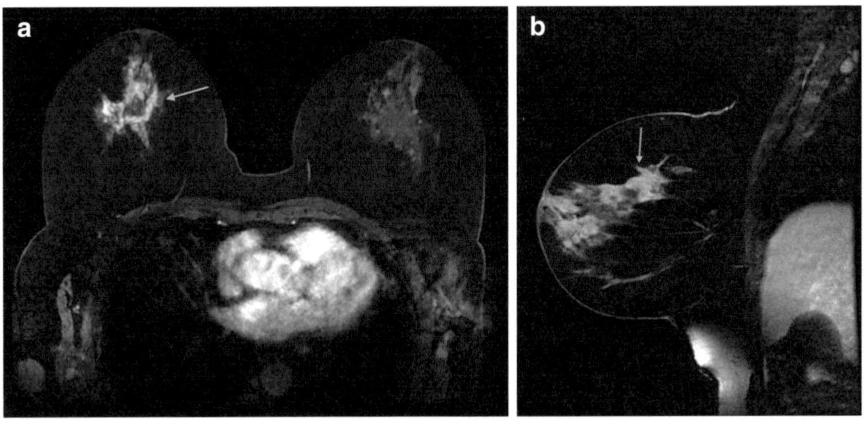

Fig. 10.2 Axial and Sagittal T1 post contrast images demonstrate an irregular mass with associated nonmass enhancement (*arrow*). Biopsy revealed HER2+ IDC

disease [6]. Clinically, this denotes a poor prognosis because tumors that are ER/PR negative do not respond to hormonal therapy. Also, targeted therapy with monoclonal antibodies against HER 2 will not work in tumors that are HER2 negative. TNBCs are typically high-grade [5]. Histologically, triple negative breast cancers are associated with the presence of a central scar, tumor necrosis, the presence of spindle cells or squamous metaplasia, high total mitotic count, and high nuclear-cytoplasmic ratio [5].

TNBCs often appear as circumscribed round or oval masses and are less likely to show distortion or calcifications [7]. Ultrasound frequently demonstrates a solid hypoechoic or mixed echogenicity oval, round or irregular mass with circumscribed or indistinct margins [5, 8]. TNBCs are generally seen as mass lesions on MRI with very few appearing as non-mass enhancement (NME) (Fig. 10.3). Masses may be round, oval or irregular with circumscribed, irregular or spiculated margins. Differentiation from benign masses can be difficult, as many features such as oval,

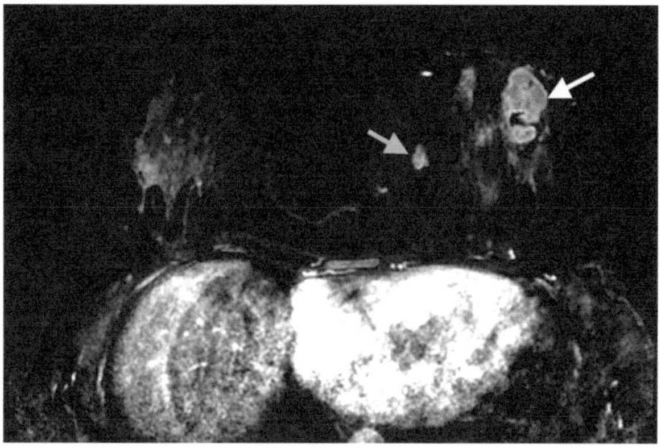

Fig. 10.3 Axial T1-weighted post contrast subtraction image demonstrates an irregularly shaped circumscribed mass with heterogeneous enhancement (*white arrow*). A smaller similar mass is noted medially (*gray arrow*). Biopsy of the large and small masses yielded triple negative cancer

circumscribed masses, persistent enhancement, and high T2 signal are seen both in benign lesions and TNBCs, although the high T2 signal in a TNBCs is often due to necrosis (Fig. 10.3). Rim-enhancement and internal, enhancing septations should increase suspicion if seen [7]. TNBCs are more likely than other cancers to have persistent enhancement kinetics [7].

10.4 MRI Tools for Detecting Invasive Cancer

10.4.1 MR-BI-RADS and Descriptors of Invasive Carcinomas

The MR-BI-RADS lexicon identifies specific morphologic and kinetic characteristics for Enhancing lesions and is discussed in Chap. 2, so will only briefly be addressed here. The combination of morphologic and kinetic features has a reported sensitivity of 90 % and a specificity of 72 % for detecting malignancy [2].

10.4.1.1 Morphologic Features of Invasive Disease

Invasive cancer may present as a mass, NME or a focus on MRI. A 2007 study reviewed MRI biopsy results found the probability of malignancy to be 34 % for masses, 27 % for NME, and 19 % for foci [9]. Certain lesion characteristics should raise suspicion for malignancy and invasive disease, in particular masses with irregular and spiculated margins [10, 11]. A 2006 study documenting the characteristics of 171 masses on MRI demonstrated the most frequent morphological finding in malignant lesions was heterogeneous internal enhancement (96 % of malignancies demonstrated in the delayed phase and 90 % in the early phase). Features with the highest positive predictive value for carcinoma were spiculated margin (100 %), delayed central enhancement (100 %), enhancing internal septations in the delayed phase (97 %), and irregular shape (97 %). Of the masses studied 25 % of smooth round or oval masses were malignant, 85 % of irregularly-shaped or marginated masses were malignant and 100 % of spiculated masses were malignant. Smooth margins were the most frequent finding in benign lesions (80 %) [11]. Regarding masses, a 2012 study of 969 patients demonstrated the highest PPV was found with irregular margins (PPV, 0.196) and spiculated margins, (PPV, 0.333). The lowest PPV was found with smooth margins (PPV, 0.052). Masses with marked internal enhancement were most likely to represent cancer (PPV, 0.231). Both plateau (PPV 0.152) and washout (PPV, 0.178) were associated with cancer [12].

10.4.1.2 Kinetic Features of Invasive Disease

Tumor enhancement may be plotted on a time-signal intensity curve. The initial contrast enhancement and the delayed contrast enhancement characteristics are calculated. These kinetic curves have become a standard component of the breast MRI exam and allow for better prediction of malignancy. Due to angiogenesis, malignancies demonstrate rapid wash-in and wash-out of the contrast agent. This is known as a type 3 time-signal intensity curve. This type 3 pattern is the most concerning curve type. However, benign entities (such as lymph nodes) may demonstrate this washout curve. In addition, a persistent or plateau curve may be seen in both benign and malignant lesions [10, 13]. A 2010 study comprised of 120 malignancies, both in situ and invasive cancers, demonstrated persistent enhancement in 10 % of masses, plateau enhancement in 48.6 %, and washout in 41 % of masses [13]. Enhancement patterns of NME were less specific for malignancy [13].

10.4.2 Evolving MRI Techniques for Imaging Invasive Disease

10.4.2.1 Diffusion Weighted Imaging

New functional MRI tools may improve the sensitivity of MRI for detecting invasive disease. Diffusion weighted imaging (DWI) is one such technology (Fig. 10.4) and is discussed in detail in Chap. 15. Malignant breast tumors have high cellularity and often demonstrate restricted water diffusion (high signal intensity) and lower apparent diffusion coefficient (Fig. 10.4). Studies demonstrate an increase in specificity compared to contrast-enhanced MRI alone [14]. A 2010 study of 84 breast lesions demonstrated 97.9 % sensitivity and 75.7 % specificity of DWI. The addition of DWI to standard MRI may be particularly helpful in increasing MRI specificity for malignancy, with one study demonstrating a 13.5 % increase in specificity [15].

10.4.2.2 MR Proton Spectroscopy

Proton MR spectroscopy (1H-MRS) is discussed in detail in Chap. 15. Spectroscopy may be used to help characterize lesions. The choline concentrations in tumors may be associated with increased membrane synthesis by replicating cells and therefore

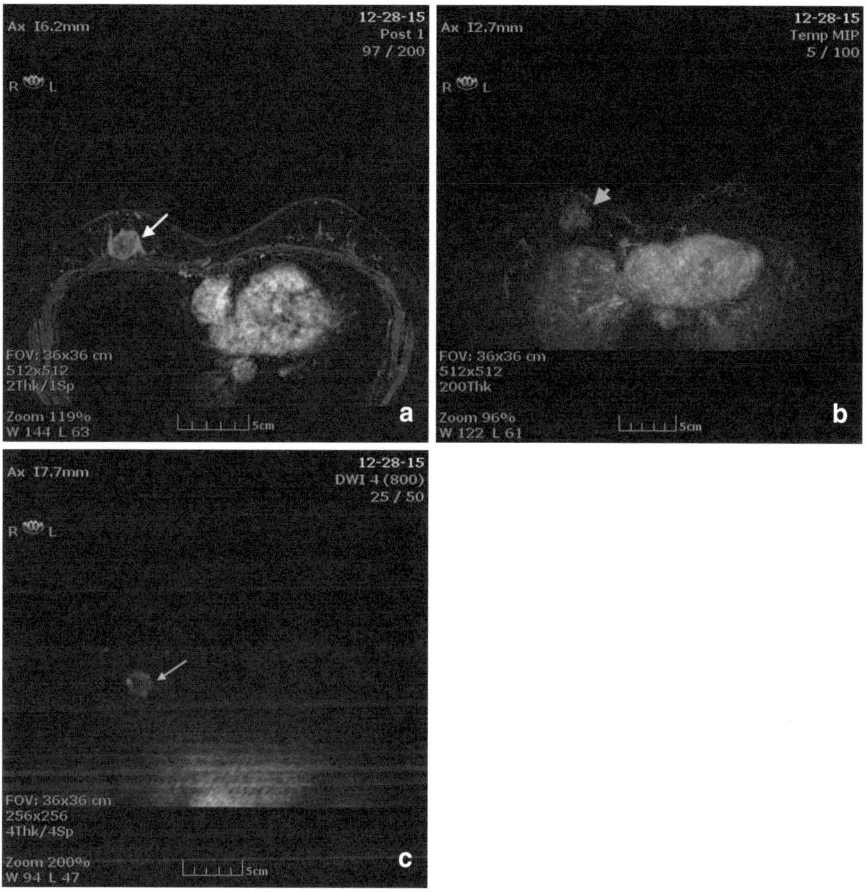

Fig. 10.4 (**a**) Axial T1 post contrast image demonstrates a round rim enhancing mass with an irregular border (*arrow*). (**b**) MIP image demonstrates enhancement within the mass (*arrowhead*). (**c**) DWI image demonstrates bright signal within the mass indicating restricted diffusion (*arrow*)

with biologic aggressiveness [16]. Increased total choline-containing compound has been associated with overexpression of the HER-2neu gene [17] and with an aggressive breast cancer phenotype [17, 18]. Studies show that tCho detection rate is higher in invasive cancer compared to DCIS, possibly associated with more aggressive behavior and/or faster cell replication.

Choline kinase overexpression has been found to be significantly associated with high histologic grade and ER-negative status [16]. These associations may be due to increased cell proliferation. ER is considered a favorable prognostic indicator in breast tumors as ER-positive tumors are more likely to be well differentiated and less aggressive. Patients with ER-positive tumors have more therapeutic options, such as ER blockers or aromatase inhibitors, than do patients with ER-negative tumors. A study of ER status and MR spectroscopic features found that the total choline-containing compound detection rate was higher in ER-negative patients [16].

HER-2/neu is associated with an aggressive tumor phenotype and reduced survival rate. The intracellular domain of HER-2 neu has tyrosine kinase activity that regulates cell growth and proliferation [19]. HER-2 neu is overexpressed in 20–25 % of invasive breast cancers and has been associated with more aggressive tumors, early relapse, and shorter survival [20]. The choline detection rate has been found to be higher in HER-2 neu- positive than in HER-2 neu-negative tumors. Additionally, triple-negative tumors showed significantly higher signal-to-noise ratio (SNR) than did non–triple-negative tumors [20]. Shin and colleagues found that on MRS, IDCs were consistently positive for choline whereas DCIS and IDC with an extensive intraductal component (EIC) were likely negative [18]. SNR was significantly higher in tumors of high histologic grade than lower histologic grade [18]. In summary, proton MRS may be an imaging biomarker for malignancy.

10.5 Radiologic-Pathologic Correlation and Invasive Disease

10.5.1 Specific Tumor Types and MRI Appearance

Traditional pathologic classification divides invasive disease into two major subtypes: invasive ductal carcinoma and invasive lobular carcinoma. Invasive ductal carcinoma not otherwise specified (IDC-NOS) is the most common. The remaining ductal cancers are further subdivided into unusual ductal carcinomas including papillary, micropapillary, mucinous, tubular, and adenoid cystic. Stromal malignancies including metaplastic carcinomas, phyllodes, and sarcomas are rarely encountered. MRI appearance varies according to histologic type; however, tremendous overlap is present.

10.5.2 Invasive Ductal Carcinoma NOS

IDC NOS comprises 85 % of breast cancers. The presence of glandular differentiation and intercellular cohesion defines ductal differentiation. However, most ductal carcinomas consist of invasive tubules and glands and have no specific type designation [21]. These tumors often elicit a scirrhous reaction, resulting in the irregular border seen on MRI. However, high-grade ductal carcinomas may grow so rapidly that there is no time for a scirrhous reaction, resulting in circumscribed borders. This circumscribed appearance is more common in BRCA related carcinomas [21].

Common MRI findings are an irregularly-shaped mass with heterogeneous enhancement and irregular or spiculated margins (Fig. 10.5). Also, peripheral or rim enhancement can be seen. Although IDC-NOS is typically not bright on T2 -weighted images, some IDC-NOS demonstrate areas of T2 hyperintensity secondary to necrosis [22]. The margins of lesions are often best characterized on nonfat saturated T1-weighted images. Surrounding breast tissue must be carefully evaluated, as small satellite masses may be present. Satellite lesions are masses with similar enhancement

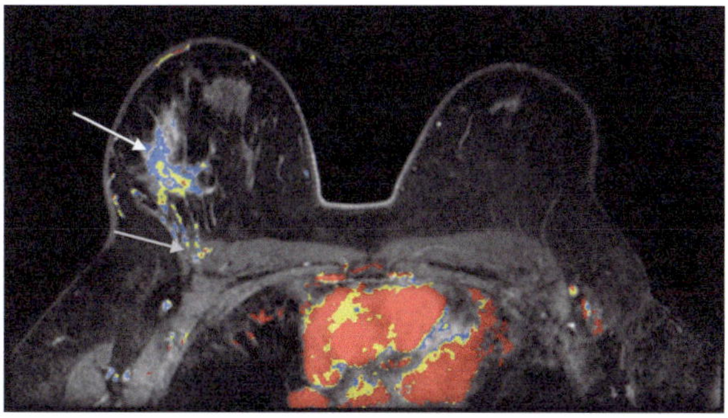

Fig. 10.5 Axial post contrast color image shows an irregular mass with heterogeneous enhancement (*white arrow*). Note the loss of a fat plane between the mass and the pectoralis muscle, as well as enhancement of the pectoralis (*gray arrow*). Biopsy revealed IDC NOS

characteristics as the primary cancer, but are smaller, and usually in close proximity. Contrast enhancement characteristics may vary but the most common pattern is rapid wash-in and rapid wash-out (type 3 curve) [22].

10.5.3 Papillary Carcinoma

10.5.3.1 Histology and Presentation

Papillary carcinoma is a rare variant of invasive ductal carcinoma accounting for less than 2 % of carcinomas and is most commonly found in postmenopausal women [23, 24]. Histologically, the epithelium proliferates into villous-like projections that eventually fill the lumen [23]. Papillary carcinoma is differentiated from a papilloma by the malignant appearing epithelial cells and an absent myoepithelial layer. Papillary carcinomas are subdivided into solid, intracystic without invasion, intracystic with a focus of invasion, and invasive papillary carcinoma [24]. This carcinoma may arise in the central ducts and is located in the retroareolar region in about 50 % of patients [24]. Bloody nipple discharge is present in 22–34 % of patients [23]. Patients with papillary carcinoma often have a better prognosis than patients with IDC-NOS. Axillary lymph nodes are involved less often in patients with papillary carcinoma than in patients with other types of ductal carcinoma [23].

10.5.3.2 Imaging

Papillary carcinomas are frequently round, oval, and circumscribed on mammography [23]. This round appearance is due to their cystic component [25]. Papillary cancers do not produce a fibrotic reaction and generally do not show spiculation by mammography. Ultrasound features are a solid hypoechoic or mixed solid and cystic mass with vascularity [23]. Differentiation from benign papillary lesions can be difficult. MRI features of papillary carcinomas are an irregular or round, enhancing mass, often near the nipple. Papillary carcinomas may be bright on both T1 and T2

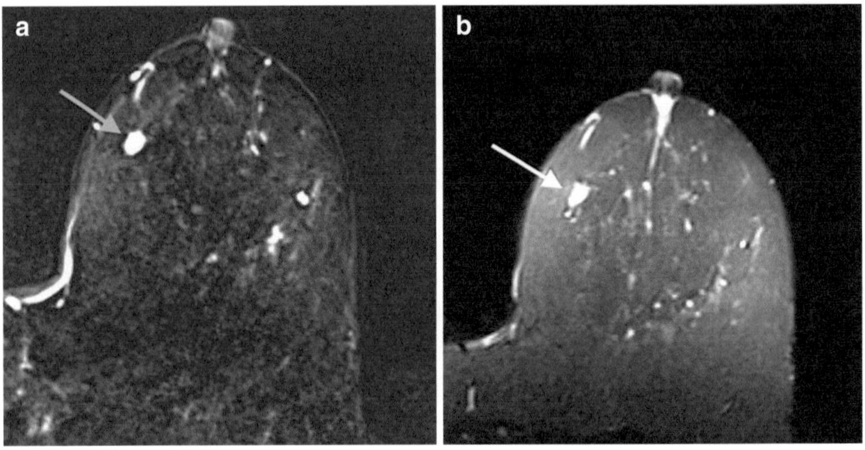

Fig. 10.6 (**a**) Axial T1 post contrast subtraction image demonstrating and oval circumscribed enhancing mass (*gray arrow*). (**b**) Axial T2 image demonstrating increased signal intensity (*white arrow*). Biopsy revealed papillary carcinoma

images. [25]. Intracystic papillary carcinoma will have hyperintensity on T2-weighted images (Fig. 10.6). Enhancement curves can vary from type 1 to type 3. MRI may be helpful in delineating multiple papillary masses [25].

10.5.4 Invasive Micropapillary Carcinoma

10.5.4.1 Histology and Presentation

Invasive micropapillary carcinoma (IMPCa) is a histologic pattern of breast cancer characterized by small, tightly cohesive groups of neoplastic cells disposed within well-delineated clear spaces resembling lymphatic vessels [26]. Micropapillary carcinomas of the breast are described pathologically as having numerous small pseudo-papillary clusters of cells without fibrovascular cores and clusters surrounded by clear spaces [23, 27]. Micropapillary carcinomas account for less than 2 % of breast cancers [23]. They have a worse overall prognosis than IDC-NOS [23]. Various studies report varying percentages of metastatic disease to axillary lymph nodes from 64 to 90 % [27, 28].

10.5.4.2 Imaging

Mammographic appearances include masses displaying a lobulated or irregular shape with spiculated or indistinct margins. Architectural distortion may also be present [23]. When calcifications are associated, they are typically fine pleormorphic or linear branching. Ultrasound features include a hypoechoic or mixed echogenicity mass with irregular shape and spiculated, microlobulated, or indistinct margins.

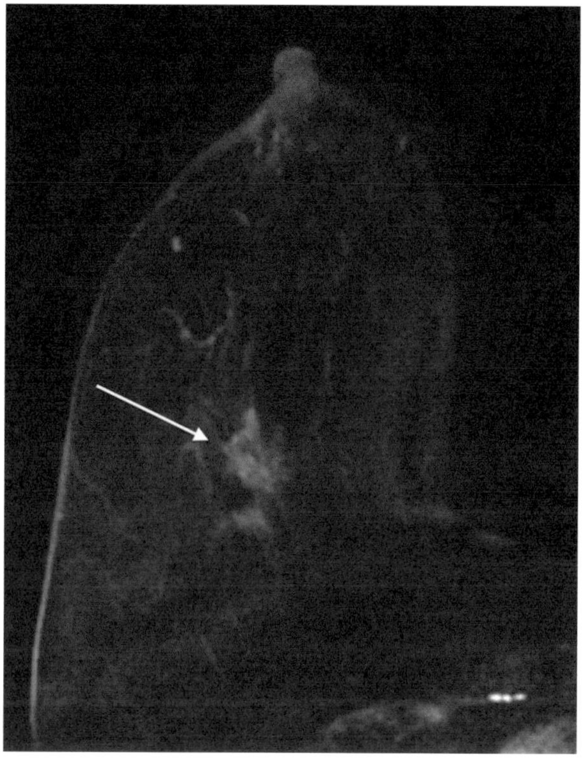

Fig. 10.7 Axial T1 subtraction image demonstrates an enhancing spiculated mass with spiculated borders (*arrow*). Biopsy revealed invasive micropapillary carcinoma

MRI findings include masses displaying an oval/round or irregular shape with irregular or spiculated margins [29] (Fig. 10.7). Initial rapid enhancement with washout or plateau kinetics in the delayed phase may be observed. Internal enhancement may be homogeneous or heterogeneous [29]. NME has also been reported. Careful attention should be paid to lymph nodes as invasive micropapillary carcinoma has a predilection for lymph node involvement [29].

10.5.5 Medullary Carcinoma

10.5.5.1 Histology and Presentation

Medullary carcinoma of the breast is rare, accounting for less than 5 % of breast cancers [30]. It is defined by the World Health Organization (WHO) classification of breast tumors as "a well-circumscribed carcinoma composed of poorly differentiated cells arranged in large sheets, with no glandular structure, scant stroma, and a prominent lymphoplasmacytic infiltrate" [30]. It is most commonly seen in women in their late 40s and early 50s and has a more favorable prognosis than IDC-NOS [30]. A higher incidence of medullary carcinoma is noted in patients with BRCA1 mutation. A series of 1490 patients managed with breast-conservation therapy that consisted of lumpectomy and radiation therapy at Yale University included 46 cases

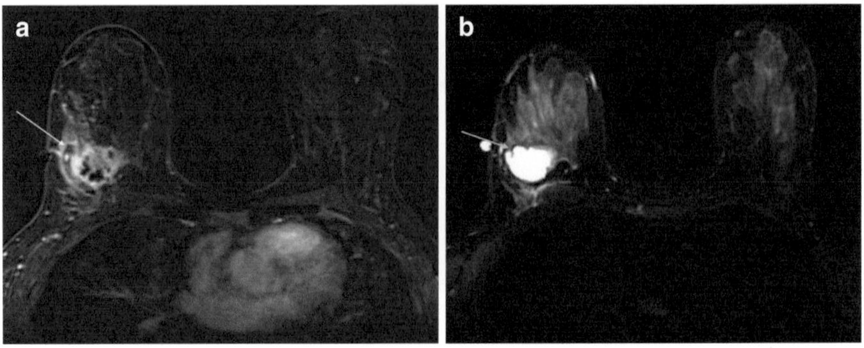

Fig. 10.8 (**a**) Axial T1 post contrast subtraction image demonstrates a mass with an irregular border and rim enhancement characteristic of medullary carcinomas (*white arrow*). (**b**) T2 image demonstrates hyperintense signal within the mass (*gray arrow*). Biopsy revealed medullary carcinoma

of medullary carcinoma. The 10-year distant relapse-free survival in the medullary cohort was significantly better than in the control group of IDC NOS (94.9 % vs. 77.5 %, $p = 0.028$) [30].

10.5.5.2 Imaging

Mammographic appearance is a dense oval or round mass with circumscribed or microlobulated margins. Ultrasound appearance may be confused with a fibroadenoma [30]. Often medullary carcinomas are circumscribed, hypoechoic, parallel masses with varying degrees of through transmission [30]. The MRI appearance has been reported as isointense on T1-weighted and isointense or slightly hyperintense on fat-saturated T2-weighted images. Medullary carcinomas have oval or round shapes and smooth margins upon contrast enhancement. Heterogeneous enhancement with delayed, peripheral enhancement on late-phase contrast MRI has been reported [30]. Rapid wash-in and rapid wash-out or plateau enhancement is often seen. The peripheral rim enhancement correlates with a peripheral compressed fibrous tissue with prominent lymphocytic infiltration noted at pathology [30] (Fig. 10.8).

10.5.6 Mucinous Carcinoma

10.5.6.1 Histology and Presentation

Mucinous carcinoma, also known as colloid, mucous, or mucoid carcinoma of the breast is a well-differentiated type of invasive adenocarcinoma characterized by large amount of extracellular epithelial mucus. Mucinous carcinoma constitutes

1–7 % of breast carcinomas. Two subtypes of mucinous carcinoma may be differentiated histologically: pure and mixed. The pure type typically has indolent growth, while the mixed type has variable biological behavior, often similar to IDC-NOS. The pure type typically demonstrates a lower histological grade (well-differentiated tumors), higher hormone receptor expression, lower incidence of adverse oncogenes, lower rate of axillary lymph node involvement at diagnosis, and longer disease-free survival [31].

10.5.6.2 Imaging

Mucinous carcinoma may present as circumscribed lesions. A multimodality approach is helpful to reach appropriate diagnosis as well as to differentiate between the two histological types of the neoplasm. Typically, a mucinous carcinoma presents as an oval or round mass with circumscribed margins. At mammography, the pure type correlates with circumscribed or microlobulated margins while the mixed type presents with more indistinct or spiculated contours secondary to a higher degree of fibrosis and peripheral desmoplasia, similar to a IDC-NOS. Microcalcifications are uncommon and may be associated with peripheral component of DCIS [32]. Sonographically, mucinous carcinomas are often heterogeneous in echogenicity and may have mixed solid and cystic components. Posterior acoustic enhancement is common [33].

Mucinous carcinoma on MRI typically has a lobular shape, homogeneous and markedly high signal intensity on T2-weighted images, and a persistent enhancement pattern on dynamic MR images (with rim-like peripheral or heterogeneous internal enhancement). Thus, it has MR imaging features of both benignity and malignancy (Fig. 10.9). The combination of MR imaging features is useful for preoperative diagnosis of the tumor [34]. High signal intensity on T2-weighted images is seen in a pure mucinous carcinoma because the entire tumor is filled by mucin. In mixed mucinous carcinomas, the solid component is identifiable by its relative signal hypointensity on the T2-weighted images [35].

High signal intensity of the mucinous cancer on T2-weighted images is not pathognomonic because other lesions such as necrosis, hemorrhage, edema, myxoid matrix or cystic component are also high signal [36]. On dynamic contrast-enhanced sequences, variable enhancement morphology may occur; however, peripheral, ring-shaped, or heterogeneous enhancement are more characteristic and progressive along time. Enhancing internal separation may also be present. The pure type of mucinous cancer generally demonstrates mild to moderate enhancement at the early phases, with type 1 (persistent) curves or type 2 (plateau) curve. The persistent enhancement pattern is related to the tumor cellularity, nuclear grading, and amount of extracellular mucin. Thus, an intense enhancement in the first 2 min after gadolinium injection, or a type 3 curve (washout) must raise suspicion of mixed-type MMC or, an even rarer pure tumor with high cellularity [37].

Compared with other subtypes of breast cancer, mucinous cancers typically demonstrate low signal intensity on diffusion-weighted images and high apparent

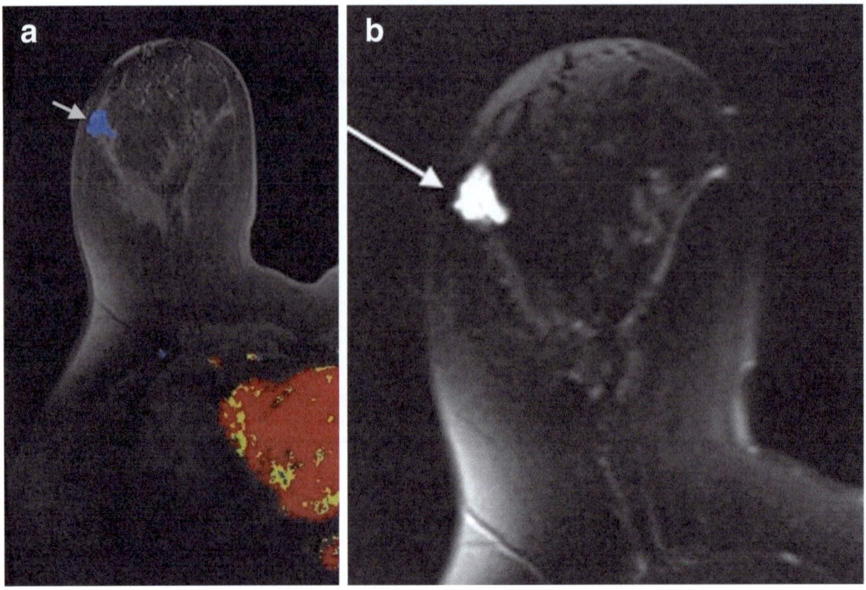

Fig. 10.9 (**a**) Axial T1 post contrast color image demonstrates an irregular mass with plateau (Type II) enhancement (*gray arrow*). (**b**) T2 image demonstrates high signal intensity (*white arrow*). Biopsy revealed mucinous carcinoma

diffusion coefficient (ADC) values in relation to IDC-NOS. High ADC values may be associated with the presence of extracellular mucin and low tumor cellularity.

10.5.7 Tubular Carcinoma

10.5.7.1 Histology and Presentation

Tubular carcinoma of the breast is a sub-type of IDC-NOS. The peak age at presentation is comparatively younger than with other types of breast cancer. Median age at diagnosis is in the mid- to late 40s. Most tubular carcinomas are non-palpable and found incidentally at screening rather than manifesting with clinical findings [38]. Although tubular carcinomas may contain other histologic elements, an excess of 75 % tubular elements is usually required for the diagnosis of tubular carcinoma [38]. A distinguishing pathological feature is a single layer of cells lining tubules with loss of lobular architecture and surrounding infiltration. The glands in tubular carcinomas lack myoepithelial cells. Lesions may be multifocal or multicentric in 10–20 % of cases [39].

Invasive cancers containing tubular elements are not uncommon; however, pure tubular carcinoma is rare and accounts for less than 2 % of all breast cancers. Less pure tubular carcinomas are referred to as mixed tubular carcinomas. A third type is tubulolobular carcinoma has both tubular and infiltrating lobular elements.

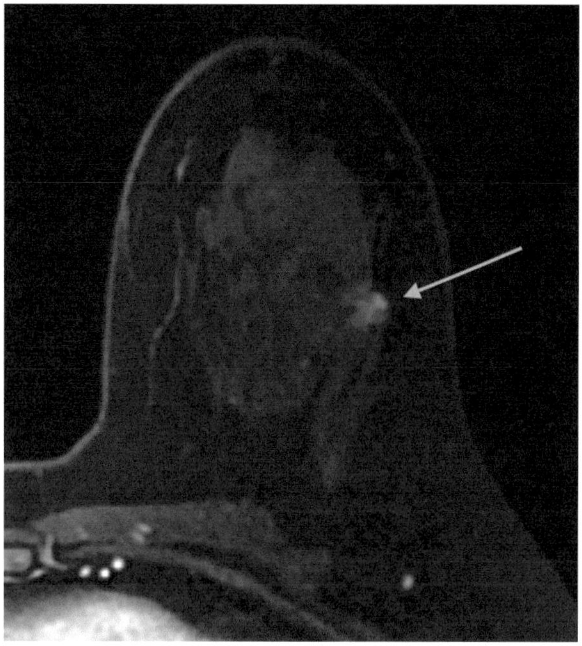

Fig. 10.10 Axial post contrast T1 image demonstrates a small left sided spiculated mass with heterogeneous enhancement (*arrow*). Biopsy revealed tubular carcinoma

10.5.7.2 Imaging

In the majority of cases, on mammography, the lesion is small (< 1 cm), spiculated, and can occur with or without calcifications. The appearance mimics typical IDC-NOS manifesting as one or more small, spiculated masses. The spicules are often longer than the central mass. Amorphous microcalcifications may be present in 10–15 % of cases [39]. On sonography, the appearance also mimics IDC-NOS, presenting as a hypoechoic solid mass with ill-defined margins and posterior acoustic shadowing. Dynamic subtraction MR-imaging might show characteristics of a malignant tumor and cannot be differentiated from IDC-NOS based on MR imaging alone (Fig. 10.10). The prognosis is usually excellent with survival of 97 % at 10 years. The pure tubular forms carry the best prognosis.

10.5.8 Adenoid Cystic Carcinoma

10.5.8.1 Histology and Presentation

Adenoid cystic (ACC) is a rare variant of IDC accounting for 0.1 % of breast cancers [40]. Histologically, ACC is characterized by small basaloid cells with a solid cribriform pattern or tubular growth patterns enclosing pseudoglandular spaces with minimal eosinophilic material [40]. The cell of origin is unknown, but may arise from the ductal epithelium and myoepithelium. Adenoid cystic carcinoma has various growth patterns: glandular, tubular, and solid [40]. Patients typically present with a painful subareolar palpable mass. Prognosis is excellent with 10 year survival around 98 %, despite being ER/PR negative.

10.5.8.2 Imaging

Mammography demonstrates an ill-defined, lobulated mass with rare calcifications. Ultrasound demonstrates a hypoechoic or mixed ecogenicity mass with irregular borders and minimal color flow [41]. MRI features can include circumscribed or spiculated margins (Fig. 10.11) [41]. Enhancement kinetics have been described from type 1 to type 3. Initial enhancement has been described as rapid and heterogeneous [41]. ACC with primarily solid features may demonstrate high signal on T2-weighted images [41].

10.5.9 Invasive Lobular Carcinoma

10.5.9.1 Histology and Presentation

Invasive lobular carcinoma (ILC) is the second most common histologic type of breast carcinoma, accounting for approximately 10–15 % of all invasive breast cancers. ILC spreads as sheets of a single-cell layer along Cooper's ligaments and other structures in the breast. Typically these tumors show a single-file infiltration of malignant cells through the breast stroma with a relative paucity of desmoplastic response, hemorrhage, necrosis, or calcification [42]. Because of this infiltrative growth pattern, ILC is more difficult to detect at clinical examination and mammography than is IDC [43]. ILC is usually larger at diagnosis than IDC and is often multifocal. [44]. ILC has a higher rate of multiplicity and bilaterality than IDC. Lymph node metastases are less common with ILC than IDC for similar size lesions, so the

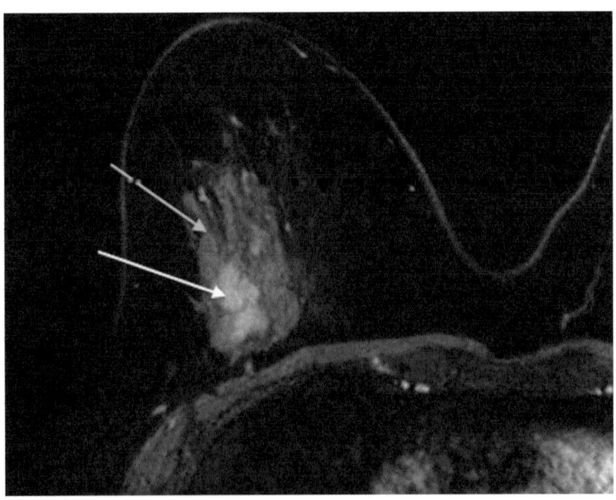

Fig. 10.11 Axial T1 post contrast image demonstrates an irregular heterogeneously enhancing mass. Biopsy revealed adenoid cystic carcinoma. It should be noted that both the central area of intense enhancement (*white arrow*) and the peripheral area of less intense enhancement (*gray arrow*) revealed carcinoma

stage at diagnosis for ILC is overall similar to that for IDC despite the larger size at diagnosis. [44, 45]. However, higher false-negative rates (up to 19 %) are reported for ILC than for other invasive cancers at mammography because ILC is often difficult to diagnose mammographically [46].

The most common clinical findings of ILC are palpable thickening and skin or nipple retraction [47]. When large, a firm palpable mass may become evident at clinical examination, often with the clinical examination findings being of greater concern for breast carcinoma than are the imaging findings. The mammogram often underestimates tumor size relative to the physical examination findings. ILC also has a propensity for metastatic spread to the peritoneum, retroperitoneum, and gynecologic organs. Therefore, metastatic ILC should be considered in women presenting with ascites, hydronephrosis, and/or pelvic masses [48].

10.5.9.2 Imaging

The sensitivity of mammography for the detection of ILC reportedly ranges between 57 and 80 %. The most frequent manifestation of ILC is architectural distortion with or without a central mass or a focal asymmetry. Calcifications are an uncommon feature of ILC. Unlike IDC, ILC is more frequently seen in only one view, most commonly in the craniocaudal view, which typically has better compression than the MLO view [49]. When ILC is large, the affected breast may appear to be decreasing in size on the mammogram, which has been termed the “shrinking breast” [50].

Sonography is a valuable adjunct to mammography, with reported sensitivities ranging from 68 to 98 % [51–54]. Sonography is superior to mammography in identifying multicentricity and multifocality and more accurately reflects the size of a mass than does mammography or clinical examination. The most common sonographic manifestation of ILC is an irregular or angular mass with hypoechoic and heterogeneous internal echoes, ill-defined or spiculated margins, and posterior acoustic shadowing, findings that are seen in 54–61 % of cases. Additional manifestations include circumscribed masses, focal shadowing without a discrete mass, as well as sonographically occult lesions. Although the US appearances of various subtypes of ILC overlap considerably, classic ILC tends to manifest as focal shadowing without a discrete mass, whereas pleomorphic type ILC is more typically seen as a shadowing mass. Signet ring, alveolar, and solid subtypes of ILC are more likely to manifest as a lobulated, well-circumscribed mass [46].

MR imaging is extremely useful for assessing the extent of the disease, with reported sensitivity of approximately 95 %. It is superior to mammography and ultrasound in estimating tumor size as well as identifying multifocal and multicentric disease. A meta-analysis by Mann et al. found that MR imaging was able to detect additional ipsilateral malignant findings not evident at mammography or US in 32 % of ILC patients. In addition, unexpected cancer in the contralateral breast was seen at MR imaging in 7 % of cases. MR imaging has been shown to affect clinical management in 50 % of patients with ILC, leading to changes in surgical management in

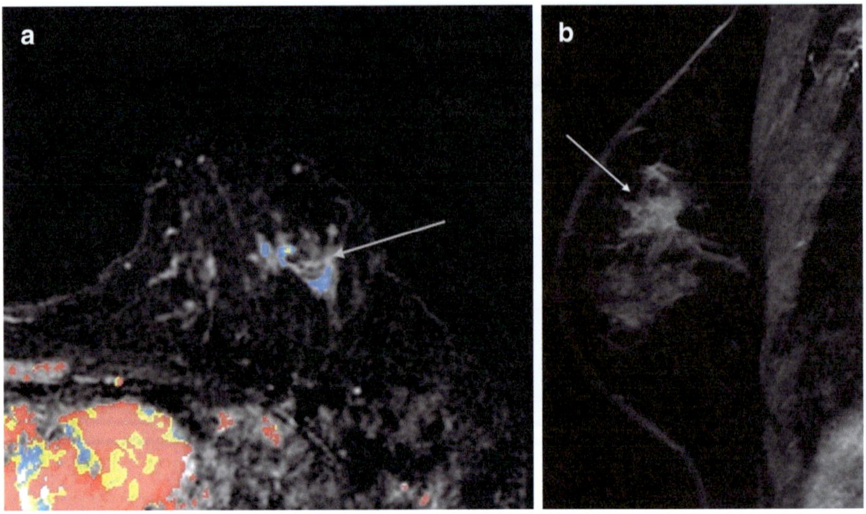

Fig. 10.12 (**a**) Axial post contrast color image demonstrates an area of nonmass enhancement with plateau kinetics (*arrow*). (**b**) Sagittal T1 post contrast image demonstrates nonmass enhancement (*arrow*). Biopsy revealed ILC at multiple sites

28 % of cases [46, 55–57]. In 39 % of women with ILC, MR imaging depicts more extensive disease than is suspected with conventional imaging [58]. On MR images, ILC may manifest as an enhancing solitary mass with irregular margins, multiple enhancing lesions, or only enhancing septations [46, 55–56, 58–59].

Additional manifestations include a dominant lesion surrounded by multiple small, enhancing foci, multiple small enhancing foci with interconnecting enhancing strands, architectural distortion, regional or focal heterogeneous NME, enhancing septa, and normal appearing breast parenchyma (Fig. 10.12). Interestingly, histopathologic findings suggest that the enhancing strands and septa correlate with tumor cells streaming within the breast stroma. Most ILC exhibit heterogeneous rather than homogeous enhancement, and some show poor enhancement [59]. ILC tends to demonstrate delayed maximum enhancement, with washout exhibited by only a minority of lesions [60]. Some ILCs may infiltrate and grow without significant angiogenesis and neovascularity, resulting in false negative MRI [60]. At MR spectroscopy, the tCho detection rate is also higher in IDC compared to ILC, which may be related to the infiltrating nature of ILC, resulting in fat contamination problem (from preserved background fat) in ILC [58].

A study assessing the impact of preoperative MRI on the re-excision rate in ILC found that patients who had an MRI had significantly lower re-excision rates compared with patients without preoperative MRI (9 % versus 27 %, respectively). This group also concluded that there was a trend towards a lower rate of final mastectomy in the ILC subgroup, although this finding did not attain significance [61]. Thus, women with ILC are among those most likely to benefit from the use of preoperative MRI for the assessment of extent of disease.

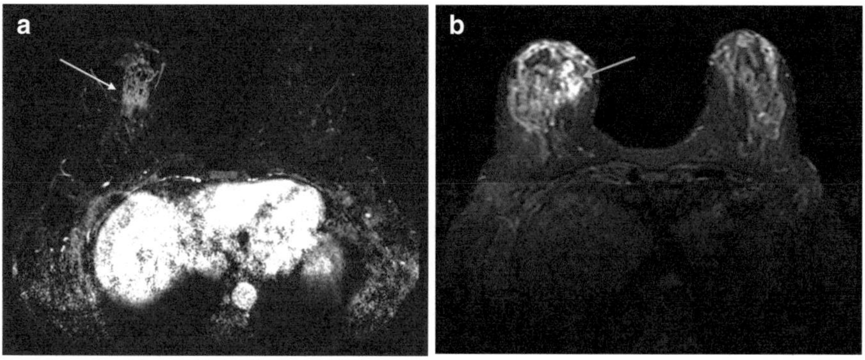

Fig. 10.13 Axial post contrast subtracted image demonstrates an irregular mass with heterogeneous enhancement (*white arrow*). T2 images demonstrate increased signal within the mass secondary to necrosis (*gray arrow*). Biopsy revealed metaplastic carcinoma

10.5.10 Metaplastic Carcinoma

10.5.10.1 Histology and Presentation

Metaplastic carcinoma is a mixed group of malignant neoplasms containing both glandular and nonglandular patterns with epithelial and/or mesenchymal components. Metaplastic carcinoma of the breast is a rare but aggressive type of breast cancer that has been recognized as a unique pathologic entity by the World Health Organization. Morphologically, it is characterized by the differentiation of neoplastic epithelium into squamous cells and/or mesenchymal-looking elements (squamous cells, spindle cells, cartilage or bone, etc.) [62]. It shares many similarities with invasive ductal carcinoma and benign lesions on mammography [62]. It is typically ER/PR/Her2 negative (triple negative).

Metaplastic carcinomas present primarily in women over 50 as a rapidly growing palpable mass [62]. Velasco et al. reported characteristics of 12 patients with metaplastic carcinoma. All masses demonstrated irregular shape and spiculated margins. T2 signal was variable but was greater that the surrounding tissue. T2 signals reported were homogeneous hypersignal(2/12), mottled hypersignal(9/12) and isointense (1/12). Contrast enhancement pattern was ringlike in 73 % and homogeneous in 27 % [63] (Fig. 10.13).

10.5.11 Phyllodes Tumors

10.5.11.1 Histology and Presentation

Phyllodes is a tumor of stromal origin. Phyllodes tumors account for fewer than 1 % of breast cancers and presents as rapidly enlarging palpable masses in middle-aged to older women [38]. Phyllodes tumors are generally benign. However 10 % of

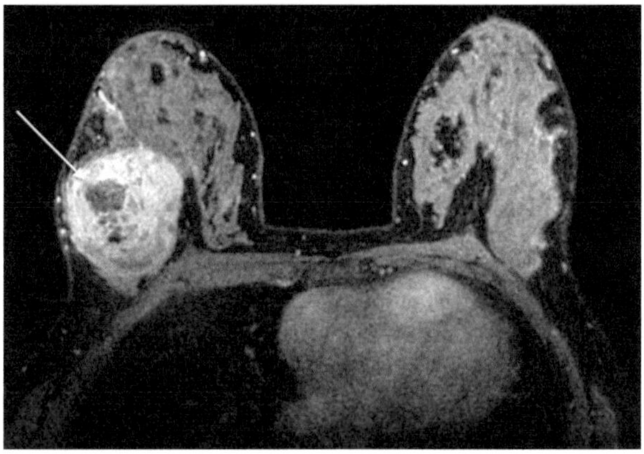

Fig. 10.14 Axial post contrast T1 image demonstrates an oval circumscribed mass with central areas of decreased enhancement (*arrow*). Biopsy revealed malignant phyllodes

phyllodes tumors are malignant. Phyllodes tumors are classified from low-grade to high-grade. Wide excision is indicated even for low-grade tumors, since a phyllodes tumor can be locally aggressive [38]. The risk of metastatic disease is very uncommon with phyllodes tumors. In the rare cases where the tumor does metastasize, these lesions spread hematogenously, most commonly to the lungs. A chest x-ray is useful in initial staging [38]. Sentinel node biopsy and axillary dissection is not helpful, since these tumors do not spread through the lymphatic system [38].

10.5.11.2 Imaging

On mammography, phyllodes tumors typically are seen as a large oval or round mass with circumscribed or ill-defined borders. Ultrasound often demonstrates an oval, hypoechoic mass similar to a fibroadenoma with multiple cystic spaces and mixed echogenicity [38]. MRI findings in a phyllodes tumor are similar to findings seen in a fibroadenoma. Findings include a well-marginated, oval or round mass with hypointense to isointense T1 signal and hyperintense T2 signal. Nonenhancing internal septations and variable enhancement curves from type 1 to type 3 may be present [64] (Fig. 10.14). High T2 signal in the surrounding breast tissue may be noted in a phyllodes. Cystic spaces with increased T2 signal may be present. Distinguishing a phyllodes from a fibroadenoma based on MRI is difficult [64].

10.6 Conclusion

In conclusion, recent understanding of the molecular nature of breast cancers has helped to explain certain imaging phenotypes seen on MRI. A variety of MR imaging characteristics can be seen with different histopathologic breast pathologies. Invasive ductal carcinoma presents most frequently as an irregular mass and often demonstrates Type 3 enhancement kinetics. Mucinous, papillary, adenoid cystic and metaplastic carcinoma may demonstrate increased T2 signal. Delayed rim enhancement is a concerning finding seen in triple negative, adenoid cystic and medullary cancers. Lobular cancers can show minimal to no enhancement and present as masses, distortion, and non-mass enhancement. Tubular carcinomas display similar characteristics to invasive ductal carcinomas NOS, often appearing as an enhancing, spiculated mass. Attention to specific morphologic and kinetic characteristics can help in differentiating types of cancers. Recent MRI multiparametric developments such as diffusion and spectroscopy may be useful in identifying biologically significant invasive disease. Additionally, MRI may help in identifying axillary nodal involvement and in surgical planning.

References

1. Sung JS, Li J, Da Costa GD, Patil S, Van Zee KJ, Dershaw DD, et al. Preoperative breast MRI for early-stage breast cancer: effects on surgical and long-term outcomes. AJR Am J Roentgenol. 2014;202(6):1376–82.
2. Peters NH, Borel Rinkes IH, Zuithoff NP, Mali WP, Moons KG, Peeters PH. Meta-analysis of MR imaging in the diagnosis of breast lesions. Radiology. 2008;246(1):116–24. PMID:18024435.
3. Lehman CD, Isaacs C, Schnall MD, Pisano ED, Ascher SM, Weatherall PT, et al. Cancer yield of mammography, MR, and US in high-risk women: prospective multi-institution breast cancer screening study. Radiology. 2007;244(2):381–8.
4. Trop I, LeBlanc SM, David J, Lalonde L, Tran-Thanh D, Labelle M, et al. Molecular classification of infiltrating breast cancer: toward personalized therapy. Radiographics. 2014;34(5): 1178–95.
5. Uematsu T, Kasami M, Yuen S. Triple-negative breast cancer: correlation between MR imaging and pathologic findings. Radiology. 2009;250(3):638–47.
6. Molleran VM. MRI features of invasive disease. In: Molleran VM, Mahoney M, editors. Breast MRI. Philadelphia: Saunders Elsevier; 2013. p. 56.
7. Dogan BE, Gonzalez-Angulo AM, Gilcrease M, Dryden MJ, Yang WT. Multimodality imaging of triple receptor-negative tumors with mammography, ultrasound, and MRI. AJR Am J Roentgenol. 2010;194(4):1160–6.
8. Krizmanich-Conniff KM, Paramagul C, Patterson SK, Helvie MA, Roubidoux MA, Myles JD, et al. Triple receptor-negative breast cancer: imaging and clinical characteristics. AJR Am J Roentgenol. 2012;199(2):458–64.
9. Boo-Kyung H, Schnall MD, Orel S, Rosen M. Outcome of MRI-guided breast biopsy. AJR Am J Roentgenol. 2008;191(6):1798–804.
10. Morris EA, Comstock CE, Lee CH, et al. ACR BI-RADS® Magnetic Resonance Imaging. In: ACR BI-RADS® Atlas, Breast Imaging Reporting and Data System. Reston: American College of Radiology; 2013.
11. Tozaki M, Igarashi T, Fukuda K. Positive and negative predictive values of BI-RADS-MRI descriptors for focal breast masses. Magn Reson Med Sci. 2006;5(1):7–15.
12. Mahoney M, Gatsonis C, Hanna L, DeMartini WB, Lehman C. Positive predictive value of BI-RADS MR Imaging. Radiology. 2012;264(1):51–61.
13. Baltzer P, Benndorf M, Dietzel M, Gajda M, Runnebaum I, Kaiser W. False- positive findings at contrast-enhanced breast MRI: a BI-RADS descriptor study. AJR Am J Roentgenol. 2010;194(6):1658–63.
14. Menezes GL, Knuttel FM, Stehouwer BL, Pijnappel RM, Van Den Bosch MA. Magnetic resonance imaging in breast cancer: a literature review and future perspectives. World J Surg Oncol. 2014;5(2):61–70.

15. Kul S, Cansu A, Alhan E, Dinc H, Gunes G, Reis A. Contribution of diffusion -weighted imaging to dynamic contrast-enhanced MRI in the characterization of breast tumors. AJR Am J Roentgenol. 2011;196(1):210–7.
16. Ramírez de Molina AR, Gutiérrez R, Ramos MA, Silva JM, Bonilla F, Sanchez JJ, et al. Increased choline kinase activity in human breast carcinomas: clinical evidence for a potential novel antitumor strategy. Oncogene. 2002;21:4317–22.
17. Yeung DK, Yang WT, Tse GM, et al. Breast cancer: in vivo proton MR spectroscopy in the characterization of histopathologic subtypes and preliminary observations in axillary node metastases 1. Radiology. 2002;225(1):190–7.
18. Shin HJ, Baek HM, Cha JH, Kim HH. Evaluation of breast cancer using proton MR spectroscopy: total choline peak integral and signal-to-noise ratio as prognostic indicators. AJR Am J Roentgenol. 2012;198(5):W488–97.
19. Burstein HJ. The distinctive nature of HER2-positive breast cancers. N Engl J Med. 2005;353(16):1652–4.
20. Stefano R, Agostara B, Calabro M, Campisi I, Ravazzolo B, Traina A, et al. Expression levels and clinical-pathological correlations of HER2/neu in primary and metastatic human breast cancer. Ann N Y Acad Sci. 2004;1028(1):463–72.
21. Rabban J. A pathologist's overview of the pathology of breast disease. In: Kopans D, editor. Breast imaging. Philadelphia: Lippincott Williams and Wilkins; 2007. p. 62.
22. Bartella L, Dershaw D. Magnetic resonance imaging of invasive breast carcinoma. In: Morris E, Liberman L, editors. Breast MRI: diagnosis and intervention. New York: Springer Science & Business Media; 2005. p. 174–5.
23. Muttarak M, Lerttumnongtum P, Chaiwun B, Peh WC. Spectrum of papillary lesions of the breast: clinical, imaging, and pathologic correlation. AJR Am J Roentgenol. 2008;191(3): 700–7.
24. Riham E, Chong J, Kulkarni S, Goldberg F, Muradali D. Papillary lesions of the breast: MRI, ultrasound, and mammographic appearances. AJR Am J Roentgenol. 2012;198:264–71.
25. Molleran V. MRI features of invasive disease. In: Molleran V, Mahoney M, editors. Breast MRI. Philadelphia: Saunders Elsevier; 2013. p. 54–6.
26. Nassar H, Wallis T, Andea A, Dey J, Adsay V, Visscher D. Clinicopathologic analysis of invasive micropapillary differentiation in breast carcinoma. Mod Pathol. 2001;14(9):836–41.
27. Kuroda H, Sakamoto G, Ohnisi K, Itoyama S. Clinical and pathologic features of invasive micropapillary carcinoma. Breast Cancer. 2004;11(2):169–74.
28. Luna-More S, Gonzalez B, Acedo C, Rodrigo I, Luna C. Invasive micropapillary carcinoma of the breast. A new special type of invasive mammary carcinoma. Pathol Res Pract. 1994;190: 668–74.
29. Lim HS, Kuzmiak CM, Jeong SI, Choi YR, Kim JW, Lee JS, et al. Invasive micropapillary carcinoma of the breast: MR imaging findings. Korean J Radiol. 2013;14(4):551–8.
30. Tominaga J, Hama H, Kimura N, Takahashi S. MR imaging of medullary carcinoma of the breast. Eur J Radiol. 2009;70(3):525–9.
31. Bae SY, Choi MY, Cho DH, Lee JE, Nam SJ, Yang JH. Mucinous carcinoma of the breast in comparison with invasive ductal carcinoma: clinicopathologic characteristics and prognosis. J Breast Cancer. 2011;14(4):308–13.
32. Conant EF, Dillon RL, Palazzo J, Ehrlich SM, Feig SA. Imaging findings in mucin-containing carcinomas of the breast: correlation with pathologic features. AJR Am J Roentgenol. 1994; 163(4):821–4.
33. Lam WW, Chu WC, Tse GM, Ma TK. Sonographic appearance of mucinous carcinoma of the breast. AJR Am J Roentgenol. 2004;182(4):1069–74.
34. Kawashima M, Tamaki Y, Nonaka T, Higuchi K, Kimura M, Koida T, et al. MR imaging of mucinous carcinoma of the breast. AJR Am J Roentgenol. 2002;179(1):179–83.
35. Santamaría G, Velasco M, Bargalló X, Caparrós X, Farrús B, Fernández PL. Radiologic and pathologic findings in breast tumors with high signal intensity on T2-weighted MR images. Radiographics. 2010;30(2):533–48.

36. Woodhams R, Kakita S, Hata H, Iwabuchi K, Shigeaki U, Mountford C, et al. Diffusion-weighted imaging of mucinous carcinoma of the breast: evaluation of apparent diffusion coefficient and signal intensity in correlation with histologic findings. AJR Am J Roentgenol. 2009;193(1):260–6.
37. Monzawa S, Yokokawa M, Sakuma T, Takao S, Hirokaga K, Hanioka K, et al. Mucinous carcinoma of the breast: MRI features of pure and mixed forms with histopathologic correlation. AJR Am J Roentgenol. 2009;192(3):W125–31.
38. Harvey JA. Unusual breast cancers: useful clues to expanding the differential diagnosis. Radiology. 2007;242(3):683–94.
39. Sheppard DG, Whitman GJ, Fornage BD, Stelling CB, Huynh PT, Sahin AA. Tubular carcinoma of the breast: mammographic and sonographic features. AJR Am J Roentgenol. 2000;174(1):253–7.
40. Thompson K, Grabowski J, Saltzstein SL, Sadler GR, Blair SL. Adenoid cystic breast carcinoma: is axillary staging necessary in all cases? Results from the California cancer registry. Breast J. 2011;17(5):485–9.
41. Glazebrook KN, Reynolds C, Smith RL, Gimenez EI, Boughey JC. Adenoid cystic carcinoma of the breast. AJR Am J Roentgenol. 2010;194(5):1391–6.
42. Razek NMA, Hassan MAF, Fattah SA, Eshak SI. Dynamic MR-Mammography as the best method for diagnosis of invasive lobular breast carcinoma: A retrospective study. Egyptian J Radiol Nucl Med. 2013;44(2):405–9.
43. Berg WA, Gutierrez L, NessAiver MS, Carter WB, Bhargavan M, Lewis RS, et al. Diagnostic accuracy of mammography, clinical examination, US, and MR imaging in preoperative assessment of breast cancer. Radiology. 2004;233:830–49.
44. Yeatman TJ, Cantor AB, Smith TJ, Smith SK, Reintgen DS, Miller MS, et al. Tumor biology of infiltrating lobular carcinoma implications for management. Ann Surg. 1995;222:549–61.
45. Newstead GM, Baute PB, Toth HK. Invasive lobular and ductal carcinoma: mammographic findings and stage at diagnosis. Radiology. 1992;184(3):623–7.
46. Mann RM, Hoogeveen YL, Blickman JG, Boetes C. MRI compared to conventional diagnostic work-up in the detection and evaluation of invasive lobular carcinoma of the breast: a review of existing literature. Breast Cancer Res Treat. 2008;107(1):1–14.
47. Le Gal M, Ollivier L, Asselain B, Meunier M, Laurent M, Vielh P, et al. Mammographic features of 455 invasive lobular carcinomas. Radiology. 1992 Dec;185(3):705–8.
48. Winston CB, Hadar O, Teitcher JB, Caravelli JF, Sklarin NT, Panicek DM, et al. Metastatic lobular carcinoma of the breast: patterns of spread in the chest, abdomen, and pelvis on CT. AJR Am J Roentgenol. 2000;175(3):795–800.
49. Porter AJ, Evans EB, Foxcroft LM, Simpson PT, Lakhani SR. Mammographic and ultrasound features of invasive lobular carcinoma of the breast. J Med Imaging Radiat Oncol. 2014;58(1):1–10.
50. Harvey JA, Fechner RE, Moore MM. Apparent ipsilateral decrease in breast size on mammography: a sign of infiltrating lobular carcinoma. Radiology. 2000;214(3):883–9.
51. Butler RS, Venta LA, Wiley EL, Ellis RL, Dempsey PJ, Rubin E. Sonographic evaluation of infiltrating lobular carcinoma. AJR Am J Roentgenol. 1999;172(2):325–30.
52. Helvie MA, Paramagul C, Oberman HA, Adler DD. Invasive lobular carcinoma: imaging features and clinical detection. Invest Radiol. 1993;28(3):202–7.
53. Paramagul CP, Helvie MA, Adler DD. Invasive lobular carcinoma: sonographic appearance and role of sonography in improving diagnostic sensitivity. Radiology. 1995;195(1):231–4.
54. Evans WP, Warren Burhenne LJ, Laurie L, O'Shaughnessy KF, Castellino RA. Invasive lobular carcinoma of the breast: mammographic characteristics and computer-aided detection. Radiology. 2002;225(1):182–9.
55. Schelfout K, Van Goethem M, Kersschot E, Verslegers I, Biltjes I, Leyman P, et al. Preoperative breast MRI in patients with invasive lobular breast cancer. Eur Radiol. 2004;14(7):1209–16.
56. Munot K, Dall B, Achuthan R, Parkin G, Lane S, Horgan K. Role of magnetic resonance imaging in the diagnosis and single-stage surgical resection of invasive lobular carcinoma of the breast. Br J Surg. 2002;89(10):1296–301.

57. Del Frate C, Borghese L, Cedolini C, Bestagno A, Puglisi F, Isola M, et al. Imaging in the diagnosis and single-stage surgical resection of invasive lobular carcinoma Role of pre-surgical breast MRI in the management of invasive breast carcinoma. Breast. 2007;16(5):469–81.
58. Weinstein SP, Orel SG, Heller R, Reyonalds C, Czerniecki B, Solin LJ, et al. MR imaging of the breast in patients with invasive lobular carcinoma. Am J Roentgenol. 2001;176(2): 399–406.
59. Qayyum A, Birdwell RL, Daniel BL, Nowels KW, Jeffrey SS, TA A, et al. MR imaging features of infiltrating lobular carcinoma of the breast: histopathologic correlation. AJR Am J Roentgenol. 2002;178(5):1227–32.
60. Yeh ED, Slanetz PJ, Edmister WB, Talele A, Monticciolo D, Kopans DB. Invasive lobular carcinoma: spectrum of enhancement and morphology on magnetic resonance imaging. Breast J. 2003;9(1):13–8.
61. Mann RM, Loo CE, Wobbes T, Bult P, Barentsz JO, Gilhuijs KG, et al. The impact of preoperative breast MRI on the re-excision rate in invasive lobular carcinoma of the breast. Breast Cancer Res Treat. 2010;119(2):415–22.
62. McKinnon E, Xiao P. Metaplastic carcinoma of the breast. Arch Pathol Lab Med. 2015;139(6): 819–22.
63. Velasco M, Santamaría G, Ganau S, Farrús B, Zanón G, Romagosa C, et al. MRI of metaplastic carcinoma of the breast. AJR Am J Roentgenol. 2005;184(4):1274–8.
64. Wurdinger S, Herzog AB, Fischer DR, Marx C, Raabe G, Schneider A, et al. Differentiation of phyllodes breast tumors from fibroadenomas on MRI. AJR Am J Roentgenol. 2005;185(5): 1317–21.

Chapter 11
Targeted Ultrasound After MRI

Chloe Chhor and Adrienne Newburg

Abstract A magnetic resonance imaging (MRI)-directed ultrasound (US), also known as second-look US or targeted US, is performed to assess for a sonographic correlate for a lesion detected by MRI that was not initially seen at mammography or ultrasound. If a correlate is seen at ultrasound, US-guided biopsy is the preferred method as it can be less expensive, faster, easier, and more comfortable for patients than MRI-guided biopsy. Understanding the differences in breast position between MRI (prone) and ultrasound (supine) in addition to knowledge of the location and morphology of the MRI-detected lesion can aid in identifying a sonographic correlate. Performing imaging-histopathologic concordance and imaging follow-up are important in patient management. In the absence of a sonographic correlate, MRI-guided biopsy is still required of any lesion deemed suspicious at MR imaging.

Keywords Magnetic Resonance Imaging • MRI • Ultrasound • US • MRI-directed ultrasound • Directed-ultrasound • Targeted-ultrasound • Second-look ultrasound • Sonographic correlate • Breast cancer • Breast lesions • Incidental breast lesions • Breast biopsy • Ultrasound-guided biopsy • MRI-guided biopsy

11.1 Introduction

Breast MRI has been shown to have a high sensitivity (up to 100 %) for the detection of breast cancer but its specificity and positive predictive value is reported to be lower [2, 9, 11, 15, 18, 20]. Unsuspected suspicious MRI-detected lesions, designated category 4 or 5 according to the American College of Radiology Breast Imaging

---

C. Chhor, MD (✉)
Department of Radiology, NYU School of Medicine, New York, NY, USA
e-mail: chloe.chhor@nyumc.org

A. Newburg, MD
Department of Radiology, University of Massachusetts Medical School, UMass Memorial Medical Center, Worcester, MA, USA

S.L. Heller, L. Moy (eds.), *Breast Oncology: Techniques, Indications, and Interpretation*, DOI 10.1007/978-3-319-42563-4_11

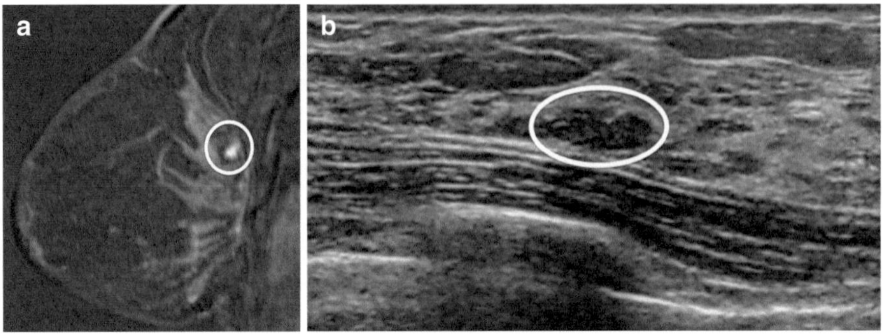

Fig. 11.1 Posteriorly located lesion that is not amenable for MRI-guided biopsy. (**a**) Subtracted sagittal T1W post-contrast image. (**b**) MRI-directed US from right breast. A 27-year-old woman with BRCA2 gene mutation found to have an oval enhancing mass (*circle* in **a**) in the right breast in the far posterior aspect, just anterior to the pectoralis major muscle. MRI-directed US identified a 9-mm oval hypoechoic mass at 10:00, 5-cm from the nipple (*circle* in **b**). US-guided FNA aspiration was performed demonstrating fibroadenoma, which is benign and concordant. This mass remained stable at 12-months follow-up

Reporting and Data System (BI-RADS) [16], therefore warrant biopsy to establish tissue diagnosis. Management options include MRI-directed wire-localization for surgical excision, proceeding directly to MRI-guided biopsy, or performing an MRI-directed ultrasound, also known as second-look or targeted US. An MRI-directed ultrasound is utilized to find a correlate for a lesion detected at MRI that was either not seen on a breast ultrasound performed antecedent to the MRI or because ultrasound had not been previously performed. Identifying a sonographic correlate enables US-guided biopsy. Compared to MRI-guided biopsy or wire-localization, US-guided biopsy is better tolerated, less expensive, more readily available, and faster [1, 5, 6, 13]. In addition, US guided biopsy also allows greater access to lesions in certain locations such as those located posteriorly (see Fig. 11.1), in the axillary tail, or in women with implants that may present a biopsy challenge under MRI guidance.

11.2 Technique in Performing MRI-Directed US

Thorough and careful review of the breast MRI is essential prior to performing an MRI-directed ultrasound. If a technologist performs the ultrasound study, it is also important to review the MRI study with the technologist. When reviewing the breast MRI study, utilization of 3D reconstructions can help make it easier to understand the location of the lesion in all 3 planes (see Fig. 11.2) and its relationship to surrounding structures [24]. The location and morphology of the MRI-detected lesion are important information to know to determine the expected location and appearance of the lesion at ultrasound.

Lesion location information to note includes the quadrant and o'clock position, distance from nipple, skin, and chest wall, anatomic relationship to surrounding tissue, and its relationship to other landmarks. It is important to keep in mind that

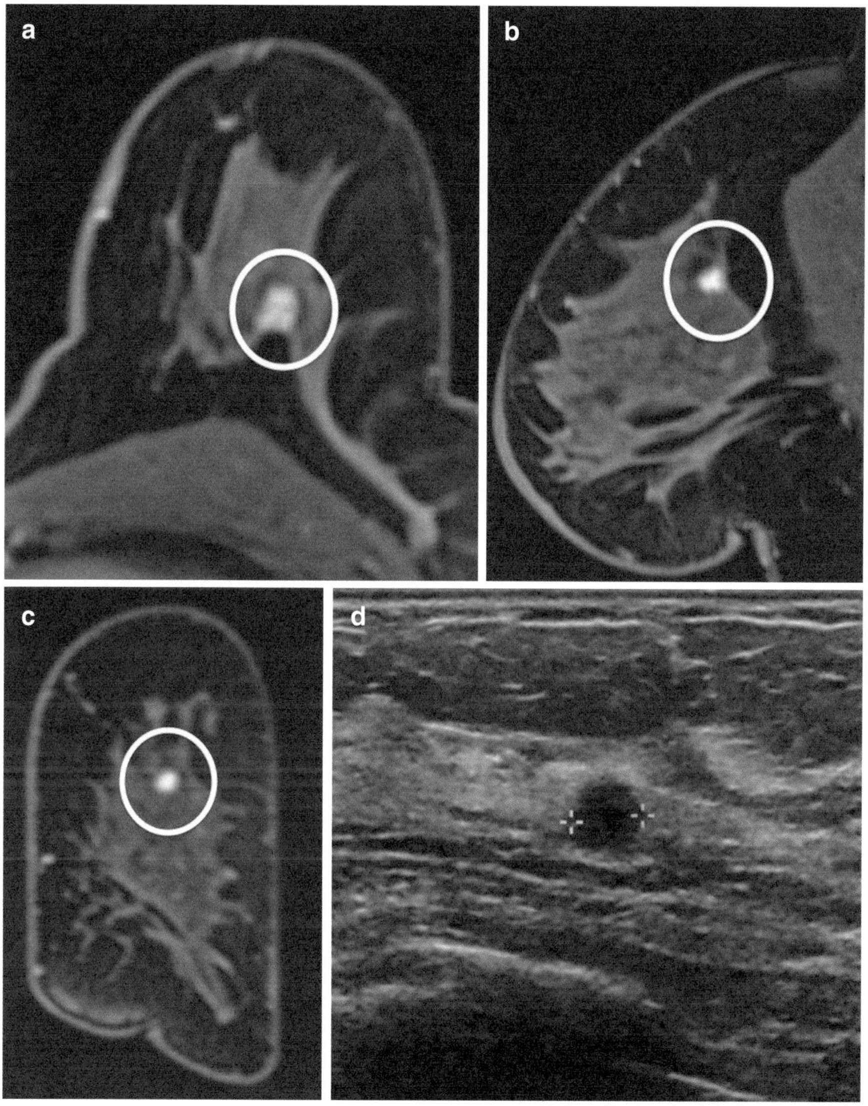

Fig. 11.2 3D reconstructions can help make it easier to understand the location of the lesion in all 3 planes. (**a**) Axial T1W post-contrast image. (**b**) Sagittal T1W post-contrast image. (**c**) Reconstructed coronal post-contrast image. (**d**) MRI-direct US from left breast. 39 year-old found on extent of disease MRI to have an enhancing round mass with irregular margin (*circle*) in the left breast at 12:00, 5-cm from the nipple. The 3 planes aided in ultrasound localization of the mass (calipers). Biopsy demonstrated invasive ductal carcinoma

the positioning of the breast is different between MRI and ultrasound [19, 24]. Breast US is performed with the patient in the supine or supine oblique position with the arm raised while breast MRI is performed with the patient in the prone position. In the supine position with the arm raised, the breast tissue is flattened and widened which makes the breast tissue, including breast lesions, appear more

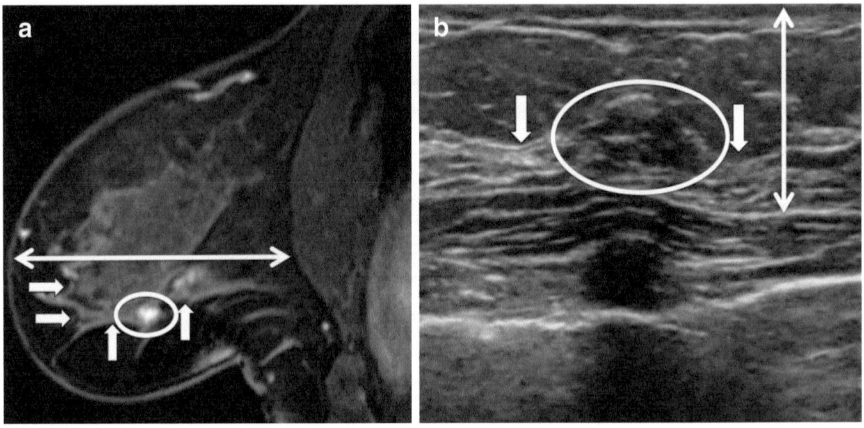

Fig. 11.3 Effects of the breast in the prone position at MRI and supine position at US and the relationship of lesion to surrounding tissue. (**a**) Subtracted sagittal T1W post-contrast image with patient in prone position. (**b**) MRI-directed US image from left breast. Breast tissue in the prone position appears more stretched in the anterior to posterior dimension (double arrowhead in **a**) while in the supine position along with compression by the ultrasound probe, the breast tissue becomes flattened and widened. In the supine position, the breast tissue, including breast lesions, appear more compact (*double arrowhead* in **b**). 41-year-old woman with a strong family history of breast cancer was found to have an oval irregular enhancing mass (*circle* in **a**) in the left breast middle depth which at ultrasound, the mass (*circle* in **b**) appears more posteriorly located due to flattening of the breast tissue. However, the lesion's relationship to surrounding tissue is maintained between the two modalities (glandular tissue indicted by *arrows*). Biopsy demonstrated fibroadenoma

compact. The distance between the chest wall and the glandular tissue is decreased on US relative to MRI (see Fig. 11.3). With MRI, the breast in the prone position is pendant with little to no compression; this results in the tissue appearing more stretched in the anterior to posterior dimension (see Fig. 11.3). The distance between the chest wall and the glandular tissue is increased and lesions can appear more anterior on MRI than on US images [19, 24]. Carbonaro et al. showed lesion displacement of about 3–6 cm along the three orthogonal directions on prone versus supine MRI [4]. The o'clock position of the lesion in ultrasound can also vary by one or two hours compared to the MRI [17]. Since lesion displacement can vary between ultrasound and MRI, the anatomic relationship of the lesion to surround tissue (subcutaneous fat, glandular tissue, or retroglandular fat) (see Fig. 11.3) can be used to help in identifying a correlate with more confidence [19]. The relationship of the lesion to surrounding tissue is maintained between the two modalities.

More reliable location information to note is the distance to the skin and nipple (see Fig. 11.4) as suggested by Carbonaro et al. [4]. The median lesion-to-skin and lesion-to-nipple displacements were less than 1 cm and that the lesion-to-nipple distance may be the most reliable measure to be used for MRI-directed US [4]. In addition to using the skin and nipple as fixed markers, the relationship of the lesion to co-existing lesions such as cysts, scars, implants, clips, known cancer (see Fig. 11.5), or known fibroadenomas may be helpful. Knowledge of co-existing lesions is

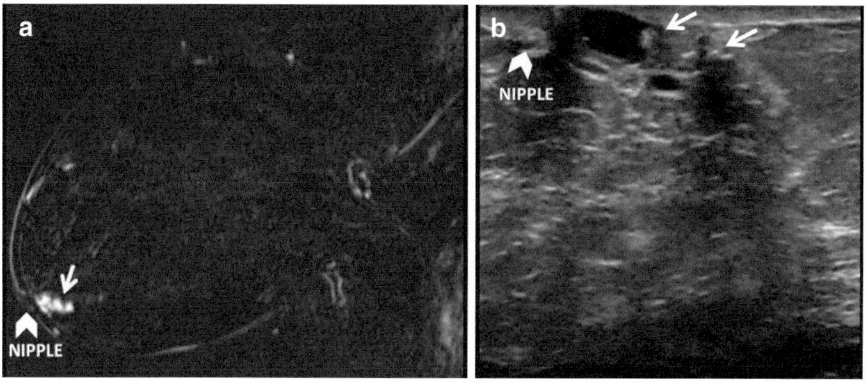

Fig. 11.4 Nipple as a fixed landmark. (**a**) Subtracted T1W post-contrast image. (**b**) MRI-directed US from left breast. Sixty-eight year-old with history of breast cancer found on surveillance MRI to have an oval mass with irregular margins (*arrow*) in the left retroareolar breast subjacent to the nipple (*arrowhead*). Using the nipple (*arrowhead*) as a fixed landmark, an irregular hypoechoic mass was identified within a focally dilated duct at US. Biopsy yielded papillary lesion

also important to prevent erroneous correlation, particularly in patients with multiple lesions within a similar region of the breast [19].

MRI lesion morphology with respect to shape, size and contours can also be useful in finding a lesion on MRI-directed ultrasound (see Fig. 11.6). Perfect morphologic agreement of lesions between the two modalities must not necessarily be expected [10]. Lesions at US tend to look smaller than at MRI as they are compressed in a vertical direction by the ultrasound probe. In addition, round lesions at MRI often appear oval or elliptical at ultrasound [19].

If no sonographic correlate is identified or confident correlation is difficult, MRI-guided biopsy must be performed on all lesions classified as BI-RADS category 4 or 5 at MRI [5, 10, 13, 19, 25].

11.3 Evidence-Based Findings

11.3.1 Frequency of Sonographic Correlate for MRI-Detected Lesions

Several studies have investigated the frequency at which MRI-directed ultrasound identifies a sonographic correlate for a lesion initially detected on MRI. These studies vary widely in rates of correlate, most likely because of heterogeneous methodologies and study populations, and also the inherently user-dependent nature of ultrasound [12, 22]. Limitations of the studies generally included retrospective design and lack of defined protocol establishing which lesions underwent MRI-directed ultrasound versus MRI-guided biopsy directly [5, 12, 13, 22]. In 2014 Spick and Baltzer published a meta-analysis of 17 studies that found a pooled detection rate for sonographic

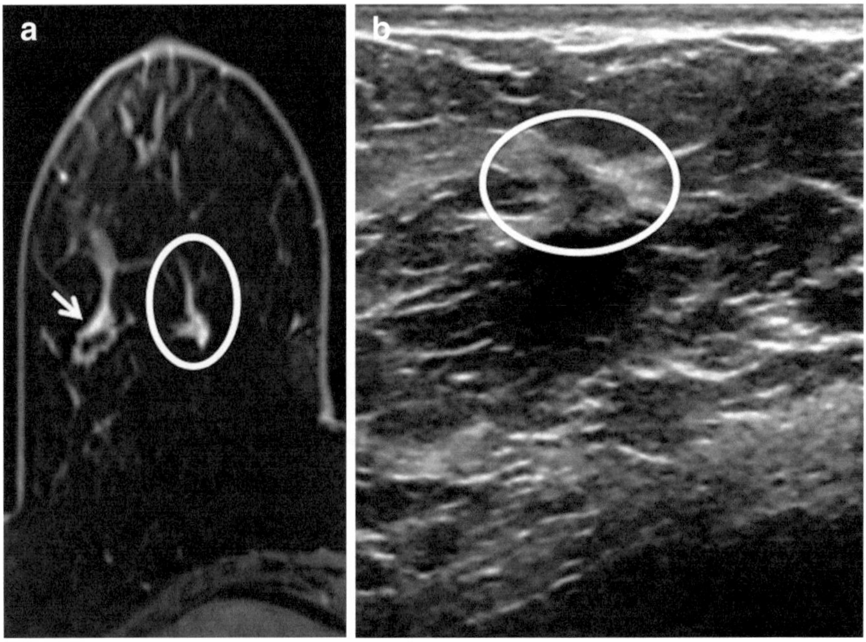

Fig. 11.5 Known cancer as a landmark. (**a**) Axial T1W post-contrast image. (**b**) MRI-directed US from right breast. Sixty-four-year-old woman with known right breast invasive ductal carcinoma (*arrow*) found on extent of disease MRI to have an irregular enhancing mass (*circle* **a**) medial to the known malignancy. Using the known malignancy as a landmark, a subtle sonographic correlate (*circle* **b**) was identified. Biopsy demonstrated a second area of invasive ductal carcinoma.

correlate of 58 %, with a wide reported range of 22–82 % [22]. Analyses of lesion characteristics have helped to understand which given MRI lesions are the most likely to have ultrasound correlates, with most studies showing masses and malignant lesions to be the most likely MRI-detected findings to also be seen on ultrasound.

11.3.2 Lesion Type

The three primary enhancing lesion types as defined by the BI-RADS lexicon [16], mass, focus and non-mass enhancement, show varying rates of sonographic correlate. Masses have been shown by many studies to be the lesion type most likely to have a correlate. In their meta-analysis, Spick and Baltzer found that mass lesions were more likely than non-mass enhancement to have a correlate ($p < .0001$) [22]. Many single studies have also demonstrated statistical significance for MRI-detected masses having a higher rate of sonographic correlate than non-mass enhancement. Meissnitzer et al. found a sonographic correlate for 62 % of masses and 31 % of

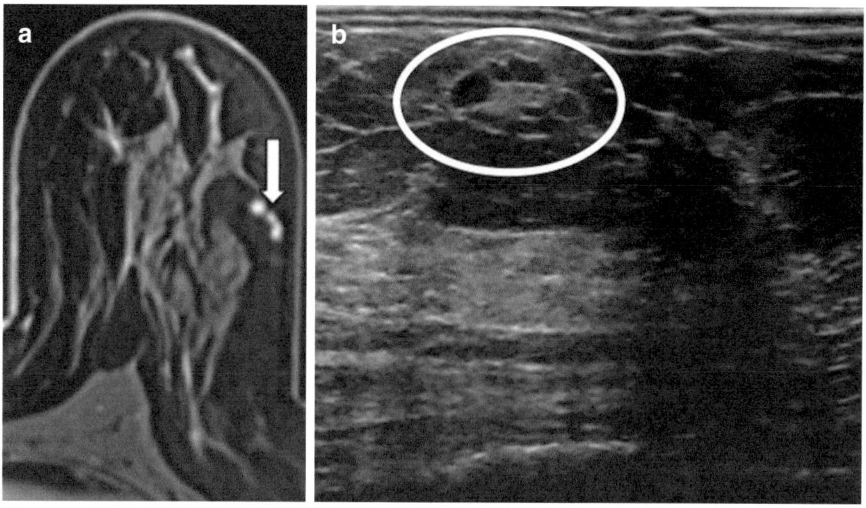

Fig. 11.6 Shape, size and contours can be useful in finding a lesion on MRI-directed ultrasound. (**a**) Axial T1W post-contrast image. (**b**) MRI-directed US from left breast. Forty-seven year-old woman with known malignancy was found on extent of disease MRI to have several enhancing contiguous masses (*arrow*) in the left breast at 2:00, 5 cm from the nipple. At ultrasound, several oval, circumscribed adjacent hypoechoic masses (*circle*) were identified similar in shape, size, and contour to the MRI lesion. At biopsy, the masses represented the lobulated cortex of a benign lymph node

non-mass enhancement ($p < 0.001$) [13]. Abe et al. found a correlate for 67 % of MRI-detected masses and 12 % of non-mass enhancement ($p < 0.005$) [1]; these authors also reported a 46 % correlate rate for foci, an intermediate rate between that of the other two lesion types [1]. Similarly, Hollowell reported a correlate rate of 49 % for masses, 42 % for foci, and 15 % for non-mass enhancement ($p = .0006$) [7]. DeMartini et al. found MRI-directed ultrasound yield to be higher for masses (58 %) than for foci (37 %) or non-mass enhancement (30 %) [5].

11.3.3 Size

Some studies have shown lesion size to affect chance of identifying an ultrasound correlate, with larger lesions more likely to have a correlate. Meissnitzer et al. found that for both masses and non-mass enhancement, increasing lesion size resulted in increasing ultrasound conspicuity that was statistically significant [13]. Wiratkapun et al. found a positive association between increasing size of MRI mass lesions and detection of ultrasound correlate (odds ratio 1.23, $p = .01$) [25]. Several other authors did not find lesion size to significantly affect frequency of detection [3, 5, 8, 10].

Spick and Baltzer also did not find size to be a significant predictor of sonographic correlate detection rate on meta-regression analysis, but recommended caution when interpreting this result because of the small number of studies that specifically reported on lesion size and lack of stratification by lesion type [22].

11.3.4 Level of Suspicion and Kinetics

Meissnitzer et al. found that BI-RADS category 5 versus 4 lesions were significantly more likely to have a correlate, both for masses (81 % versus 59 %, $p = 0.005$) and for non-mass enhancement (75 % versus 26 %, $p = 0.009$) [13]. However, level of suspicion was not reported upon or not found to be statistically significant in many other studies. Similarly, there is limited reported data regarding MRI lesion enhancement kinetics and rate of correlate. Meissnitzer et al. found no significant effect of enhancement kinetics on correlate detection rate [13].

11.3.5 Histology

Many studies have shown malignant lesions to be statistically more likely than benign lesions to have a sonographic correlate [1, 7, 10, 13, 21], including on meta-analysis ($p < .0001$) [22]. However, investigators have shown that malignancy is not excluded if a sonographic correlate is not found, with rate of sonographically occult malignancy reported at 12 % in pooled estimate on meta-analysis [22] and with a wide range on single studies, up to 53 % [1, 5, 6, 10, 13, 25]. Thus, there is consensus among numerous authors who endorse that absence of a correlate does not obviate biopsy, such that suspicious MRI-detected lesions without sonographic correlate should go on to MRI-guided biopsy [5–7, 10, 12, 13, 21, 22, 25].

11.4 Potential Limitations of MRI-Directed US

With increasing availability of breast MRI, some facilities proceed directly to MRI-guided biopsy, as there are some potential disadvantages for performing MRI-directed US rather than proceeding directly to MRI-guided biopsy. MRI-directed ultrasound may prolonged work-up time resulting in delay of diagnosis, added expense of performing the ultrasound prior to MRI-guided biopsy, and patients may experience a false sense of reassurance in the setting of a negative ultrasound [5, 10, 12, 13, 21]. In addition, confident correlation on MRI-directed US can be challenging and can result in inaccurate correlations. In one study it was reported that the follow-up imaging in 80 benign, concordant ultrasound-guided biopsies, 10 of the sonographic lesion did not correspond to the MRI finding [13]. Five cancers were diagnosed in 9/10 lesions that underwent MRI-guided biopsy.

11.5 Imaging-Histopathologic Correlation

Determining concordance between imaging findings and histologic results is important and is the responsibility of the radiologist who performed the biopsy. Whether the histolopathologic diagnosis correlates with the imaging findings will determine patient management with respect to recommendation for surgical excision or short-term follow-up. In the case of MRI-directed ultrasound, imaging-histopathologic correlation should be made based on the level of suspicion with both the presumed ultrasound correlate and the lesion initially detected on MRI.

Following ultrasound-guided biopsy, a clip should be routinely placed at the site of biopsy with a post-procedure mammogram performed to help facilitate assessment of concordance and for subsequent imaging follow-up (see Fig. 11.7). Breast-MRI imaging in more than one plane or reformatting MR images into more than one plane can help assess correlation of lesion location marked by the biopsy clip on the post-ultrasound guided biopsy mammogram and the location of the lesion on MRI [12, 17, 19, 24]. Immediate action for the MRI-detected lesion is often prompted by histopathologic discordance but will not typically occur if the result is benign concordant. For benign concordant results, some practices will wait for MRI follow-up, typically 6 months after ultrasound biopsy which may delay management of the MRI detected lesion if the presumed ultrasound correlate is not the same as the MRI lesion [17, 23, 24]. To minimize delay in patient care, a more definitive confirmation of MRI-sonographic correlation can be obtained on the same day as the US-guided core biopsy by getting a fast single T1 weighted gradient echo (GE) sequence without fat saturation [14, 17, 24]. The T1 weighted GE sequence (3D rapid EG, TR/TE, 8/4.6; matrix, 276×464; flip angle 16° voxel size, $0.8 \times 0.8 \times 0.8$ mm) [17, 24] is sensitive to artifacts with magnetic susceptibility and will help verify MRI-sonographic correlate. The acquisition time is between 2 and 4 min. A biopsy under MRI should be recommended if there is disagreement between the biopsy performed with ultrasound and the MRI lesion. Depending on the practice workflow and availability of the MRI scanner, MRI-guided biopsy can be done on the same day if the US-guided biopsy site is found not to correlate with location of MRI lesion. It is important to keep in mind that evaluation of the biopsy site and targeted lesion may be limited because of hematoma and other post-biopsy changes. For any benign concordant result after ultrasound-guided biopsy of a sonographic correlate to a lesion initially detected on MRI a 6-month follow-up MRI is recommended [23].

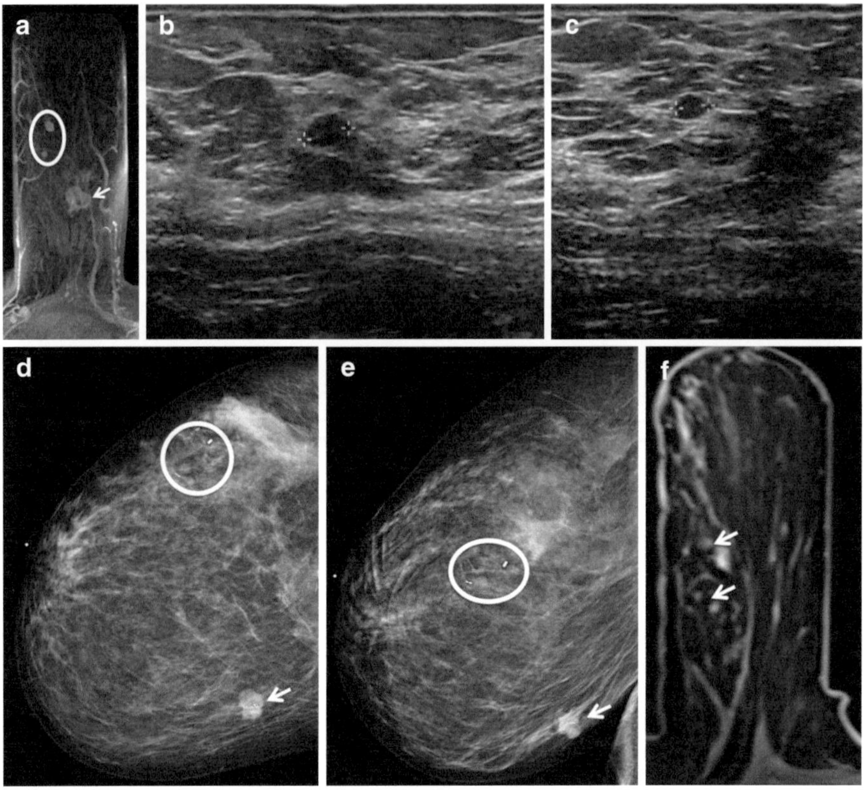

Fig. 11.7 Imaging correlation after biopsy of MRI-detected lesion with sonographic guidance. (**a**) Axial T1W post-contrast MIP image. (**b**) MRI-US from right breast at 9:30, 6-cm from the nipple. (**c**) Targeted US of right breast at 10:00, 7-cm from the nipple. (**d**) Right CC view after US-guided biopsy. (**e**) Right LM view after US-guided biopsy. (**f**) Axial T1W post contrast image. Forty-two-year-old female with recent diagnosis of invasive ductal carcinoma (*arrow*) in the lower inner quadrant posterior depth. At extent of disease MRI, 2 additional lesions (*circle*) were seen. Possible correlates (calipers) were identified at ultrasound with biopsy and clip placement yielding fibroadenoma for the 9:30 6-cm from the nipple 0.6-cm mass and papillary lesion for the 10:00, 7-cm from the nipple 0.5-cm mass. Post-US guided biopsy mammogram (CC and LM views) shows the biopsy clips (*circle*) to be within expected location of the MRI lesions. This was confirmed on MRI showing susceptibility artifacts (*arrows* in **f**) associated with lesions of interest

11.6 Conclusion

MRI-directed ultrasound is an important adjunctive tool in the evaluation of lesions detected at MR imaging. Identification of a sonographic correlate enables US-guided biopsy of the MRI-detected lesions which is the preferred method as it can be less expensive, faster, easier, and more comfortable for patients than MRI-guided biopsy. To help facilitate identifying an MRI-sonographic correlate, it is important to thoroughly review the breast MRI prior to performing the targeted ultrasound and understand the differences in breast position between the two modalities. Lesion location, depth, and characteristics, as well as the appearance of the surrounding tissue and relationship to other focal lesions that may be present, must be considered. The likelihood of finding a correlate to an MRI lesion varies depending on lesion size and morphology with larger lesions and masses being easier to identify at US. Following biopsy, it is important to confirm accuracy of MRI-ultrasound correlation and perform imaging-histopathologic correlation. MRI-guided biopsy needs to be performed for any MRI-US discordant cases. Also for benign concordant MRI-US cases, a follow-up breast MRI must be carried out 6 months after the biopsy.

Not all MRI-detected lesions will be seen at ultrasound. Absence of a sonographic correlate for a MRI-detected lesion with suspicious imaging features does not preclude the need for biopsy under MRI-guidance.

References

1. Abe H, Schmidt R, Shah R, Shimauchi A, Kulkarni K, Sennett C, et al. MR-directed ("second-look") ultrasound examination for breast lesions detected initially on MRI: MR and sonographic findings. AJR. 2010;194(2):370–7.
2. Bluemke DA, Gatsonis CA, Chen MH, DeAngelis GA, DeBruhl N, Harms S, et al. Magnetic resonance imaging of the breast prior to biopsy. JAMA. 2004;292(22):2735.
3. Candelaria R, Fornage BD. Second-look US examination of MR-detected breast lesions. J Clin Ultrasound. 2011;39:115–21.
4. Carbonaro L, Tannaphai P, Trimboli R, Verardi N, Fedeli M, Sardanelli F. Contrast enhanced breast MRI: spatial displacement from prone to supine patient's position. Preliminary results. Eur J Radiol. 2012;81(6):e771–4.
5. DeMartini W, Eby P, Peacock S, Lehman C. Utility of targeted sonography for breast lesions that were suspicious on MRI. AJR. 2009;192(4):1128–34.
6. Destounis S, Arieno A, Somerville PA, Seifert PJ, Murphy P, Morgan R, et al. Community-based practice experience of unsuspected breast magnetic resonance imaging abnormalities evaluated with second-look sonography. J Ultrasound Med. 2009;28:1337–46.
7. Hollowell L, Price E, Arasu V, Wisner D, Hylton N, Joe B. Lesion morphology on breast MRI affects targeted ultrasound correlation rate. Eur Radiol. 2015;25:1279–84.
8. Hong M, Cha J, Kim H, Shin H, Chae E, Shin J, et al. Second-look ultrasonography for MRI-detected suspicious breast lesions in patients with breast cancer. Ultrasonography. 2014; 34(2):125–32.
9. Kuhl CK, Schrading S, Leutner CC, Morakkabati-Spitz N, Wardelmann E, Fimmers R, et al. Mammography, breast ultrasound, and magnetic resonance imaging for surveillance of women at high familial risk for breast cancer. J Clin Oncol. 2005;23(33):8469–76.
10. LaTrenta LR, Menell JH, Morris EA, Abramson AF, Dershaw DD, Liberman L. Breast lesions detected with MR imaging: utility and histopathologic importance of identification with US. Radiology. 2003;227:856–61.
11. Lehman C, Isaacs C, Schnall M, Pisano E, Ascher S, Weatherall P, et al. Cancer yield of mammography, MR, and US in high-risk women: prospective multi-institution breast cancer screening study 1. Radiology. 2007;244(2):381–8.
12. Leung J. Utility of second-look ultrasound in the evaluation of MRI-detected breast lesions. Semin Roentgenol. 2011;46(4):260–74.
13. Meissnitzer M, Dershaw D, Lee C, Morris E. Targeted ultrasound of the breast in women with abnormal MRI findings for whom biopsy has been recommended. AJR. 2009;193(4):1025–9.

14. Monticciolo D. Postbiopsy confirmation of MR-detected lesions biopsied using ultrasound. AJR. 2012;198(6):W618–20.
15. Morris E, Liberman L, Ballon D, Robson M, Abramson A, Heerdt A, et al. MRI of occult breast carcinoma in a high-risk population. AJR. 2003;181(3):619–26.
16. Morris EA, Comstock CE, Lee CH, et al. ACR BI-RADS® Magnetic Resonance Imaging. In: ACR BI-RADS® Atlas, Breast Imaging Reporting and Data System. Reston: American College of Radiology; 2013.
17. Nouri-Neuville M, de Rocquancourt A, Cohen-Zarade S, Chapellier-Canaud M, Albiter M, Hamy A, et al. Correlation between MRI and biopsies under second look ultrasound. Diagn Interv Radiol. 2014;95(2):197–211.
18. Orel S, Schnall M. MR imaging of the breast for the detection, diagnosis, and staging of breast cancer. Radiology. 2001;220(1):13–30.
19. Park V, Kim M, Kim E, Moon H. Second-look US: how to find breast lesions with a suspicious MR imaging appearance. Radiographics. 2013;33(5):1361–75.
20. Sardanelli F, Podo F, D'Agnolo G, Verdecchia A, Santaquilani M, Musumeci R, et al. Multicenter comparative multimodality surveillance of women at genetic-familial high risk for breast cancer (HIBCRIT study): interim results 1. Radiology. 2007;242(3):698–715.
21. Sim L, Hendriks J, Bult P, Fook-Chong S. US correlation for MRI-detected breast lesions in women with familial risk of breast cancer. Clin Radiol. 2005;60(7):801–6.
22. Spick C, Baltzer P. Diagnostic utility of second-look US for breast lesions identified at MR imaging: systematic review and meta-analysis. Radiology. 2014;273(2):401–9.
23. Sung J, Lee C, Morris E, Comstock C, Dershaw D. Patient follow-up after concordant histologically benign imaging-guided biopsy of MRI-detected lesions. AJR. 2012;198(6):1464–9.
24. Trop I, Labelle M, David J, Mayrand M, Lalonde L. Second-look targeted studies after breast magnetic resonance imaging: practical tips to improve lesion identification. Curr Probl Diagn Radiol. 2010;39(5):200–11.
25. Wiratkapun C, Duke D, Nordmann A, Lertsithichai P, Narra V, Barton P, et al. Indeterminate or suspicious breast lesions detected initially with MR imaging. Acad Radiol. 2008;15(5):618–25.

Chapter 12
Breast Biopsy and Breast MRI Wire Localization

Steven Allen

Abstract Breast MRI guided intervention has become an increasingly important technique for breast radiologists largely due to increasing diagnostic breast MRI examination volumes. Alongside this there has been improved diagnostic image quality with a resulting number of breast lesions detected only on MRI requiring further clarification. International guidelines now insist that institutions performing breast MRI should provide the option of an MRI-guided intervention for further lesional work up, whether in their own unit or at a local center that can be referred to. This chapter covers the indications for these interventions, in particular which lesions require biopsy and when a lesion can just be managed with imaging follow up. Technical aspects are considered such as MRI scanner hardware and software requirements, as well as which biopsy needles are most appropriate. Limitations and complications are covered including "tips and tricks" that may be of use in certain specific clinical situations. Outcomes of MRI-guided biopsies are discussed based on current literature with a final view taken on future directions.

Keywords Breast • Biopsy • Diagnostic • Intervention • Magnetic resonance imaging • Wire • Localisation • Vacuum • Diagnosis • Therapy

12.1 Background and Indications

Breast MRI has controversially found increasing use as a diagnostic imaging investigation over the last decade or so [1, 2]. While its sensitivity is unquestionably high in cancer detection, this unfortunately comes at the expense of a lower specificity [3–5]. Where additional lesions are demonstrated on MRI, the initial follow up investigation is a focused ultrasound exam but unfortunately this has variable accuracy at

S. Allen, MBBS, MRCS, FRCR
Department of Imaging, Royal Marsden Hospital, London, UK
e-mail: stevenallen@nhs.net

S.L. Heller, L. Moy (eds.), *Breast Oncology: Techniques, Indications, and Interpretation*, DOI 10.1007/978-3-319-42563-4_12

locating and characterizing the abnormality [6, 7]. There are sometimes landmarks in the breast such as cysts or scars that will allow correlation on follow up imaging but clearly this is not always the case. Larger lesions are reportedly easier to locate as well as lesions characterized as BIRADs 5 [8–10]. Non mass enhancement is less commonly delineated and overall a "MRI-directed second look" ultrasound will detect an area of MRI abnormality in just over half of cases (16–65 %) [9–11]. The second look or MRI-directed US will be further discussed in chapter 11.

Where lesions are characterized by the MRI BIRADs lexicon as 3 or above, the reported final malignancy rate is 20–62 % [10–14]. There are several MRI characteristics such as lesional enhancement pattern, shape and size that may predict the likelihood of malignancy.

Where ultrasound or indeed mammography shows a lesion, then a targeted biopsy should be performed stereotactically or under ultrasound guidance as these are the most accessible, fast and least expensive guidance methods. A marker clip is then ideally left in place. A repeat MRI after a time interval (typically 6 months) may be recommended if the imaging pathological correlation is good and the histological result is non malignant.

If no concordant abnormalities are seen in a low risk situation and enhancement is not suspicious, then once again a follow up MRI exam could be performed at 6 months. Where ultrasound is negative, the malignancy rate falls but lesions that are suspicious on MRI and lack a correlate on "MRI-directed second look" ultrasound are malignant in 13–22 % of cases [11–17]; these should also be histologically verified via an MRI-guided biopsy. Lesions that should be considered suspicious include BI-RADS 4 or 5 abnormalities (Fig. 12.1). BI-RADS 3 lesions in high risk women undergoing MRI screening or those with an index primary breast cancer (ipsilateral or contralateral) may also be indicated for biopsy. Where there is uncertainty, and indeed wherever possible, the decision for MRI guided biopsy is made following a multidisciplinary team discussion where all the imaging can be considered alongside clinical and pathological factors in order that the correct recommendation can be made on a case by case basis.

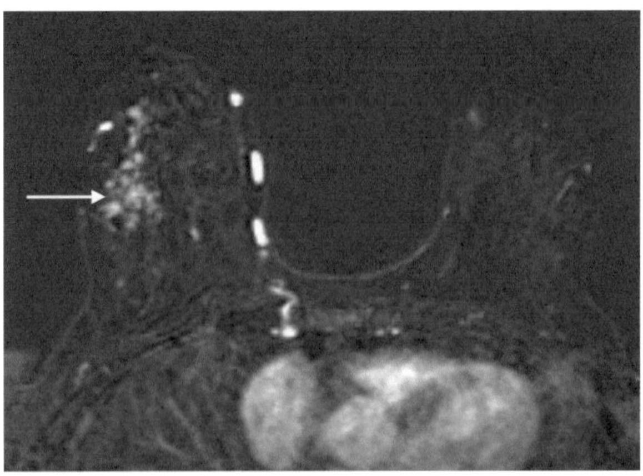

Fig. 12.1 An axial fat saturated contrast enhanced subtraction image showing a focal area of non mass-like enhancement in the outer right breast (*arrow*). This was not demonstrated mammographically or on ultrasound and was considered indeterminate. An MRI guided biopsy was recommended

Contraindications for breast MRI biopsy are the same as those for a diagnostic MRI (pacemaker, other implantable devices etc.), contrast medium injections (allergy, severe renal impairment) and biopsies (poor coagulation, allergy to local anesthesia) [18, 19]. These contraindications may be relative and careful consultation with clinical colleagues such as cardiologists and hematologists may facilitate the biopsy procedure depending on each individual case. Radiofrequency excisional biopsy devices (Intact®) cannot be used because of interference with the electromagnetic wave.

MRI-guided biopsies should only be carried out in experienced breast centers where these are preformed regularly [20–22]. The team must have suitable experience in performing both breast MRI and vacuum-assisted breast biopsy, although the exact training requirements in MRI-guided vacuum-assisted biopsies varies enormously internationally. In some countries where access to MRI is more limited, the initial training involves only a few procedures, but 15 procedures are required according to the European guidelines [20].

12.2 Technical Aspects

Most MRI scanners currently used in clinical practice have a field strength of either 1.5 T or 3 T. In the latter system the sensitivity of detecting the cancer is greater for the same specificity [23], although artefacts are generally increased. Susceptibility artifact is more than double in size at 3 T vs 1.5 T [24].

Open MRI scanners in theory provide easier access to the breast and real time monitoring of insertion of the cannula. However, to date these scanners utilize a low field (0.2–0.5 T), which is not of sufficient quality imaging for breast imaging [25].

The coils used for biopsy should if possible be the same as those used for diagnosis in order to reproduce the diagnostic scan (and hence lesion requiring biopsy) as close as is possible. It must be possible to access the breast to take the samples, which assumes that the coil is open. Current dual breast coils allow either external, internal or even superior access although the lateral approach is preferred as this is technically the most straightforward as shall be discussed (Fig. 12.2).

As an alternative to biopsy coils, perforated plate systems can be used together with flexible ring coils placed around the breast. Perforated plate systems are sometimes advantageous for reaching findings close to the thoracic wall. Compared to multi-channel breast biopsy coils, however, a ring coil is associated with a reduced signal-to-noise ratio and thus inferior image quality. This is true particularly for findings far from the coil (for example near the nipple).

Internal access is limited for deep (medial) lesions and this is technically more challenging. However historically where the whole breast would be traversed by the biopsy system, the contralateral breast can now be positioned on a board and the radiologist works from beneath in a tunnel. In principle, the shortest possible access should be selected and newer generation coils allow for medial and lateral access for biopsy. The medial access may be more difficult due to the longer distance in

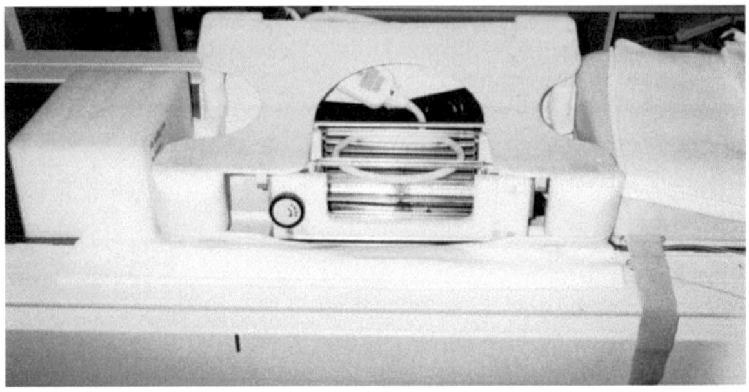

Fig. 12.2 An image showing a breast biopsy compatible MRI coil

conjunction with the reduced light and operating space beneath the patient. As a general principal post-biopsy, a clip insertion is recommended to ensure the ability for localization through subsequent ultrasound or mammographic guided wire marking of the clip.

Regardless of targeting method, an opaque landmark such as a vitamin E capsule is attached to the compression plate. The end of this is positioned in contact with the breast and used as the landmark for the three spatial planes and to allow subsequent targeting. This appears as a focal area of hyperintensity on the unenhanced T1 weighted views.

The MRI scanner itself will likely have a targeting software package or this can be obtained separately depending on the manufacturer. These are particularly useful for posterior contrast enhancement. Computer aided detection software (CAD) purchased usually as a stand alone software package can facilitate better lesion delineation particularly in relation to the subtraction imaging. The biopsy system used is then computed with calculation of the necessary depth taking account of the materials and thickness of the grid.

The principle used is that the same image is taken on four occasions: before biopsy (target identification), after positioning a guide (checking correct position of the biopsy system), after taking the biopsy (confirming that the biopsy cavity is consistent with the target) and after positioning the clip (checking the correct position of the marker).

Initial and then dynamic images are preferably taken in high- resolution T1 weighted sequences. This could be a 2D exam but is preferably a 3D echo gradient with fat saturation [26]. It is ideally the highest possible spatial resolution at a temporal resolution of 60–120 s per series, with either transverse or sagittal slice orientation. The acquisition may be taken through axial sections although resolution is often better in sagittal sections [27]. For reliable lesion imaging, subtraction series of every contrast enhanced series should be acquired. Rapid T1 W spin echo (TSE) images are preferable in order to reduce artifact from the needles [27].

The maximum intravenous contrast dose (0.2 ml/kg) or a half dose is injected depending on whether or not a repeat end of procedure injection is planned. This is performed at an injection rate of 2–3 ml/s and the contrast agent is then washed out with a subsequent bolus injection of 20 mls of physiological saline solution (0.9 % NaCl).

The Mammotome® (Devicor Inc., Cincinnati, USA) was the earliest available vacuum biopsy system and was used for MRI-assisted biopsy in the late 1990s. However currently there are several manufacturers that now produce equipment for MRI-guided VAB of the breast. In Europe the EnCorTM (Senorx or Enspire, Bard GmbH, Karlsruhe, Germany) and the ATEC® (Hologic Inc., Bedford, USA) are now widely popular and have superseded the less automated Vacora® (Bard GmbH, Karlsruhe, Germany) system.

MRI-guided VAB was initially performed using an 11-gauge needle, but as with mammogram guided VAB, MRI-guided vacuum-assisted biopsy have trended toward larger needle gauges (up to 7G). These allow the collection of the same tissue volume with fewer samples in a shorter examination time. There are no specific guidelines defining the number of samples for MRI-VAB, but a European consensus paper on the use of MRI-VAB recommends taking at least 24 11G samples or an equivalent tissue volume if larger needle gauges are used [21]. However, the recommended sample here is based on very limited evidence. The number of samples reported in the literature ranges from 2 to 75 with a median of 12 [28–33].

Most VAB devices have a cable connection to the vacuum source located outside the MRI examination room. Non-magnetic materials should be used in preference to ferromagnetic materials (needles, biopsy guns, etc.) in order to minimize the chances of an accident from magnetic attraction. As these various guns are non-magnetic (Vacora® less than the others), they are not attracted by the magnet although interference with their operation does occur if they come too close to the magnet.

The Vacora® is a battery-operated system and thus a true handheld system. The disadvantage of this system is that the device has to be removed from the breast after each sample is taken. This causes more difficulty from blood [30] and air and it is essential to use a support for the gun in order to reduce the risk of displacing the cannula. The vacuum aspirate is reported to be less powerful and the sampling process slower (69 min vs 39 min). Automated coaxial systems are reported to be able to biopsy smaller lesions (10 mm vs 19 mm) in a shorter exam time [34]. While the automated devices mentioned also take individual samples, the biopsy system remains in the breast during the entire intervention. The samples are then automatically transported to a chamber in the handle, where they can later be removed. The ATEC® and EnCorTM provide the advantage of the automated removal of multiple samples in immediate succession. The ATEC® additionally provides the option of rinsing the biopsy cavity with saline.

12.3 The Procedure

Efficiency and speed are of particular importance during this type of biopsy procedure. Because of the transient nature of contrast enhancement on MRI. there is a narrow window of time in which to perform the procedure and verify needle placement. Although variable to some extent, a 15–20 min time frame is expected. The more prolonged the procedure becomes, the more likely the contrast will wash out and also the more likely the patient is to move, resulting in motion artifact and potentially leading to incorrect targeting.

Patient positioning may vary slightly depending on institutional practice. The patient may be positioned on her side with her head turned to the opposite side and her arm above her head. Alternatively, the patient's head may be placed on a head rest or positional device so that the patient is looking straight down. A venous line with long connection tubing is in place. The breast is wedged in the surface coil and the guiding system is set up from the beginning. The skin marker is positioned in contact with the skin as close as possible to the projection of the lesion if no CAD system is being used, or further away in order to avoid obstruction of it if one is being used. Vitamin E capsules are often used as fiducial markers and are taped over the expected site of the lesion.

Modest compression is used to avoid masking the enhancement [35] and to reduce the accordion effect (decompression of the breast may cause displacement of a clip or coil). Accessibility of the presumed site of the lesion is then checked and positioned in the effective grid compression area (Fig. 12.3).

The patient is brought into the magnet and an initial contrast enhanced image is taken to find the lesion and locate it against the opaque landmark (this usually appears as a T1 weighted hyperintensity on the unenhanced image) (Fig. 12.4). Distances are measured manually or by software in the 3 spatial planes between this reference point ("zero") and the lesion.

After sterile preparation the local anesthesia is administered. In the absence of a contraindication, this usually consists of a large volume of lidocaine with epinephrine (lidocaine HCL 1 % and epinephrine 1:100,000). 20–40 cm^3 is commonly infiltrated in split doses, with 10–20 cm^3 administered before insertion of the biopsy device, and 10–20 cm^3 is administered by the device just prior to and during sampling. Epinephrine may sometimes minimise parenchymal hematoma formation, which amongst other things could potentially obscure the biopsy site. Initial subcutaneous anesthesia, however, is ideally obtained by using a small volume of lidocaine only with epinephrine not administered to the skin. It is of particular importance to ensure that no air bubbles are present within the syringe at the time of administration as even small air bubbles can cause significant artifact on the MRI.

Following the anesthetic, a skin incision is made. Depth is then adjusted by adding 20 mm for Senorx®, 10 mm for Vacora®, but nothing for Mammotome®. Once in place the metal sheath is replaced with a silicone sheath or with the position marker. The patient is returned inside the magnet and a rapid image is then taken to check the correct position of the introducer (Figs. 12.5, 12.6, 12.7, and 12.8).

The introducer is replaced by the cannula and then a series of samples are taken. The number of samples depends on the size of the lesion and quality of targeting. The ability to sample in a designated direction is a major advantage to performing this test with a vacuum biopsy needle. Prior to sampling it may be obvious that the lesion is slightly eccentrically site in relation to the needle tip. In this situation, the biopsy window can be targeted towards the lesion rather than just sweeping a full 360 degree circle. Early rounds of sampling usually produce the highest yield and the more samples that are obtained, the more likely it is that there will be hematoma formation in the target area. The result of this is that the biopsy device becomes

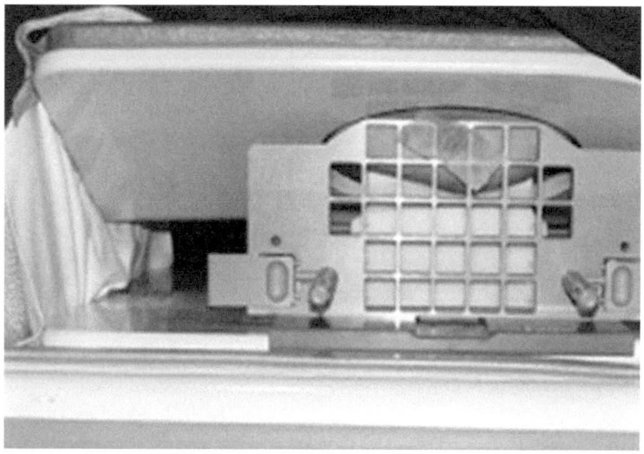

Fig. 12.3 An image showing a patient within the breast biopsy coil and demonstrating the grid localisation system

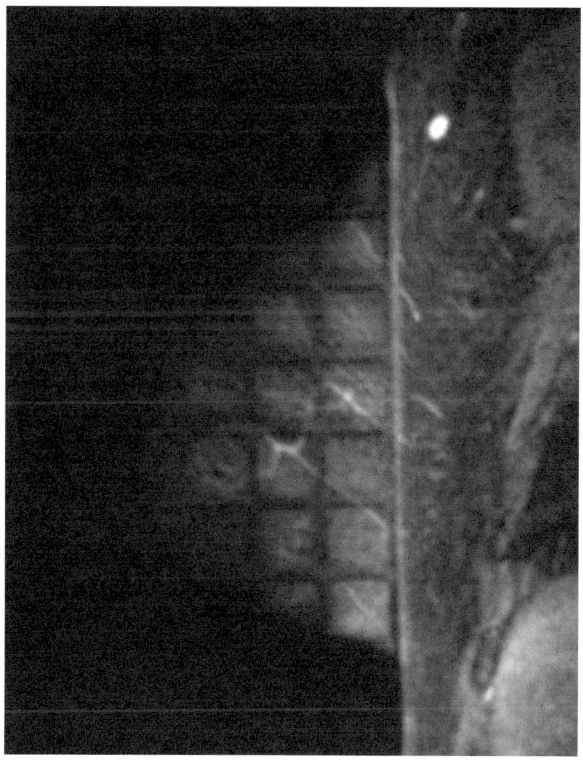

Fig. 12.4 A pre biopsy fat saturated contrast enhanced sagittal image showing the grid system over the skin allowing appropriate skin marking for needle entry point

more distant from the target lesion and there are thus diminishing returns of later and continued sampling in this scenario. For MRI guided biopsies, it is important to remember that the clock face is relative to the grid and not to the breast or to the patient. The aperture of the vacuum needle needs to be adjusted to reflect this. The samples are then placed in formalin and sent to pathology. The specimens are fixed and then sectioned and interpreted by an experienced breast histopathologist.

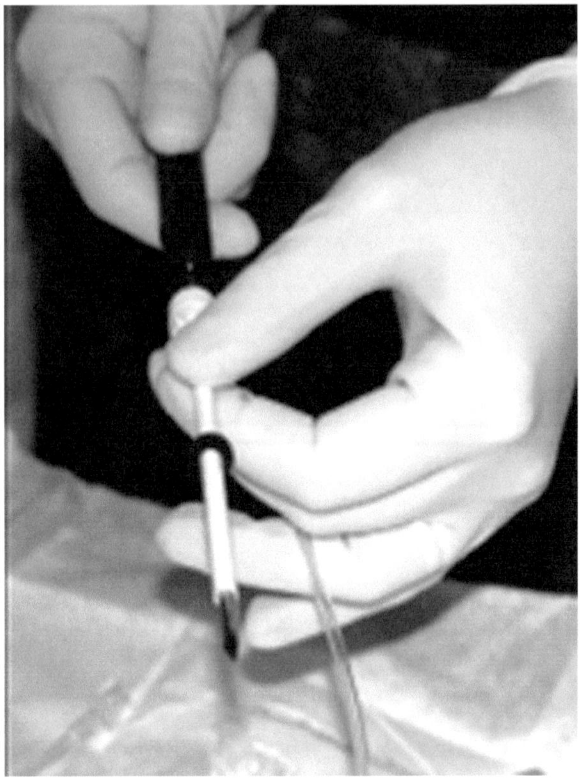

Fig. 12.5 An image showing the needle introducer being assembled prior to MRI guided biopsy

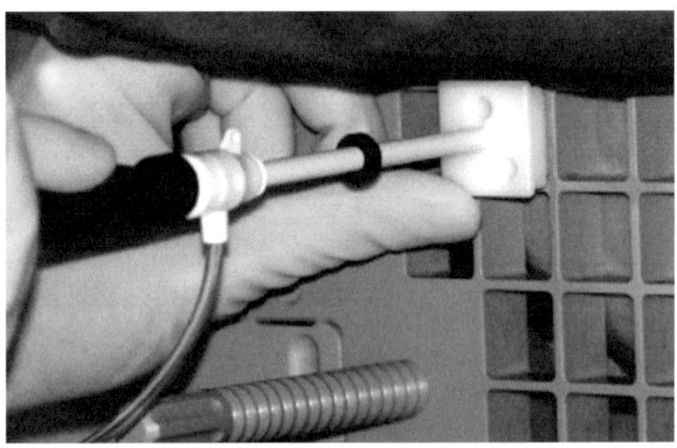

Fig. 12.6 An image showing a patient within the breast biopsy coil and demonstrating the introducer being passed through the grid localisation system

A marker clip is routinely positioned as this may be only landmark, which could be used to guide any subsequent surgery if required [29, 36–39]. It is ideally placed through the cannula prior to its removal or alternatively following the check image, through the introducer. The patient is repositioned in the tunnel for a final sequence in order to determine whether the contrast uptake dissipated although it is often sufficient to check that the biopsy area is correctly centered on the lesion (by comparing with the pre-biopsy image) and that the clip has been deployed. This sequence is

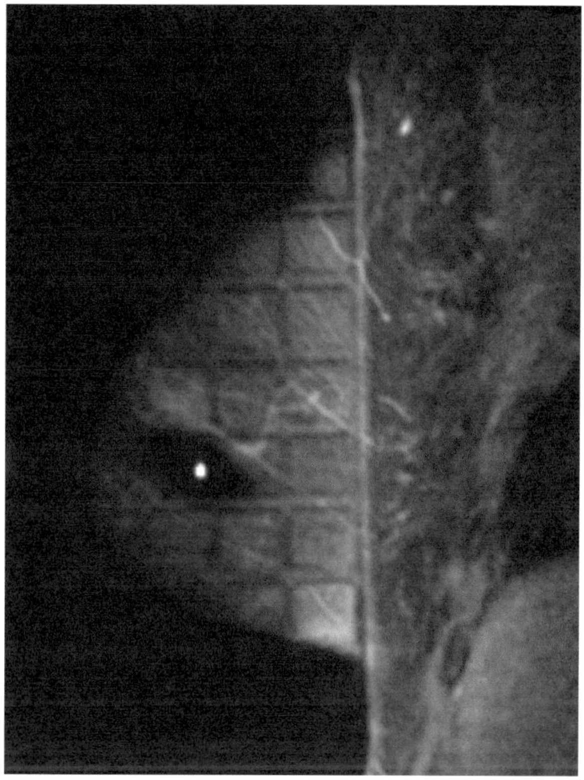

Fig. 12.7 A pre biopsy fat saturated contrast enhanced sagittal image showing the grid system over the skin with the biopsy needle passing through the image in position for biopsy

carried out with or without contrast enhancement and may facilitate further sampling or lesion retargeting (Fig. 12.9).

At the termination of the procedure, the patient is removed from the tunnel, placed flat on her back and manual compression to the breast biopsy site is applied followed by a compressive dressing. Monitoring following the procedure should be as per local protocols for a vacuum biopsy and be dependent on various patient factors as well as the degree of hematoma that has formed.

Signal void from the marker clip may be indistinguishable from signal void from air introduced during the procedure and so in order to ensure that the marker has deployed correctly, a post biopsy mammogram is usually recommended. A craniocaudal and mediolateral mammogram would typically be obtained. The position of the marker clip on the mammogram should be compared with the expected site of the lesion based on the diagnostic MRI examination. Any marker displacement needs to be clearly noted as a future wire localization may be required dependent on the histopathology from the biopsy.

Multiple lesions can be attempted at a single appointment although this may be challenging even for the most tolerant patient. As with any biopsy procedure, the most suspicious lesion should undergo intervention first, in case the later sites are not visualized or the patient is unable to continue. When dealing with multiple lesions in the same breast, the most favourable scenario is if the lesions can be positioned

Fig. 12.8 A prelocalisation fat saturated contrast enhanced sagittal image demonstrates the lesion persists (*arrow*) and therefore a MRI biopsy was performed

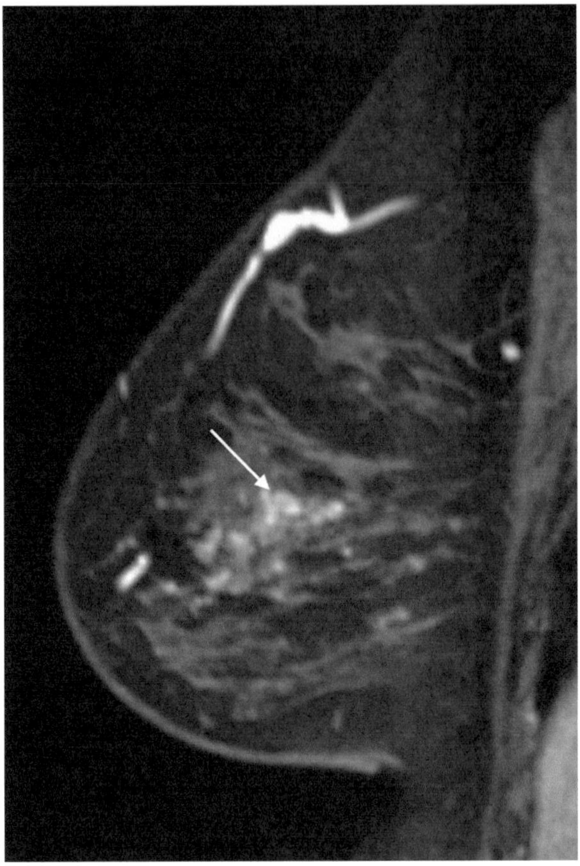

beneath the grid surface simultaneously so that access to both sites can be obtained without the need to reposition. In succession, both lesions are localised, anesthetized and then introducer stylets inserted prior to biopsies. If multiple lesions within a single breast cannot be positioned at the same time (or indeed there are bilateral lesions), then the more suspicious lesion is sampled first and sampling at this site completed (including marker deployment). If washout does occur because of the time elapsed between the gadolinium injection and biopsy at the second site, then landmarks may be adequate to guide the procedure.

12.4 Pitfalls and Limitations

Unfortunately despite the latest MRI technical developments there is a procedural failure rate. This rather varies in the literature as to the frequency but may be up to 25 % [40–44]. This will occur most commonly due to either non visualisation of the target lesion or an inaccessible target area. The target may not be seen because it has

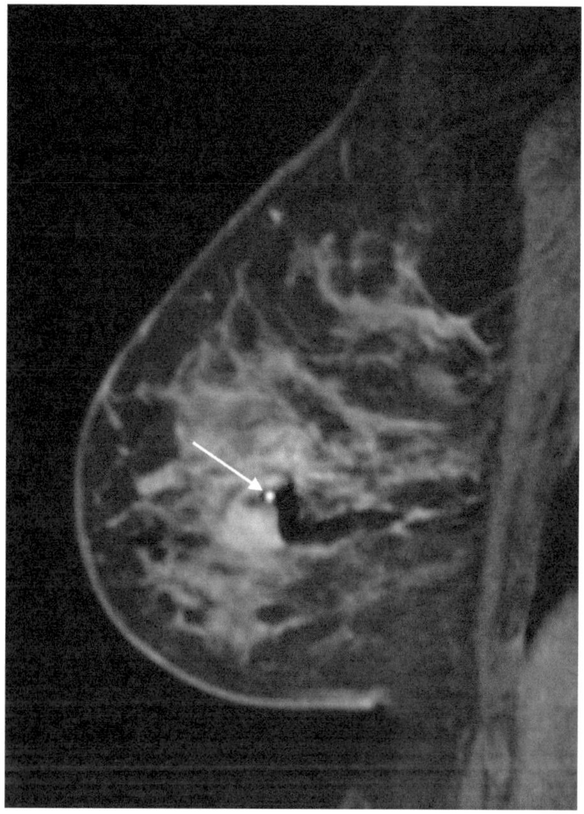

Fig. 12.9 A mid biopsy contrast enhanced sagittal image showing the needle within the target lesion (*arrow*). Biopsy related hematoma is demonstrated as signal dropout (*black* areas around the needle)

disappeared due to excessive compression. In this situation a further image could be performed with less breast compression. Alternatively the initial MRI may have been performed at the wrong time of the menstrual cycle and as such the target is no longer identifiable. This masking effect is more common in smaller sized targets (<5 mm), and where background enhancement may also obscure the area [40, 45]. If indeed the target demonstrates a clear decrease in size at the time of the procedure compared to the original MRI scan then that is an indication not to perform the biopsy.

Motion artefacts can also cause false positive findings on MRI in particular on subtraction images of the T1-weighted contrast enhanced series, where they result in hyperintense findings that could be interpreted as lesions of increased contrast enhancement. To avoid these false positives, the unsubtracted series should also be evaluated [17, 28]. Overly forceful breast compression may result in reduced contrast enhancement. If there is suspicion of this, then a repeat MRI with less breast compression would be recommended. Alternatively a delayed MRI sequence may sometimes be valuable in demonstrating the target even if the early subtraction views do not [33, 46].

Benign contrast uptake in premenopausal patients that are examined at a time other than during the second week of their menstrual cycle may increase the false positivity by 17 % [12]. If a hormonal cause for the contrast enhancement in the target lesion is suspected, an alternative approach would be to perform a follow up MRI examination [47, 48]. The malignancy rate of lesions that are not visible on a subsequent interventional MRI is low. A rate of 2 % has been reported relatively recently [22]. When lesions are no longer visible at the time of the procedure, a follow-up examination tuned to the menstrual cycle in a premenopausal woman may be performed, ideally at a 6-month interval [49]. It is more difficult to do this in patients undergoing MRI for local staging of a known breast carcinoma, as a delayed scan would undoubtedly interfere with their treatment pathway.

Superficial lesions and lesions near the nipple may be in a difficult location for biopsy. Also lesions that are far posterior in the breast near the chest wall or very lateral in the axillary tail may be inaccessible despite the best attempts at positioning. Placing the patient in the prone oblique position may allow access to the axillary tail and posterior breast tissue [36]. Lesions located posteromedially may sometimes be accessed by placing the affected breast in a contralateral coil. Minimizing padding on the coil may also be useful to reduce elevation of posterior breast tissue in certain situations [49].

Some breasts are too thin to accommodate the sampling aperture, even with the use of the reverse compression paddle. An alternative approach in these patients is an MRI guided needle localization followed by surgical excision.

The morbidity of MRI-guided vacuum-assisted biopsy is low [29, 37, 43, 50]. This is a similar rate to stereotactic procedures though higher than for ultrasound guided biopsies [51]. The most common complication is a hematoma and although generally minor, 10 % of procedures, however, have to be stopped because of adverse effects [29, 37, 52]. Bleeding requiring surgery only occurs in less than 1 % of procedures [29, 37]. Lack of significant breast compression during a sometimes prolonged procedure makes this more likely than with an ultrasound guided biopsy. In the largest multicenter study published to date, Perlet et al. [41] reported that complications occurred in only 17 of 538 (3 %) MRI-VABs using an 11G needle. Specifically, these cases involved five vasovagal reactions, one infected hematoma, six large hematomas (>3 cm) and five cases of significant bleeding during the intervention, two of which required surgical hemostasis. A more recent study involving 389 MRI-VABs using 9G and 10G needles [28] reports an even lower complication rate of 1 % (n = 4) [53].

12.5 Accuracy

Overall, MRI guided biopsy has a technical success rate of over 96 % in the larger studies regardless of lesion size and needle size [52, 54]. The malignancy rate varies widely (between 18 and 61 %) with a mean of 28 %, and this likely reflects patient cohort and local MRI evaluation variations across the world. The incidence of benign lesions exhibits a similar range of 18–70 %, with a mean of 62 %. Concordance between imaging and histopathology is as an essential component of

MRI-guided biopsies as it is with other image guided methods. Lee et al. found 7 % of MRI-guided vacuum-assisted biopsy results to be discordant, and of the discordant lesions that were surgically removed, malignancy was identified in 30 % [55]. This demonstrates the importance of imaging pathological correlation and implies a small but significant number of false negative MRI-guided biopsies although seemingly considerably higher than from breast biopsies on other imaging targeting methods. This elevated false negative rate on MRI biopsy likely relates to sampling not performed under real-time direct visualization and that lesion targeting cannot be as easily verified [56]. It may in part relate to the small size of many of the target lesions that are seen on MRI but are occult on all other imaging modalities. Another issue is patient cohort in that patients undergoing breast MRI and then subsequent MRI biopsy generally have a significantly higher prior probability of malignancy. Histology may show a specific concordant benign diagnosis such as lymph gland or fibroadenoma and no further action may be needed. Alternatively a follow up diagnostic MRI could be performed at 6 months particularly where no definitive concordant pathological diagnosis is obtained (for instance normal breast tissue). Lesions that are sufficiently suspicious on the diagnostic imaging can still be recommended for surgical excision if it is believed that there is lack of histological concordance.

Undersampling as with other image guided biopsies can occur with subsequent cancer found at surgery. In a study of 557 MRI guided biopsies, there was an increased upgrade rate after histological analysis of open surgical excision compared to stereotaxis and ultrasound guidance. The number of false negatives was 3 %, 1 % and 0.4 VAB procedures, respectively. Benign and high-risk lesions were also upgraded at a significantly higher rate after open surgical excision for the MRI-guided procedure than was the case for the other modalities [51]. A further recent retrospective review of 147 high risk lesions sampled at MRI guided 9G vacuum biopsy showed 20.4 % (n = 30) were upgraded at subsequent surgery. The upgrade rate was highest for atypical ductal hyperplasia, lobular carcinoma in situ, and radial scar. No imaging features were predictive of upgrade but this was significantly higher for women with a personal cancer history than for other indications combined ($p = 0.0114$) [57].

MRI guided wire localisation is very infrequently performed. The reasons for this are simple. Lesions that are identifiable only by breast MRI will invariably have been sampled by MRI guided biopsy and as has been discussed, a marker clip is deployed at the termination of this procedure and subsequently checked mammographically. Thus if the patient has an unfavourable histology from the biopsy and subsequently requires surgery, then the target can in all likelihood be localised at the very least by stereotaxis or mammographic guidance or may be even by ultrasound (if the clip is correctly sited and is identifiable on ultrasound). On the rare occasions that a patient has a suspicious MRI abnormality and has a specific contraindication to biopsy (or indeed refuses biopsy) then an MRI wire localisation may be required. Additionally an MRI guided bracketing wire localisation of a large target may better define the target volume in cases of extensive disease seen mainly on MRI but less well on mammography and sonographically (commonly invasive lobular breast cancer in women with relatively high breast density). In a similar way to performing an

MRI biopsy, the patient is consented, positioned and an MRI exam performed. The lesion is localised and local anesthesia is administered. A smaller volume is required as the needle guide for most wires are only 18–19.5G. An MRI compatible needle and wire are then inserted through the introducer and prior to deployment of the wire itself and removal of the needle, a check sequence is performed in order to verify position of the wire tip [58–60]. Following this the needle guide is repositioned (or removed if the wire tip location is optimal). The patient will then have the wire carefully secured and bandaged in order to prevent displacement prior to heading to surgery. In practice this procedure may be more easy to perform than an MRI guided biopsy and most certainly is often of shorter duration. Historically units that were just embarking on a breast MRI biopsy service commenced by performing these in a few cases, although nowadays breast MRI biopsy experience is far more widespread that new units should be able to get adequate exposure and thus commence a full MRI biopsy without performing localisations first. Due to the infrequent nature of these localisation procedures there is relatively little published data on their outcomes, although complication rates and accuracy appear similar to other modalities [58–60].

12.6 Conclusion

Suspicious breast lesions detectable only by MRI require an MRI-guided vacuum assisted breast biopsy. As well as clarifying that the other standard image-guided methods do not demonstrate the target, presence of a false positive abnormality should be excluded. A follow-up MRI typically at six months will be required in most cases where the procedure fails to identify the target seen on the original diagnostic MRI. For premenopausal women the procedure as well as any follow-up exams should optimally be scheduled during the second week of the menstrual cycle. MRI guided biopsy is a very safe procedure with a low complication rate and MRI guided wire localisation with subsequent surgical biopsy should be used only in rare cases. In the future, tools such as spectroscopy, newer software developments and higher magnetic strength fields may increase the specificity of MRI allowing better target selection for biopsy as well as possibly the detection of post-biopsy residual tumor. Breast MRI guided biopsy is an important skill for the breast radiologist in units with a significant breast MRI workload and will allow more optimal management of their patients.

References

1. Sardanelli F, Boetes C, Borisch B, Decker T, Federico M, Gilbert F, et al. Magnetic resonance imaging of the breast: recommendations from the EUSOMA working group. Eur J Cancer. 2010;46:1296–316.

2. Peters N, Borel R, Zuithoff N, Mali W, Moons K, Peeters P. Meta-analysis of MR imaging in the diagnosis of breast lesions. Radiology. 2008;246:116–24.
3. Orel SG, Schnall MD, LiVolsi VA, et al. Suspicious breast lesions: MR imaging with radiologie-pathologie correlation. Radiology. 1994;190:485–93.
4. Fischer U, Kopka L, Grabbe E. Breast carcinoma: effect of preoperative contrast-enhanced MR imaging on the therapeutic approach. Radiology. 1999;213:881–8.
5. American College of Radiology, ACR practice guideline for the performance of contrast-enhanced magnetic resonance imaging (MRI) of the breast, October 2004, Revised 2008, Available at: http://www.acr.org/SecondaryMainMenuCategories/qualitysafety/guidelines/breast/mribreast.aspx. Accessed 15 March 2010.
6. La Trenta LR, Menell J, Morris E, Abramson A, Dershaw D, Liberman L. Breast lesions detected with MR imaging: utility and histopathologic importance of identification with US. Radiology. 2003;227:856–61.
7. Thomassin-Naggara I, Chopier J, Trop I. Non mass-like enhancement at breast MR imaging: the added value of mammography and US for lesion categorization. Radiology. 2011;261:69—79.
8. Meissnitzer M, Dershaw D, Lee C, Morris E. Targeted ultrasound of the breast in women with abnormal MRI findings for whom biopsy has been recommended. Am J Roentgenol. 2009; 193:1025–9.
9. Fiaschetti V, Salimbeni C, Gaspari E, Dembele G, Bolacchi F, Cossu E, et al. The role of second-look ultrasound of BI-RADS-3 mammary lesions detected by breast MR imaging. Eur J Radiol. 2012;81:3178–84.
10. Ha G, Yi M, Lee K, Youn H, Jung S. Clinical outcome of magnetic resonance imaging-detected additional lesions in breast cancer patients. J Breast Cancer. 2011;14:213–8.
11. Park V, Kim M, Kim E, Moon H. Second-look US: how to find breast lesions with a suspicious MR-imaging appearance. Radiographics. 2013;33:1361–75.
12. Demartini WB, Eby PR, Peacock S, et al. Utility of targeted sonography for breast lesions that were suspicious on MRI. Am J Roentgenol. 2009;192:1128–34.
13. Abe H, Schmidt RA, Shah RN, et al. MR-directed ("second-look") ultra-sound examination for breast lesions detected initially on MRI: MR and sonographic findings. Am J Roentgenol. 2010;194:370–7.
14. Dietzel M, Baltzer PA, Vag T, et al. Magnetic resonance mammography in small vs. advanced breast lesions – systematic comparison reveals significant impact of lesion size on diagnostic accuracy in 936 histologically verified breast lesions. Fortschr Röntgenstr. 2011;183:126–35.
15. Hefler L, Casselman J, Amaya B, et al. Follow-up of breast lesions detected by MRI not biopsied due to absent enhancement of contrast medium. Eur Radiol. 2003;13:344–6.
16. Sadowski E, Kelez F. Frequency of malignancy in lesions classified as probably benign after dynamic contrast- enhanced breast MRI examination. J Magn Reson Imaging. 2005;21:556–64.
17. Liberman L, Mason G, Morris E, Dershaw D. Does size matter? Positive predictive value of MRI-detected breast lesions as a function of lesion size. Am J Roentgenol. 2006;186:426–30.
18. Potet J, Weber-Donat G, Thome A, Valbousquet L, Peroux E, Konopacki J, et al. Periprocedural management of hemostasis risk in interventional radiology. J Radiol. 2011;92:659–70.
19. Somerville P, Seifert P, Destounis S, Murphy P, Young W. Anti- coagulation and bleeding risk after core needle biopsy. Am J Roentgenol. 2008;191:1194–7.
20. Wallis M, Tardivon A, Helbich T, Scheer I, European Society of Breast Imaging. Guidelines from the European Society of Breast Imaging for diagnostic interventional breast proce- dures. Eur Radiol. 2007;17:581–8.
21. Heywang-Köbrunner S, Sinnatamby R, Lebeau A, Lebrecht A, Britton P, Scheer I, et al. Interdisciplinary consensus on the uses and technique of MR-guided vacuum-assisted breast biopsy (VAB): results of a European consensus meeting. Eur J Radiol. 2009;72:289–94.
22. Brennan SB, Sung JS, Dershaw DD, et al. Cancellation of MR imaging- guided breast biopsy due to lesion nonvisualization: frequency and follow-up. Radiology. 2011;261:92–9.
23. Elsamaloty H, Elzawawi M, Mohammad S, Herial N. Increasing accuracy of detection of breast cancer with 3-T MRI. Am J Roentgenol. 2009;192:1142–8.

24. Fischer U, Vosshenrich R, Keating D, Bruhn H, Döler W, Oestmann J, et al. MR-guided biopsy of suspect breast lesions with a simple stereotaxic add-on device for surface coils. Radiology. 1994;192:272–3.
25. Viehweg P, Heinig A, Amya B, et al. MR-guided interventional breast procedures considering vacuum biopsy in particular. Eur J Radiol. 2002;42:32–9.
26. Trop I, Labelle M, David J, Mayrand M, Lalonde L. Second-look targeted studies after breast magnetic resonance imaging: pratical tips to improve lesion identification. Curr Probl Diagn Radiol. 2010;39:200–11.
27. Kuhl C. The current status of breast MR imaging. Part I. Choice of tech- nique, image interpretation, diagnostic accuracy, and transfer to clinical practice. Radiology. 2007;244:356–78.
28. Han B, Schnall M, Orel S, Rosen M. Outcome of MRI-guided breast biopsies. Am J Roentgenol. 2008;191:1798–804.
29. Liberman L, Bracero N, Morris E, Thornton C, Dershaw D. MRI- guided 9-gauge vacuum-assisted breast biopsy: initial clinical experience. Am J Roentgenol. 2005;185:183–93.
30. Hauth E, Jaeger H, Lubnau J, Maderwald S, Otterbach F, Kimmig R, et al. MR-guided vacuum-assisted breast biopsy with a handheld biopsy system: clinical experience and results in postinterventional MR mammography after 24 h. Eur Radiol. 2008;18:168–76.
31. Malhaire C, El Khoury C, Thibault F, Athanasiou A, Petrow P, Ollivier L, et al. Vacuum-assisted biopsies under MR guidance: results of 72 procedures. Eur Radiol. 2010;20:1554–62.
32. Heywang-Köbrunner S, Heinig A, Schaumloeffel-Schulze U, Viehweg P, Buchmann J, Lampe D, et al. MR-guided percutaneous excisional and incisional biopsy of breast lesions. Eur Radiol. 1999;9:1656–65.
33. Lee J, Kaplan J, Murray M, Liberman L. Complete excision of the MRI target lesion at MRI-guided vacuum-assisted biopsy of breast cancer. Am J Roentgenol. 2008;191:1198–202.
34. Schrading S, Simon B, Braun M, Wardelmann E, Schild H, Kuhl C. MRI-guided breast biopsy: influence of choise of vacuum biopsy system on the mode of biopsy of MRI-only suspicious breast lesions. Am J Roentgenol. 2010;194:1650–7.
35. Kuhl C, Elevelt A, Leutner C, Gieseke J, Pakos E, Schild H. Interventional breast MR imaging: clinical use of a stereotactic localization and biopsy device. Radiology. 1997;204:667–75.
36. Liberman L, Morris E, Dershaw D, Thornton C, Van Zee K, Tan L. Fast MRI-guided vacuum-assisted breast biopsy: initial experience. Am J Roentgenol. 2003;181:1283–93.
37. Orel S, Rosen M, Mies C, Schnall M. MR imaging-guided 9-gauge vacuum-assisted core-needle breast biopsy: initial experience. Radiology. 2006;238:54–61.
38. Thomassin-Naggara I, Lalonde L, David J, Darai E, Uzan S, Trop I. A plea for biopsy marker: how, why and why not clipping after breast biopsy? Breast Cancer Res Treat. 2012;132:881–93.
39. Perretta T, Pistolese C, Bolacchi F, Cossu E, Fiaschetti V, Simonetti G. MR imaging-guided 10-gauge vacuum-assisted breast biopsy: histological characterisation. Radiol Med. 2008; 113:830–40.
40. Viehweg P, Bernerth T, Kiechle M, Buchmann J, Heinig A, Koelbl H, et al. MR-guided intervention in women with a family history of breast cancer. Eur J Radiol. 2006;57:81–9.
41. Perlet C, Heinig A, Prat S, Casselman J, Baath L, Sittek H, et al. Multicenter study for the evaluation of a dedicated breast biopsy device for MR-guided vacuum biopsy of the breast. Eur Radiol. 2002;12:1463–70.
42. Tozaki M, Yamashiro N, Sakamoto M, Sakamoto N, Mizuuchi N, Fukuma E. Magnetic resonance-guided vacuum-assisted breast biopsy: results in 100 japanese women. Jpn J Radiol. 2010;28:527–33.
43. Perlet C, Schneider P, Amaya B, Grosse A, Sittek H, Reiser M, et al. MR-guided vacuum biopsy of 206 contrast-enhancing breast lesions. Rofo. 2002;174:88–95.
44. Oxner CR, Vora L, Yim J, et al. Magnetic resonance imaging-guided breast biopsy in lesions not visualized by mammogram or ultrasound. Am Surg. 2012;78:1087–90.
45. Hefler L, Casselman J, Amaya B, Heinig A, Alberich T, Koelbl H, et al. Follow-up of breast lesions detected by MRI not biopsied due to absent enhancement of contrast medium. Eur Radiol. 2003;13:344–6.

46. Kuhl CK, Leutner C, Mielcarek P, et al. Breast compression interferes with lesion enhancement in contrast-enhanced breast MR imaging [abstract]. Radiology. 1997;205:538.
47. Morris E, Liberman L, Dershaw D, Kaplan J, La Trenta L, Abramson A, et al. Preoperative MR imaging-guided needle localization of breast lesions. Am J Roentgenol. 2002;178:1211–20.
48. Deurloo E, Peterse J, Rutgers E, Besnard A, Muller S, Gilhuijs K. Additional breast lesions in patients eligible for breast-conserving therapy by MRI: impact on preoperative management and potential benefit of computerised analysis. Eur J Cancer. 2005;41:1393–401.
49. Ikeda D. Progress report from the American College of Radiology Breast MR Imaging Lexicon Committee. Magn Reson Imaging Clin N Am. 2001;9:295–302.
50. Lehman C, Deperi E, Peacok S, McDonough M, De Martini W, Shook J. Clinical experience with MRI-guided vacuum-assisted breast biopsy. Am J Roentgenol. 2005;184:1782–7.
51. Imschweiler T, Haueisen H, Kampmann G, Rageth L, Seifert B, Rageth C, et al. MRI-guided vacuum-assisted breast biopsy: comparison with stereotactically guided and ultrasound-guided techniques. Eur Radiol. 2014;24:128–35.
52. Gebauer B, Bostanjogio M, Moesta K, Schneider W, Schlag P, Felix R. Magnetic resonance-guided biopsy of suspicious breast lesions with a hand-held vacuum biopsy device. Acta Radiol. 2006;47:907–13.
53. Plantade R, Thomassin-Naggara I. MRI vacuum-assisted breast biopsies. Diagn Interv Imaging. 2014 Sep;95(9):779–801. doi:10.1016/j.diii.2013.12.023.
54. Linda A, Zuiani C, Londero V, Bazzocchi M. Outcome of initially only magnetic resonance mammography-detected findings with and without correlate at second-look sonography: distribution according to patient history of breast cancer and lesion size. Breast. 2008;17:51–7.
55. Lee J-M, Kaplan JB, Murray MP, et al. Imaging-histologic discordance at MRI-guided 9-gauge vacuum-assisted breast biopsy. AJR Am J Roentgenol. 2007;189:852–9.
56. Sim L, Hendricks J, Bult P, Fook-Chong S. US correlation for MRI-detected breast lesions in women with familial risk of breast cancer. Clin Radiol. 2005;60:801–6.
57. Heller SL, Elias K, Gupta A, Greenwood HI, Mercado CL, Moy L. Outcome of high-risk lesions at MRI-guided 9-gauge vacuum- assisted breast biopsy. AJR Am J Roentgenol. 2014 Jan;202(1):237–45. doi:10.2214/AJR.13.10600.
58. Fischer U, Rodenwaldt J, Hundermark C, Döler W, Grabbe E. MRI-assisted biopsy and localization of the breast. Radiologie. 1997;37:692–701.
59. Lampe D, Hefler L, Alberich T, Sittek H, Perlet C, Prat X, et al. The clinical value of preoperative wire localization of breast lesions by magnetic resonance imaging: a multicenter study. Breast Cancer Res Treat. 2002;75:175–9.
60. Eby P, Lehman C. Magnetic resonance image-guided breast interventions. Top Magn Reson Imaging. 2008;19:151–62.

Chapter 13
Breast MRI and the Benign Breast Biopsy

Amy M. Fowler and Wendy B. DeMartini

Abstract This chapter, appearing in the section on MRI Findings, Interpretation, and Management, reviews the issues relevant to benign MRI-guided biopsy results. The discussion includes challenges in assessing radiologic-pathologic concordance specific to MRI, approaches for discordant biopsy results, and a review of the literature on appropriate imaging follow-up recommendations for benign concordant MRI-guided breast biopsy results. High risk lesions from MRI-guided biopsy are addressed in a separate chapter.

Keywords Benign • MRI-guided biopsy • Radiologic-pathologic concordance • Discordance • Management • Recommendations • Follow-up imaging

Abbreviations

ACR	American College of Radiology
BI-RADS®	Breast Imaging-Reporting and Data System
ER+	Estrogen receptor-positive
HER2	Human epidermal growth factor receptor 2
MRI	Magnetic resonance imaging
PACS	Picture archiving and communication systems
PPV	Positive predictive value
PR+	Progesterone receptor-positive

A.M. Fowler, MD, PhD (✉)
Department of Radiology, University of Wisconsin School of Medicine and Public Health, 600 Highland Avenue, MC 3252, Madison, WI 53792-3252, USA
e-mail: afowler@uwhealth.org

W.B. DeMartini, MD
Department of Radiology, Stanford University School of Medicine, 300 Pasteur Drive, Palo Alto, CA 94305, USA

S.L. Heller, L. Moy (eds.), *Breast Oncology: Techniques, Indications, and Interpretation*, DOI 10.1007/978-3-319-42563-4_13

13.1 Introduction

Breast MRI utilization is increasing in clinical practice in the United States. Nearly 11.5 breast MRI examinations per 1000 women undergoing breast imaging were reported to have occurred in 2009 [1]. Clinical indications for contrast-enhanced breast MRI include supplemental screening for women with greater than 20 % lifetime risk of breast cancer, preoperative planning for women with newly diagnosed breast cancer, evaluation of response to neoadjuvant chemotherapy, and occult primary tumor localization in women presenting with biopsy-proven metastatic axillary lymphadenopathy [2].

Breast MRI is the most sensitive modality for breast cancer detection [3]. When used as a supplement to mammography for high risk screening, the cancer detection rate increases from approximately 8.2 to 26.1 per 1000 women [4]. However, breast MRI is not a perfect test and its specificity is lower than its sensitivity due to overlapping imaging features of benign and malignant lesions [3]. For example, the current American College of Radiology (ACR) Breast Imaging-Reporting and Data System (BI-RADS®) practice benchmark for positive predictive value of biopsies performed (PPV_3) is 20–50 % for breast MRI screening programs [5]. Thus, many biopsies will yield benign results. It is imperative that radiologists have a solid understanding of the management of benign results, including the assessment of adequate tissue sampling, the process for determining whether the histopathologic result appropriately explains the imaging finding, and recommendations for follow-up imaging. This chapter focuses on these important issues surrounding benign MRI-guided breast biopsy results. The management of high risk lesions identified at MRI-guided biopsy is not addressed in this chapter.

13.2 Radiologic-Pathologic Concordance for MRI-Guided Breast Biopsies

Percutaneous biopsy is preferred over needle localization and surgical excision for findings visualized only on MRI [6, 7]. If percutaneous biopsy results are benign and concordant, unnecessary surgical excisional biopsy and its associated greater cost, time, morbidity, and cosmetic changes can be avoided. For patients with malignant results, surgical planning can be optimized reducing the total number of surgeries required for complete breast cancer treatment. MRI-guided breast biopsy has been shown to be a safe alternative to MRI-guided wire localization and excisional biopsy with comparable diagnostic accuracy [8–11].

A critical component that is essential for robust diagnostic accuracy of MRI-guided breast biopsy procedures is determination of radiologic-pathologic concordance. A biopsy result is defined as concordant when the histopathology sufficiently explains the imaging findings that prompted the recommendation for biopsy (see Fig. 13.1) [12]. A discordant result is one in which the histopathology

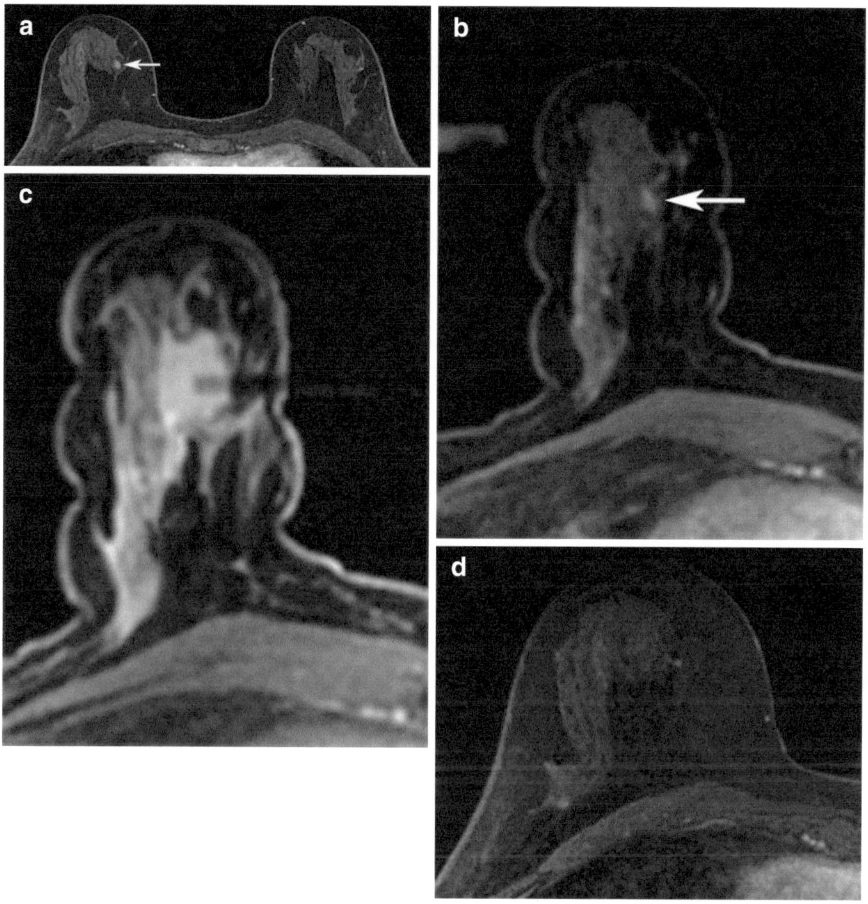

Fig. 13.1 Fifty-five-year-old asymptomatic woman undergoing screening breast MRI for elevated lifetime risk of breast cancer due to family history. (**a**) Axial T1-weighted post-contrast images demonstrated a 5 mm oval mass (*white arrow*) with circumscribed margins and heterogeneous internal enhancement in the right breast at 5 o'clock middle depth with initial rapid and delayed washout kinetics (BI-RADS® 4A). Targeted ultrasound showed no correlate. (**b**) MRI-guided biopsy was performed of the right breast mass (*white arrow*) using a medial approach with ten specimens obtained from a 9 gauge vacuum-assisted device. (**c**) Axial contrast-enhanced post-biopsy sequences demonstrated hematoma at the expected site of biopsy. Histopathology results were benign (breast tissue with cysts, fibrosis, apocrine metaplasia, and usual ductal hyperplasia) and concordant. (**d**) Six-month follow-up MRI was recommended which demonstrated susceptibility artifact from the biopsy clip and no residual enhancing mass (BI-RADS® 2)

does not explain the imaging findings and most often occurs when a benign pathology is reported for a highly suspicious imaging finding.

The purpose of determining concordance is to minimize the potential for false-negative biopsies resulting from inadequate sampling or inaccurate targeting and to avoid a delayed diagnosis of cancer. The frequency of inadequate tissue sampling of

MRI lesions has been reported as 6–14 % [13–15]. Use of vacuum-assisted devices, typically with 9 gauge needles, are encouraged which yield generous amounts of tissue for thorough histopathologic examination [7]. As for other breast imaging modalities, when a malignancy is detected within one year at the site of a benign MRI-guided biopsy it is considered a false-negative [5]. False-negative rates for MRI-guided breast biopsies range from 0.9 to 11.7 % [10, 13–17]. Accurate determination of a program's false-negative biopsy rate is inherently challenging due to the potential lack of patient follow-up at the same institution. Audit data linkage with state or regional cancer registries can be helpful to improve the accuracy of false-negative biopsy rate.

Information used in determination of radiologic-pathologic concordance starts at the time of the diagnostic examination. A BI-RADS® assessment of 5 (highly suggestive of malignancy) indicates that a benign biopsy result should, in most instances, be deemed discordant. Furthermore, subcategorization of BI-RADS® 4 assessments into 4A, 4B, and 4C (low, moderate, and high suspicion for malignancy, respectively) is also informative. In contrast to mammography and ultrasound, subcategories for BI-RADS® 4 assessments are not included for MRI in the most current edition of the BI-RADS® Atlas [5]. However, subcategorization of BI-RADS® 4 assessments can be particularly useful for breast MRI radiologic-pathologic correlation because the level of concern for malignancy is more stratified. For example, a lesion with a 4C assessment that yields benign biopsy results should be reviewed with particular scrutiny. Particular benign pathologies that are well-known to present as suspicious imaging findings, such as fat necrosis, could be considered concordant in these instances.

Assessing the adequacy of tissue sampling at the time of biopsy also contributes to concordance determination. Immediate post-biopsy images are obtained and reviewed during the procedure to allow for adjustment and additional sampling if needed. Some practices perform a second injection of contrast to revisualize the lesion [11]. However, the presence of blood and air in the biopsy cavity frequently limits the utility of this approach.

Adequate communication with the interpreting pathologist is another key factor in optimizing radiologic-pathologic concordance. Inclusion of key clinical information, indication for biopsy, imaging features of the biopsied lesion, potential differential diagnoses based on imaging, and the BI-RADS® assessment on the pathology requisition form provides a quick and focused method for conveying this important information. For complicated cases or those with unusual or unexpected histopathologic results, the pathologist may contact the radiologist who performed the procedure with specific questions before issuing their final report. Being available and engaged in these conversations further improves radiologic-pathologic concordance and strengthens the multi-disciplinary approach to patient care.

Once biopsy results are issued by pathology, the methods used for assessing radiologic-pathologic concordance vary by institution and practice type. One approach involves a dedicated multidisciplinary clinical conference. The radiologist presents the clinical history and imaging studies performed before, during, and after the biopsy to demonstrate initial findings and level of suspicion for malignancy, adequate targeting and sampling, and appropriate marker clip placement. This is followed by presentation of the histopathologic results by the pathologist. Group consensus is reached regarding concordance, and management recommendations are determined. This method can foster interdepartmental professional relationships and can be achieved in this modern electronic era through remote Picture archiving and communication systems (PACS) and scanned histology slides through programs available on the internet and/or video-conferencing. An approach such as this may be more amenable to implementation at teaching institutions. For settings in which it might not be practical for a physical radiology-pathology correlation conference such as high-volume clinical services, the radiologist may perform dedicated review of imaging findings independently or together with other radiologists in the group using the written pathology report.

Determining radiologic-pathologic concordance relies upon knowledge of the acceptable histopathology for particular imaging findings. For breast MRI, most of the research has focused on the imaging features that are predictive of malignancy. For example, foci have been shown to have lower probabilities of malignancy compared to masses or non-mass enhancement [18]. For masses on MRI, margins have been found to be an important imaging predictor [19, 20]. However, there are relatively few data regarding the MRI features that are associated with particular benign histopathology outcomes. Biopsies of breast MRI findings have been shown to result in a spectrum of benign, concordant histopathology results. These include nonspecific findings such as fibrocystic change, sclerosing adenosis, fibrosis, pseudoangiomatous stromal hyperplasia, and normal breast parenchyma [20, 21]. More specific benign and concordant results include fibroadenoma, papilloma, and lymph node. In general, nonspecific results have been more frequently associated with non-mass enhancement [20, 21], but further studies are warranted to clarify acceptable MRI lesion and histopathology outcomes.

Once radiologic-pathologic correlation has been performed and concordance has been determined, management recommendations are made and communicated to the referring physician and the patient. Patients with malignant results are referred to a breast surgeon and/or medical oncologist for treatment. Management of patients with benign results that are discordant and those with benign results that are concordant are discussed in the subsequent sections of this chapter. Importantly, an addendum is made to the original biopsy report with the histopathologic results, radiologic-pathologic concordance, and management recommendations.

Practice guidelines regarding MRI-guided breast biopsy procedures have been published by the American College of Radiology (ACR) and as a report from a European interdisciplinary consensus meeting [6, 7]. The ACR states that the physician who performed the procedure "is responsible for obtaining results of the histopathologic sampling to determine if the lesion has been adequately biopsied and is concordant or discordant with the imaging findings" [7]. The European interdisciplinary consensus report recommends "all available clinical and imaging information and VAB results be compared and discussed in an interdisciplinary conference to achieve a consensus recommendation in each case" [6]. These reports reinforce the importance of assessing concordance.

For several reasons, radiologic-pathologic concordance is more challenging for MRI-guided biopsies compared to stereotactic- and ultrasound-guided biopsies. First, there is no specimen radiograph to confirm adequate sampling due to the lack of tissue enhancement *ex vivo*. Second, there is no "real-time" visualization of the needle at the time of tissue sampling since the biopsy is performed when the patient is outside of the magnet. Determining whether the targeted finding has been appropriately sampled on post-biopsy MRI sequences has limitations as lesions with washout contrast kinetics become less conspicuous over time while enhancement of normal breast parenchyma increases. Also, lesions can be obscured by hematoma and air on post-biopsy sequences. These factors together with the higher pre-test probability of malignancy in women undergoing breast MRI support adopting a careful approach to radiologic-pathologic concordance to avoid a delayed cancer diagnosis.

13.3 Discordant MRI-Guided Breast Biopsy Results

A discordant biopsy result is one in which the histopathology does not sufficiently explain the imaging findings [12]. The discordance rates for MRI-guided breast biopsies using vacuum-assisted devices range from 0 to 9 % [9, 10, 22–26]. The rates of discordant biopsies are higher for MRI-guided biopsies compared with stereotactic- or ultrasound-guided biopsies (approximately 3 %) [12, 24]. Interestingly, discordance has not been shown to occur more often with BI-RADS® category 5 compared with category 4 lesions or to occur more often for radiologists with less experience with MRI-guided biopsies, factors that are known to affect discordance rates for stereotactic- and ultrasound-guided biopsies [24].

Further tissue sampling is warranted in cases of discordant MRI-guided biopsy results (see Fig. 13.2) [6, 7]. Options include repeat MRI-guided biopsy or surgical excision. The method used for preoperative wire localization prior to surgical excision includes mammographic-guidance if the marker clip placement is deemed appropriate. If there is significant clip displacement and mammographic landmarks are lacking, MRI-guided wire localization can be performed. The malignancy rate for discordant lesions that subsequently undergo surgical excision is 30–50 % [22, 24]. Thus, appropriate recognition and management of discordant lesions is clinically significant.

For discordant lesions undergoing repeat MRI-guided biopsy, radiologic-pathologic concordance should again be determined. Similarly, review of final histopathologic results for cases recommended for surgical excision are informative and recommended [6]. Important factors to note include the presence or absence of prior biopsy site changes in the excised specimen and whether any residual lesion exists in the specimen as well as final histopathologic size since small lesions may be completely removed during the biopsy procedure.

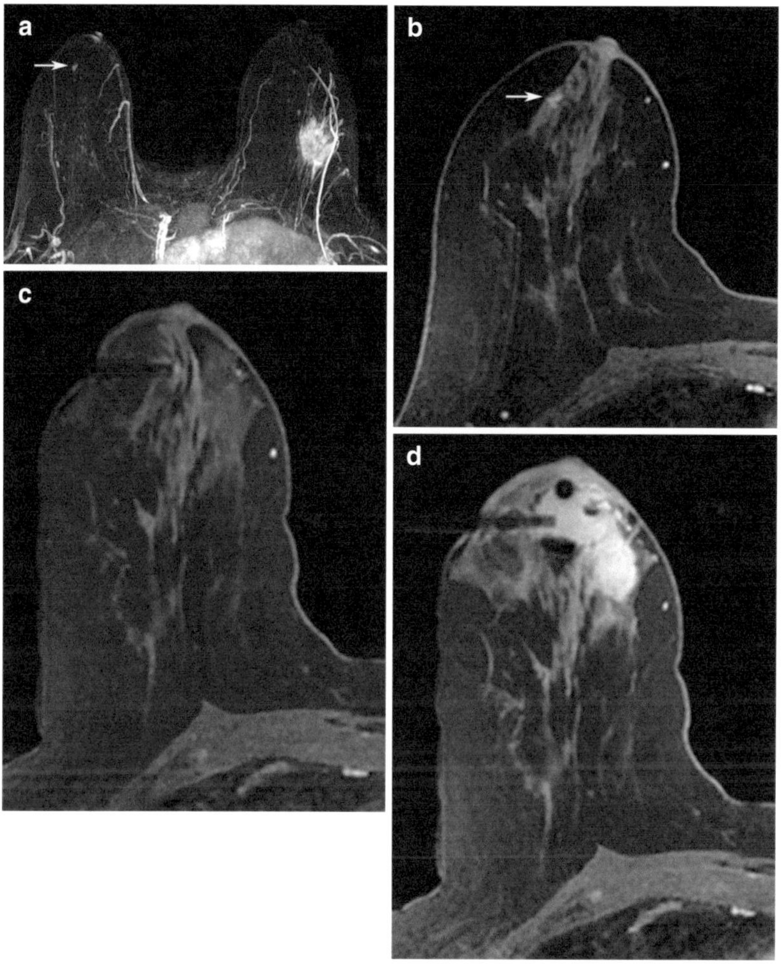

Fig. 13.2 Forty-nine-year-old woman with newly diagnosed left breast cancer undergoing preoperative breast MRI for extent of disease evaluation. (**a**) Maximum intensity projection images demonstrate the biopsy-proven malignant mass in the left breast and a 6 mm irregular mass (*white arrow*) with irregular margins and homogeneous internal enhancement in the right breast at 9 o'clock anterior depth with initial rapid and delayed plateau kinetics (BI-RADS® 4B). Axial T1-weighted post-contrast images of the right breast mass (*white arrow*) are shown in (**b**). (**c**) MRI-guided biopsy was performed of the right breast mass using a lateral approach with 8 specimens obtained from a 9 gauge vacuum-assisted device. Preferential sampling was performed in the superior and lateral directions to account for patient motion noted after targeting. (**d**) Post-biopsy hematoma was located in the expected site of biopsy. Histopathology results were benign breast tissue. The anterior location of the lesion and relative lack of sufficient compression to prevent motion were inherent technical challenges encountered since the patient was undergoing bilateral MRI-guided breast biopsies for an additional lesion in the left breast located at middle to posterior depth. (**e**) Review of post-biopsy images demonstrated a persistent enhancing mass (*white arrow*) indicating insufficient tissue sampling. The benign biopsy result was deemed discordant and repeat MRI-guided biopsy of the right breast was performed with more anterior compression. Histopathology results were ductal carcinoma in situ, low grade, ER+PR+

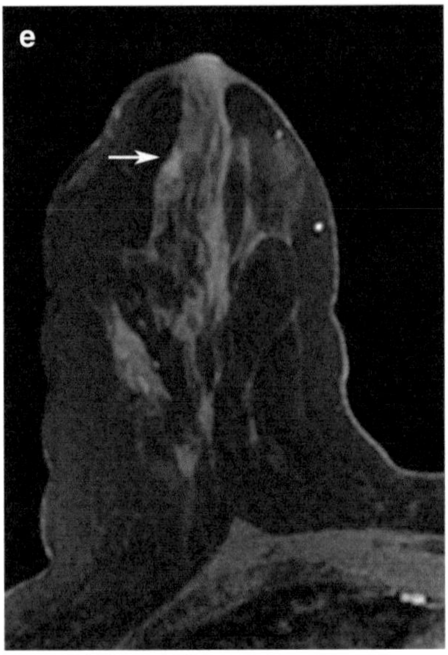

Fig. 13.2 (continued)

13.4 Management Recommendations for Patients with Benign Concordant Biopsy Results

Due to the challenges involved in confirming adequate sampling at the time of the MRI-guided biopsy procedure, a follow-up MRI examination is recommended for patients with benign concordant biopsy results to identify any delayed false-negative cases. The overall cancer yield at follow up-MRI has been reported as 0.9–2.3 % [13, 16, 17, 20]. The recommendation for follow-up MRI also includes when biopsies of suspicious MRI findings are performed using ultrasound guidance of presumed correlates identified on MRI-targeted ultrasound. The rationale for this recommendation is based on the results of Meissnitzer et al. which demonstrated that the presumed correlate on ultrasound did not correspond to the MRI finding of concern in 12.5 % of cases (10/80) with 5 cancers diagnosed in 9 lesions that underwent subsequent MRI-guided biopsy [27].

Ideally, the follow-up examination should be performed at the same institution using the same imaging acquisition protocol to best evaluate for potential interval change. Two studies have described an increase in the largest lesion dimension by 10 % as evidence of an interval size change, but there is no standardized definition for what constitutes clinically significant change [13, 16]. Lesions demonstrating concerning enlargement or development of more suspicious imaging features should undergo repeat biopsy or surgical excision (see Fig. 13.3) [16]. If the biopsied lesion decreases in size or resolves completely on the follow-up MRI, adequate sampling

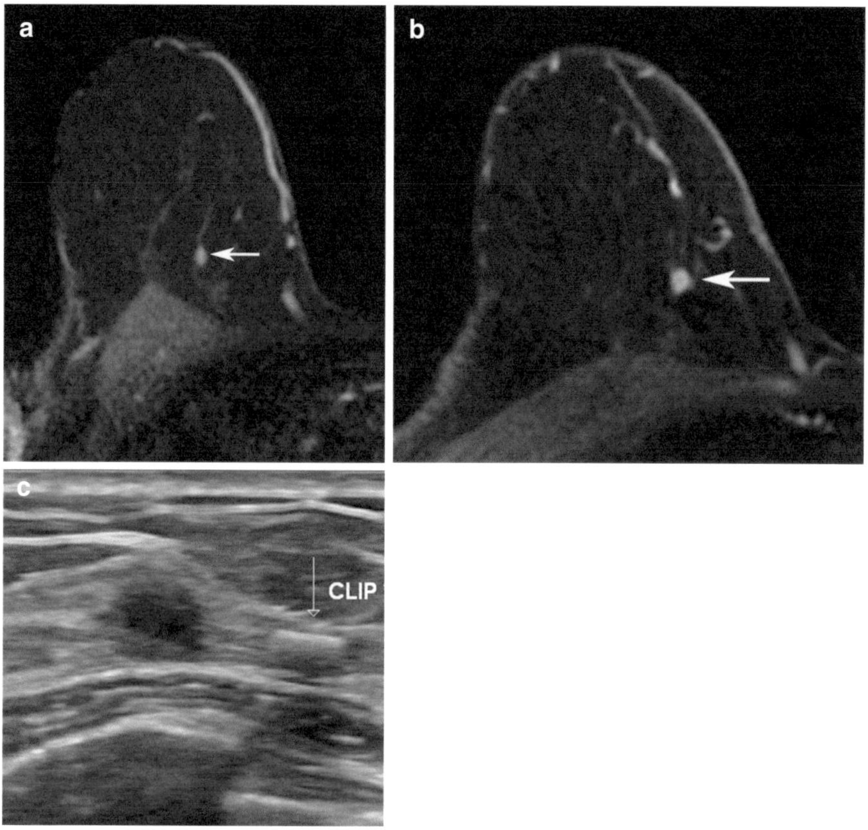

Fig. 13.3 Seventy-four-year-old woman with a personal history of prior treated right breast cancer and BRCA1 gene mutation undergoing asymptomatic screening breast MRI. (**a**) Axial T1-weighted post-contrast images demonstrated a new 3 mm focus of enhancement (*white arrow*) in the right breast at 1 o'clock posterior depth with initial rapid and delayed plateau kinetics (BI-RADS® 4A). MRI-guided biopsy was performed and ten specimens were obtained using a 9 gauge vacuum-assisted device. Histopathology results were benign and concordant. Six-month follow-up MRI was recommended. (**b**) Axial T1-weighted post-contrast images demonstrated a 6 mm round mass with a circumscribed margin and homogeneous enhancement (*white arrow*) in the right breast at 1 o'clock posterior depth with initial rapid and delayed plateau kinetics (BI-RADS® 4B). Susceptibility artifact from the previous placed MRI-guided biopsy clip was present along the posterior aspect of the mass. (**c**) Targeted ultrasound demonstrated an irregular hypoechoic mass with indistinct margins which correlated with the mass seen on MRI. A biopsy clip was noted adjacent to the mass. Histopathology results from ultrasound-guided biopsy were invasive ductal carcinoma, grade 2, ER-PR-HER2-

is confirmed and no further surveillance is required [15, 16]. This approach is supported by data of Dratwa et al. that showed no interval change at a 12 month follow-up MRI for 117 benign concordant lesions that had decreased or resolved at the initial 6 month examination [20].

There is currently no consensus on the optimal interval for the initial follow-up MRI nor the duration of follow-up imaging. In general, initial follow-up MRI is performed at 6–12 months after the index MRI [7, 28]. Several studies have been reported that recommend 6 month follow-up for all benign concordant lesions [9, 14, 15, 23, 25, 26, 28, 29]. Others base the follow-up interval on the specificity of the histopathologic result. For example, follow-up MRI is recommended at 6 months and 12 months after a nonspecific benign concordant biopsy result and at 12 months for a specific result such as a fibroadenoma, fat necrosis, or benign lymph node [11]. One study proposes that specific benign concordant diagnoses may not require further follow-up MRI [10]. Further evidence is necessary to support guidelines for optimal follow-up MRI interval.

For lesions that are stable on the initial follow-up MRI (see Fig. 13.4), recommendations for subsequent imaging are mixed. Some recommend returning to routine screening [9]. Given the potential uncertainty of adequate sampling during the biopsy procedure, others recommend continued follow-up MRI in 6–12 months [15, 16].

Studies investigating the short-term and long-term outcomes of benign concordant biopsy results are increasing in number [13–17]. Li et al. reported results from a retrospective review of 177 lesions with benign concordant MRI-guided biopsy results. Although the follow-up recommendations varied at the discretion of the procedure radiologist, all cases had follow-up MRI within 12 months [13]. Most of the lesions (155/177) had decreased in size or resolved at the initial follow-up MRI with no subsequent cancer diagnosis. Seventeen lesions were felt to warrant a second biopsy and four were found to be cancers, for an overall cancer yield of 2.3 % (4/177). All cancers detected were ≤1.0 cm in pathologic size, lymph node negative, and occurred in women with a personal history of breast cancer. Two cancers presented as enlarging non-mass enhancement at 6 and 12 months after the initial benign concordant biopsies. Given the potential for detection of false negatives, a 6 month follow-up interval was deemed most appropriate by this research group [30, 31].

A recent retrospective study by Dratwa et al. reported that 1.7 % (2/119) of benign concordant lesions displayed interval increase in size at the 6 month follow-up MRI [20]. Both lesions underwent surgical excision and yielded malignancy. These results also support an initial 6 month follow-up MRI recommendation.

While a 6 month follow-up MRI is a conservative method for minimizing delayed false-negative biopsies, some disadvantages exist to this approach. New lesions requiring further workup can occur on the follow-up MRI. While new cancers can be discovered (3/12, 25 %) as in Li et al. [13], additional false-positive findings may also occur. Furthermore, patient compliance is integral for the effectiveness of short-interval follow-up imaging. Rates of compliance for 6 month follow-up MRI are 43–63 % [16, 17, 29, 32]. Women with the indication of high-risk screening for the initial MRI are more likely to return for follow-up imaging compared to women having MRI for problem-solving or for extent of disease [17]. Women referred from outside institutions are less likely to be compliant with recommended follow-up

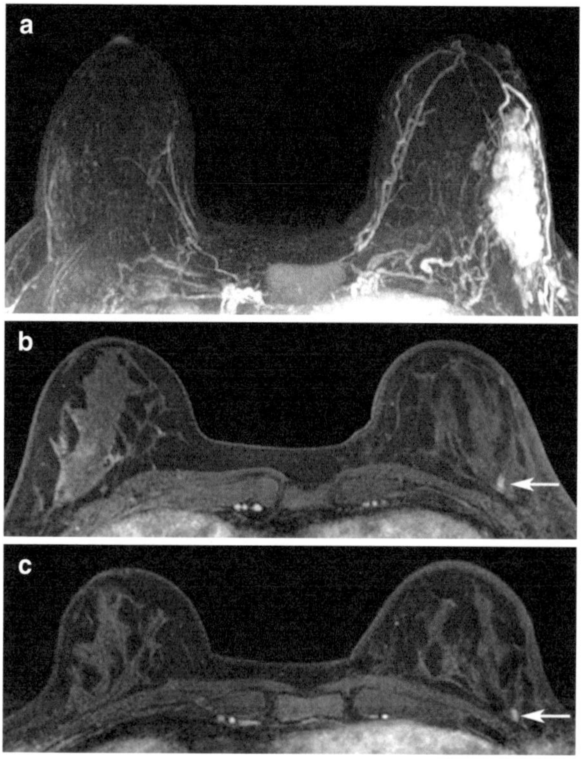

Fig. 13.4 Thirty-two-year-old woman undergoing asymptomatic screening breast MRI for a personal history of treated left breast cancer. (**a**) Maximum intensity projection images from the initial MRI examination performed for extent of disease evaluation demonstrate the biopsy-proven malignant mass in the left breast. The patient underwent left breast lumpectomy with oncoplastic reduction, radiation therapy, and right breast reduction surgery. Final surgical margins were negative for carcinoma. (**b**) The patient's first screening MRI was performed 10 months following surgery and demonstrated an 8 mm area of focal non-mass enhancement (*white arrow*) in the left breast at 4 o'clock posterior depth with initial rapid and delayed plateau kinetics (BI-RADS® 4B). Diagnostic mammogram and targeted ultrasound showed no correlate. Histopathology results from MRI-guided biopsy were benign (breast tissue with radiation changes and focal changes from prior surgery) and concordant. (**c**) Six-month follow-up MRI was recommended which demonstrated no significant interval change (*white arrow*). An additional short-interval follow-up MRI was recommended in 6 months (BI-RADS® 3)

compared to those within the same institution [32]. Potential deterrents to compliance include the relatively high cost and variable insurance coverage for short-interval follow-up breast MRI.

Two studies have been subsequently published suggesting that 6 month follow-up MRI may not be necessary and that initial MRI follow-up at 12 months is acceptable [16, 17]. Shaylor et al. reported results from a retrospective review of 113 benign concordant lesions with follow-up MRI [17]. One malignancy (ductal carcinoma in situ) was detected 2 years after the initial benign biopsy for an overall cancer yield of 0.9 % (1/113). Since no cancers were detected at the 6 month follow-up MRI examination, the authors propose that annual screening MRI is a reasonable approach.

Similarly, results from Lee et al. suggest that the initial follow-up MRI examination can be deferred to 12 months without reducing cancer detection rates [16]. This study was a retrospective review of 85 eligible cases of benign concordant MRI-guided biopsies with a minimal follow-up of 2 years. Most of the lesions (57/70) had decreased in size or resolved at the initial 6 month follow-up MRI and all of these were confirmed as benign with ≥2 years of imaging and clinical follow-up. No cancers were detected at the 6-month or 12-month follow-up MRI. One malignancy (invasive ductal carcinoma with a micrometastatic sentinel lymph node) was detected after the biopsied mass enlarged at 24 months post biopsy despite being stable on the MRI performed at 10 months. The overall cancer yield was 1.2 % (1/85). The authors concluded that deferring the initial follow-up MRI to 12 months after biopsy is acceptable and that follow-MRI examinations should be continued for a minimum of 2 years to confirm benignity.

Some studies have reported no malignancies during their follow-up imaging period, also supporting that short-interval follow-up MRI may not be necessary. Perlet et al. reported results from a multicenter European study of 316 of 362 benign MRI-guided biopsies followed for a median of 32 months [11]. Subsequent repeat biopsy occurred in 3 patients; however, no malignancies were detected. Similarly, no cancers were found at follow-up MRI in 12 of 20 benign lesions followed for a mean of 7.5 months (range 3–14 months) reported by Hauth *et al.* or during the follow-up period of Bahrs et al. (mean 13 months; range 5–22 months) [14, 15]. It is important to note that these latter two studies performed immediate follow-up MRI 24–48 h after biopsy and resampled any lesions that appeared unchanged and that the study reported by Perlet et al. performed a second contrast injection at the time of biopsy and resampled any lesions remaining visible with minimal to no change. These important technical differences limit the generalizability of the follow-up results. Recently, Rauch et al. reported no malignancies during follow-up of 133 of 218 benign concordant lesions for a mean of 39 months (range 6–69 months) [29]. The biopsy protocol performed by this group more closely reflects the majority of practices in the United States which typically do not perform a second contrast injection or immediate follow-up MRI 24–48 h after biopsy.

Overall, a follow-up MRI in 6–12 months is typically warranted after benign concordant MRI-guided biopsies, particularly for histopathology results that are nonspecific [7]. In the future, imaging follow-up in this scenario may evolve to be less intensive, as has occurred for other image-guided percutaneous biopsies [33–36]. It is important, however, to recognize that patients undergoing MRI-guided biopsies have a higher risk of malignancy than those undergoing stereotactic- or ultrasound-guided biopsies. Accordingly, management recommendations should be based on the scientific evidence available and should be specific to the patient populations undergoing MRI-guided biopsies.

13.5 Summary

Clinical issues relevant to the care of patients undergoing MRI-guided biopsy have been reviewed. Assessment of radiologic-pathologic concordance is critical in cases of benign results to avoid a delayed diagnosis of cancer and can be more challenging for MRI-guided biopsies compared to other image-guided techniques. Discordant biopsy results are typically managed with repeat biopsy or MRI-guided wire localization and surgical excision. Evidence-based recommendations for optimal follow-up of benign concordant MRI-guided breast biopsy results continue to evolve.

References

1. Wernli KJ, DeMartini WB, Ichikawa L, Lehman CD, Onega T, Kerlikowske K, et al. Patterns of breast magnetic resonance imaging use in community practice. JAMA Intern Med. 2014;174(1):125–32.
2. ACR Practice Parameter for the Performance of Contrast-Enhanced Magnetic Resonance Imaging (MRI) of the Breast. 2014. Available from: http://www.acr.org/~/media/2a0eb28eb59041e2825179afb72ef624.pdf. Accessed 22 Dec 2015.
3. DeMartini W, Lehman C. A review of current evidence-based clinical applications for breast magnetic resonance imaging. Top Magn Reson Imaging. 2008;19(3):143–50.
4. Berg WA, Zhang Z, Lehrer D, Jong RA, Pisano ED, Barr RG, et al. Detection of breast cancer with addition of annual screening ultrasound or a single screening MRI to mammography in women with elevated breast cancer risk. JAMA. 2012;307(13):1394–404.
5. D'Orsi CJ, Sickles EA, Mendelson EB, Morris EA. ACR BI-RADS® Atlas, Breast Imaging Reporting and Data System. 5th ed. Reston: American College of Radiology; 2013.
6. Heywang-Kobrunner SH, Sinnatamby R, Lebeau A, Lebrecht A, Britton PD, Schreer I. Interdisciplinary consensus on the uses and technique of MR-guided vacuum-assisted breast biopsy (VAB): results of a European consensus meeting. Eur J Radiol. 2009;72(2):289–94.
7. ACR Practice Parameter for the Performance of Magnetic Resonance Imaging-Guided Breast Interventional Procedures. 2014. Available from: http://www.acr.org/~/media/ACR/Documents/PGTS/guidelines/MRI_Guided_Breast.pdf. Accessed 21 Dec 2015.
8. Liberman L, Morris EA, Dershaw DD, Thornton CM, Van Zee KJ, Tan LK. Fast MRI-guided vacuum-assisted breast biopsy: initial experience. AJR Am J Roentgenol. 2003;181(5):1283–93.
9. Lehman CD, Deperi ER, Peacock S, McDonough MD, Demartini WB, Shook J. Clinical experience with MRI-guided vacuum-assisted breast biopsy. AJR Am J Roentgenol. 2005;184(6):1782–7.
10. Orel SG, Rosen M, Mies C, Schnall MD. MR imaging-guided 9-gauge vacuum-assisted core-needle breast biopsy: initial experience. Radiology. 2006;238(1):54–61.
11. Perlet C, Heywang-Kobrunner SH, Heinig A, Sittek H, Casselman J, Anderson I, et al. Magnetic resonance-guided, vacuum-assisted breast biopsy: results from a European multicenter study of 538 lesions. Cancer. 2006;106(5):982–90.
12. Liberman L, Drotman M, Morris EA, LaTrenta LR, Abramson AF, Zakowski MF, et al. Imaging-histologic discordance at percutaneous breast biopsy. Cancer. 2000;89(12):2538–46.
13. Li J, Dershaw DD, Lee CH, Kaplan J, Morris EA. MRI follow-up after concordant, histologically benign diagnosis of breast lesions sampled by MRI-guided biopsy. AJR Am J Roentgenol. 2009;193(3):850–5.

14. Hauth EA, Jaeger HJ, Lubnau J, Maderwald S, Otterbach F, Kimmig R, et al. MR-guided vacuum-assisted breast biopsy with a handheld biopsy system: clinical experience and results in postinterventional MR mammography after 24 h. Eur Radiol. 2008;18(1):168–76.
15. Bahrs SD, Hattermann V, Preibsch H, Hahn M, Staebler A, Claussen CD, et al. MR imaging-guided vacuum-assisted breast biopsy: reduction of false-negative biopsies by short-term control MRI 24-48 h after biopsy. Clin Radiol. 2014;69(7):695–702.
16. Lee SJ, Mahoney MC, Redus Z. The management of benign concordant MRI-guided breast biopsies: lessons learned. Breast J. 2015;21(6):665–8.
17. Shaylor SD, Heller SL, Melsaether AN, Gupta D, Gupta A, Babb J, et al. Short interval follow-up after a benign concordant MR-guided vacuum assisted breast biopsy–is it worthwhile? Eur Radiol. 2014;24(6):1176–85.
18. Mahoney MC, Gatsonis C, Hanna L, DeMartini WB, Lehman C. Positive predictive value of BI-RADS MR imaging. Radiology. 2012;264(1):51–8.
19. Gutierrez RL, DeMartini WB, Eby PR, Kurland BF, Peacock S, Lehman CD. BI-RADS lesion characteristics predict likelihood of malignancy in breast MRI for masses but not for nonmass-like enhancement. AJR Am J Roentgenol. 2009;193(4):994–1000.
20. Dratwa C, Jalaguier-Coudray A, Thomassin-Piana J, Gonin J, Chopier J, Antoine M, et al. Breast MR biopsy: pathological and radiological correlation. Eur Radiol. 2015;26(8):2510–9 [Epub ahead of print].
21. Johnson KS, Baker JA, Lee SS, Soo MS. Suspicious breast lesions detected at 3.0 T magnetic resonance imaging: clinical and histological outcomes. Acad Radiol. 2012;19(6):667–74.
22. Liberman L, Bracero N, Morris E, Thornton C, Dershaw DD. MRI-guided 9-gauge vacuum-assisted breast biopsy: initial clinical experience. AJR Am J Roentgenol. 2005;185(1): 183–93.
23. Mahoney MC. Initial clinical experience with a new MRI vacuum-assisted breast biopsy device. J Magn Reson Imaging. 2008;28(4):900–5.
24. Lee JM, Kaplan JB, Murray MP, Bartella L, Morris EA, Joo S, et al. Imaging histologic discordance at MRI-guided 9-gauge vacuum-assisted breast biopsy. AJR Am J Roentgenol. 2007;189(4):852–9.
25. Ghate SV, Rosen EL, Soo MS, Baker JA. MRI-guided vacuum-assisted breast biopsy with a handheld portable biopsy system. AJR Am J Roentgenol. 2006;186(6):1733–6.
26. Gebauer B, Bostanjoglo M, Moesta KT, Schneider W, Schlag PM, Felix R. Magnetic resonance-guided biopsy of suspicious breast lesions with a handheld vacuum biopsy device. Acta Radiol. 2006;47(9):907–13.
27. Meissnitzer M, Dershaw DD, Lee CH, Morris EA. Targeted ultrasound of the breast in women with abnormal MRI findings for whom biopsy has been recommended. AJR Am J Roentgenol. 2009;193(4):1025–9.
28. Heywang-Kobrunner SH, Heinig A, Schaumloffel U, Viehweg P, Buchmann J, Lampe D, et al. MR-guided percutaneous excisional and incisional biopsy of breast lesions. Eur Radiol. 1999;9(8):1656–65.
29. Rauch GM, Dogan BE, Smith TB, Liu P, Yang WT. Outcome analysis of 9-gauge MRI-guided vacuum-assisted core needle breast biopsies. AJR Am J Roentgenol. 2012;198(2):292–9.
30. Brennan SB, Sung J, Lee C, Dershaw DD, Morris E. Lessons learned from MR-guided breast-biopsy. Eur J Radiol. 2012;81(Suppl 1):S10.
31. Sung JS, Lee CH, Morris EA, Comstock CE, Dershaw DD. Patient follow-up after concordant histologically benign imaging-guided biopsy of MRI-detected lesions. AJR Am J Roentgenol. 2012;198(6):1464–9.
32. Thompson MO, Lipson J, Daniel B, Harrigal C, Mullarkey P, Pal S, et al. Why are patients noncompliant with follow-up recommendations after MRI-guided core needle biopsy of suspicious breast lesions? AJR Am J Roentgenol. 2013;201(6):1391–400.
33. Salkowski LR, Fowler AM, Burnside ES, Sisney GA. Utility of 6-month follow-up imaging after a concordant benign breast biopsy result. Radiology. 2011;258(2):380–7.

34. Johnson JM, Johnson AK, O'Meara ES, Miglioretti DL, Geller BM, Hotaling EN, et al. Breast cancer detection with short-interval follow-up compared with return to annual screening in patients with benign stereotactic or US-guided breast biopsy results. Radiology. 2015;275(1):54–60.
35. Manjoros DT, Collett AE, Alberty-Oller JJ, Frazier TG, Barrio AV. The value of 6-month interval imaging after benign radiologic-pathologic concordant minimally invasive breast biopsy. Ann Surg Oncol. 2013;20(10):3163–8.
36. Youk JH, Jung I, Kim EK, Kim MJ, Son EJ, Moon HJ, et al. US follow-up protocol in concordant benign result after US-guided 14-gauge core needle breast biopsy. Breast Cancer Res Treat. 2012;132(3):1089–97.

Chapter 14
BI-RADS 3 Lesions on MRI

Pascal A. Baltzer and Claudio Spick

Abstract Probably benign (BI-RADS 3) lesions on MRI are an empirically assigned category that lack specific criteria that could be used for an objective diagnosis. In this chapter, we describe the probably benign BI-RADS 3 category on MRI and report frequency and malignancy rates. The rate of malignancy in BI-RADS 3 lesions on MRI is below 2 % in the majority of studies. It is lowest in foci (0.9 %) and highest in non-mass enhancements (4 %). Malignant BI-RADS 3 lesions diagnosed by immediate MR-directed ultrasound or a single MRI follow-up in 6–12 months (in case a lesion is not visible by MR-directed ultrasound or MR-directed ultrasound was not performed) support the recommendation of these two management approaches. Finally, in accordance with published data we discuss imaging criteria for those breast lesions that might or might not be appropriately be assigned BI-RADS 3 on MRI.

Keywords Probably benign • BI-RADS 3 • Breast MRI • Breast cancer • Magnetic resonance imaging • Breast Imaging Reporting and Data System • Breast • Breast lesion • Breast disease

14.1 Introduction

The Breast Imaging and Reporting Data System (BI-RADS) of the American College of Radiology provides a lexicon of criteria for the description and categorization of breast lesions on mammography, ultrasound, and magnetic resonance imaging (MRI) [1].

The traditional definition of breast lesions categorized as BI-RADS 3 (probably benign) comes from mammography: these lesions are supposed to harbor a <2 % risk of malignancy. Consequently, immediate biopsy is not recommended and these

P.A. Baltzer, MD (✉) • C. Spick, MD
Department of Biomedical Imaging and Image-Guided Therapy,
Medical University of Vienna, Vienna, Austria
e-mail: pascal.baltzer@meduniwien.ac.at;
claudio.spick@meduniwien.ac.at

S.L. Heller, L. Moy (eds.), *Breast Oncology: Techniques, Indications, and Interpretation*, DOI 10.1007/978-3-319-42563-4_14

lesions should undergo short-interval follow-up after 6 months, followed by additional examinations to establish long-term (2 years or more) lesion stability [2]. This approach ensures that the low proportion of lesions that might progress to cancer can be diagnosed early enough (short-interval follow-up) while the prognosis remains unaffected. Following the establishment of the BI-RADS 3 category on mammography, a reduction of unnecessary biopsies and decrease in health care costs has been achieved [2].

The BI-RADS 3 category on MRI has been adapted from the mammography BI-RADS 3 category [1]. However, several differences have to be considered. First, in contrast to the well-established criteria of BI-RADS 3 lesions on mammography and ultrasound, similar (imaging) criteria have not been established for MRI findings. Categorizing findings on breast MRI as probably benign (BI-RADS 3) has been modified primarily from the categorization of mammographic lesions (morphology, distribution, and symmetry). Nevertheless, the evaluation of breast MRI also includes additional information such as water content from (T2 signal), extracellular microstructure (Diffusion Weighted Imaging-DWI) and dynamic contrast-enhanced (DCE) analysis.

Second, short-interval follow-up MRI is not equivalent to short-interval follow-up mammography. Costs and interpretation times of MRI usually exceed those of mammography. Short-interval follow-up MRI is considered probably useful, but there are no established recommendations [1].

Third, the population undergoing MRI (e.g. for screening due to higher breast cancer risk, or staging due to known breast cancer) is different from that undergoing screening or diagnostic mammography [3]. Evaluation of a patient's breast cancer risk and history, including planned and ongoing therapeutic interventions, is highly important when categorizing BI-RADS 3 lesions on MRI.

In this chapter, we describe the probably benign BI-RADS 3 category on MRI and report its frequency and malignancy rate (Table 14.1) [4–20]. We also review the published data and discuss management strategies and imaging criteria for those breast lesion types that might appropriately be classified as BI-RADS 3 on MRI.

14.2 Literature Data and Evidence-Based Recommendations

As outlined in the previous section, the probably benign category (BI-RADS 3) in breast MRI is based on subjective decision without standardized and established imaging criteria. Most published studies that evaluated the frequency of a BI-RADS 3 assessment (recommendation for short-interval follow-up) on MRI report a rate between 6 and 12 % (Table 14.1). The range of different frequency rates can be partly explained by the study populations. Indications for MRI in these studies showed a wide range from high-risk screening, to problem solving and breast cancer staging. In 17 studies published between 2000 and 2016 and comprising 2608 lesions, 51 cancers were finally diagnosed (Table 14.1). Only 24 of these 51 (47 %) lesions were diagnosed by MRI follow-up. Eight (16 %) lesions were immediately

Table 14.1 Frequency of BI-RADS 3 lesions on MRI and malignancy rate

First author, year	Study design	Study population	BI-RADS 3 assessment, n (%)	BI-RADS 3 patients, n (%)	Malignancy rate, n (%)
Kuhl [4], 2000	Prospective	High risk	45/363 (12.4)	44/192 (22.9)	1/26 (3.8)
Liberman [5], 2003	Retrospective	High risk	89/367 (24.2)	89/367 (24.2)	9/89 (10.1)
Hartman [6], 2004	Prospective	High risk	19/75 (25)	14/41 (34.1)	0/14 (0.0)
Kriege [7], 2004	Prospective	High risk	275/4169 (6.6)	NR/1909	3/275 (1.1)
Sadowski [8], 2005	Retrospective	BI-RADS 0 mammogram	NR	79/473 (16.7)	4/79 (5)
Kuhl [9], 2005	Prospective	High risk	167/1452 (11.5)	NR/529	NR/167
Eby [10], 2007	Retrospective	Mixed	160/809 (20)	160/678 (23.6)	1/160 (0.6)
Eby [11], 2009	Retrospective	Mixed	260/2569 (10.1)	236/1735 (13.6)	2/362 (0.6)
Weinstein [12], 2010	Prospective	Known contralateral cancer	106/969 (10.9)	106/969 (10.9)	1/143 (0.7)
Hauth [13], 2010	Retrospective	Mixed	44/698 (6.3)	44/698 (6.3)	1/56 (1.8)
Marshall [14], 2012	Retrospective	Mixed	132/NR	132/NR	2/132 (1.5)
Mahoney [15], 2012	Prospective	Known contralateral cancer	106/969 (10.9)	106/969 (10.9)	1/106 (0.9)
Lourenco [16], 2014	Retrospective	Mixed	348/4370 (8.0)	345/4370 (7.9)	5/348 (1.5)
Bahrs [17], 2014	Retrospective	Mixed	182/666 (27.3)	117/NR (17.6)	3/163 (1.8)
Spick [18], 2014	Retrospective	Not high risk, no history of breast cancer	108/1265 (8.5)	108/1265 (8.5)	1/108 (0.9)
Grimm [19], 2015	Retrospective	Mixed	282/4279 (6.6)	265/3131 (8.4)	12/280 (4.3)
Guillaume [20], 2016	Retrospective	Mixed	100/820 (12)	75/820 (9)	5/100 (5)

Abbreviations: NR, not reported

upgraded after MRI-directed ultrasound examinations were performed [16, 19, 20]. Other malignancies were either detected as incidental findings after prophylactic mastectomy, interval cancers by palpation or mammography after 24 months. Finally, information regarding time to and method of diagnosis was missing in a number of cases. Considering a time frame of 24 months as adequate to differentiate new interval cancers from real lesion progression (change in follow-up), only the 24 malignant findings identified by MRI follow-up constitute the basis for doing MRI follow-up examinations. These correspond to a 0.9 % rate of false negative BI-RADS 3 lesions on MRI. It seems to be evident from these numbers, that MRI follow-up over 24 months in 6 months intervals may not be justified considering the low likelihood of malignancy, examination costs and patient compliance. Considering these data, we can recommend the following management of MRI BI-RADS 3 lesions:

First, immediate MR-directed ultrasound (also known as second look ultrasound or targeted ultrasound) of the MRI-detected lesion. Despite the fact that MR-directed ultrasound is not yet standard of care to check BI-RADS 3 findings, this approach is justified by the substantial number of second look ultrasound upgrades of MRI BI-RADS 3 lesions reported in the literature [16, 19, 20]. The value of MR-directed ultrasound is corroborated by a recent meta-analysis reporting a substantial pooled detection rate of MRI detected malignant findings of 79 % (95 % CI 71–87 %) [21]. The same publication reports a pooled detection rate of benign findings of 52 % (95 % CI 44–60 %), suggesting that a substantial rate of benign MRI BI-RADS 3 lesions may be identified and followed up by ultrasound [21].

Second, a single MRI follow-up in 6–12 months should be performed in case the BI-RADS 3 lesion is not visible on MRI-directed ultrasound. As the majority of breast cancer screening programs apply 2 year screening intervals, the additional value of a 2 year MRI follow-up does not seem to be justified considering the low likelihood of malignancy after the aforementioned workup.

These considerations do not take into account the possibility of a misclassification of BI-RADS 3 lesions that demonstrate the criteria for malignancy. Although data on this topic is sparse, such misclassification has been described in up to 80 % of false negative MRI BI-RADS 3 lesions that should have been called BI-RADS 4 [20].

BI-RADS 3 lesions that undergo follow-up MRI should be histopathologically verified if they show any change in size or morphology. If, however, the lesion demonstrates stability as compared to prior MRI examinations, a decrease in size, or shows a resolution at any point during follow-up, the lesion should be considered benign.

In the following sections, we will discuss imaging features for those breast lesion types that might appropriately be assigned BI-RADS 3 on MRI.

14.2.1 Diagnostic Criteria in BI-RADS 3 Lesions

In short, there is no definite set of features that define BI-RADS 3 lesions. While the literature reports on malignancy rates in different types (e.g. mass, non-mass, foci) of BI-RADS 3 lesions, no definite data on diagnostic criteria defining the BI-RADS 3 category are given. BI-RADS 3 category should be assigned to lesions presenting benign appearing imaging features in case the radiologist feels the need for further confirmation. Presence of suspicious morphologic features that are unlikely associated with a benign diagnosis should always be called BI-RADS 4 and not BI-RADS 3. Specific features will be discussed in the respective lesion type sections.

Care should be taken in transferring conventional mammography and ultrasound criteria directly to breast MRI. For instance, a newly diagnosed lesion showing only benign features does not necessarily need to be followed-up. This holds true especially for mass lesions with circumscribed margins and persistent or plateau enhancement curves. These findings are generally benign, especially when additional T2w and DWI features are considered (Fig. 14.1).

Fibroadenomata, the most common benign lesions in the breast, usually show a circumscribed T2w correlate and high diffusivity on Apparent Diffusion Coefficient

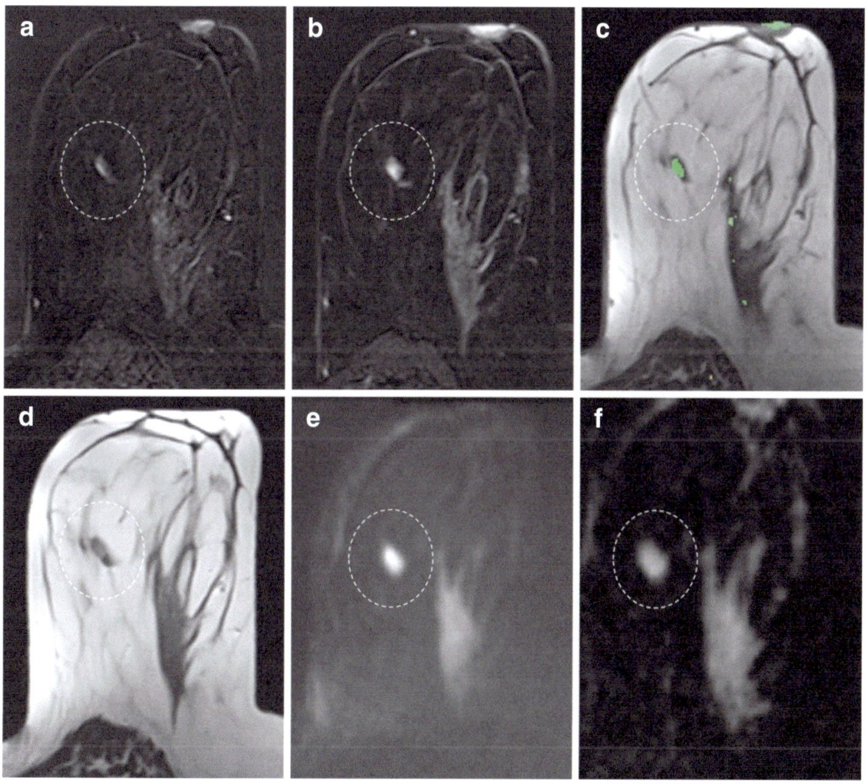

Fig. 14.1 Incidental lesion (*dashed circle*) on breast MRI of a 47-year-old woman performed for other reasons. Slow initial (**a**) and persistent late (**b**) enhancement, coded green on a parametric enhancement map (**c**). The lesion has a hyperintense and circumscribed T2w correlate (**d**) and shows high signal on the DWI image (**e**) and on the apparent diffusion coefficient (ADC) map (**f**). The quantitative ADC value was measured as 1.8×10^{-3} mm^2/s. This finding fulfills all the criteria for a benign lesion and should rather be called BI-RADS 2 (benign finding) than BI-RADS 3 (probably benign finding). MR-directed ultrasound should be attempted in order to have documented the lesion for subsequent conventional screening rounds

(ADC) maps [22]. The latter constitutes the juvenile myxoid or fluid-rich fibroadenoma type. These lesions can even show wash-out curve types, but the combination of high ADC and circumscribed margins excludes the only malignant lesion with high ADC values: invasive mucinous cancer. Fibroadenomata do mature, leading to a loss of water content and an increased hypovascularized stroma component over time. This loss of water may even cause low ADC values that are due to the low T2-signal rather than a real diffusion restriction. Although Schrading et al. have coined the term of fibroadenoma-like appearing cancers in high-risk patients [23], others have not confirmed this finding, and the authors' conclusions are likely due to the reading method applied at that time (alternator views on printed films, visual assessment of signal intensity time curves). In our own clinical experience, we have never encountered a cancer lacking all three MRI hallmarks of malignancy: non-circumscribed or spiculated margins, plateau or wash-out curve types and restricted diffusivity. Moreover, basic consideration of tumor biology implies that dangerous, fast growing tumors may appear with circumscribed margins but their fast growth requires strong and typical hypervascularization and restricted diffusivity due to high cellularity. Again, the combination of circumscribed margins with low and persistent contrast medium uptake excludes any malignant diagnosis: invasive cancer is either not circumscribed or, if circumscribed, presents a highly proliferative lesion that will always show strong contrast uptake followed by wash-out or plateau curves.

The MRI BI-RADS lexicon is characterized by the lack of a clinical decision rule—a precise description of which diagnostic criteria constitute a specific diagnosis, e.g. BI-RADS 3. Although there are several classification systems in breast MRI, such as the Göttingen score [24] or the Jena Tree [25, 26], these systems do not provide rules to differentiate between benign and probably benign lesions. However, they assign levels of suspicion to specific feature combinations, allowing the user to assess whether a lesion is benign or whether the lesion is still benign but may need further follow-up. Still, the decision to differentiate between benign and probably benign lesions is largely a decision based on the clinical background, including patient age, individual breast cancer risk and prior imaging findings. That said, we can conclude the following: first, a lesion that is already known and does not show any imaging progression over time should generally not be assigned as BI-RADS 3 on MRI. Second, a newly diagnosed lesion should not be called BI-RADS 3 if unambiguous benign imaging features are present. This does also hold true for the high-risk screening situation. Here, many authors and colleagues prefer immediate biopsy of newly diagnosed lesions. However, considering the variety of MR imaging protocols and their sensitivity for contrast media, new or stronger enhancing lesions may show such characteristics either due to protocol differences or the cyclical physiologic enhancement in premenopausal women.

The clinical indication for the breast MRI should also be considered in evaluation of BIRADS 3 lesions. If a patient is referred to MRI, e.g., due to an asymmetric density in mammography without remarkable findings on ultrasound, the pretest probability for breast cancer is very low and the indication for the examination questionable. If an incidental lesion, that is a lesion not corresponding to the mammographic asymmetry, shows only benign characteristics, the likelihood of malignancy is negligible, and the lesion should be termed benign and not probably benign. The high sensitivity of MRI implies that many lesions detected by MRI may have been already present but were not seen on conventional imaging.

However, lesions identified on MRI's performed for preoperative staging in breast cancer should be considered differently than those found on MRI's performed for other indications. Here, breast MRI may identify additional lesions, a substantial number of them malignant [27]. DCIS components, in particular, may cause subtle enhancements of non-mass character, lacking the typical features of malignancy [22]. In this setting, a BI-RADS 3 category should be restricted to findings that show benign features only. It is our clinical practice to perform biopsy on all enhancing lesions in cancer patients when typical feature combinations of benign lesions (such as fibroadenoma) are lacking, if that particular lesion would potentially change patient management. Our interdisciplinary communication in these cases has led to a very low number of BI-RADS 3 findings in preoperative cancer staging MRIs, as definite diagnoses are warranted in this setting. A BI-RADS 3 categorization is of little use in the setting of newly diagnosed cancer both in ipsilateral and contralateral breast. Short-interval follow-up for patients who will undergo breast cancer treatment is of little clinical use. If a lesion resolves during short-interval follow-up on a breast cancer patient receiving therapy (e.g. chemotherapy, hormonal therapy), it will remain unclear whether this lesion represented successfully treated breast cancer or suppressed benign proliferative activity.

14.2.2 BI-RADS 3 Masses on MRI

The literature reports 10 out of 564 masses classified as BI-RADS 3 with a final diagnosis of malignancy (1.8 %) [5, 11–13, 16–19]. These studies did not perform dedicated comparisons of feature combinations in benign and malignant lesions, thus, an evidence based recommendation on which specific criteria in masses should lead to a BI-RADS 3 categorization cannot be given. As discussed above, a mass lesion presenting with benign imaging criteria should not be called BI-RADS 3 but rather BI-RADS 2. A mass is a three-dimensional lesion that occupies a space within the breast. A mass should be evaluated by its shape, its margins and its internal characteristics (T1-weighted and T2-weighted characteristics and kinetic behavior, ADC if available). Further evaluations for a mass seen on MRI include a comparison to other breast imaging methods, previous MRIs, clinical history and breast cancer risk. Prior investigations have shown that masses with irregular shapes and those with irregular or spiculated borders have the highest likelihood of malignancy [15, 28–30]. This has also been supported by a study that revealed that the single most predictive imaging feature for malignancy was the margin [31]. Therefore, masses with irregular shape or irregular margins should not be assessed as probably benign. The arguably most important diagnostic criteria in mass lesions are margins, enhancement curve type, T2-weighted correlate and ADC values. Circumscribed margins, slow and persistent enhancement and high ADC values practically exclude cancer in mass lesions. Low ADC values and wash-out curves may be seen in benign fibroadenoma lesions; however, these findings do not present simultaneously in an individual fibroadenoma. A juvenile fibroadenoma is usually highly vascularized and demonstrates a high water content, thus presenting with wash-out and high ADC values whereas a fibroadenoma in an elderly woman presents with slow and persistent enhancement and mixed high, intermediate or even low ADC values. Non-circumscribed margins and rim enhancement are atypical in benign mass lesions and should not be assessed as BI-RADS 3 but rather categorized BI-RADS 4 [22, 24–26, 28, 29, 31]. An example of a BI-RADS 3 mass lesion is given in Fig. 14.2.

14.2.3 BI-RADS 3 Foci on MRI

Foci classified BI-RADS 3 have the lowest probability of malignancy in all BI-RADS 3 lesions. The literature lists 5 malignant foci out of 518 BI-RADS 3 foci (0.9 %) [11, 12, 16, 17, 19]. Similar to reports on BI-RADS 3 masses, no dedicated feature combinations that should lead to a BI-RADS 3 categorization in foci can be extracted from the literature. A focus (foci) is an enhancing area of less than 5 mm in diameter and is not space-occupying like a mass. Although, foci are traditionally considered to be too small to allow evaluation of margins or internal enhancement, the possibility of applying morphologic and dynamic features in foci for diagnostic purposes has been demonstrated [32].

Foci have been described as comprising up to 48 % of MRI BI-RADS 3 lesions [11, 17]. On the other hand, the likelihood for malignancy in foci is rather low as they are regularly part of normal background parenchymal enhancement. In a histologically verified series, suspicious foci detected on MRI had a 3 % (1/37) frequency of malignancy [33]. One study evaluating foci on follow-up reported that a single BI-RADS 3 focus (1.5 %, 1/67) with 4 mm (on baseline examination) increased to 7 mm on follow-up MRI and biopsy revealed a DCIS [17]. Similarly, another study identified a single focus (0.6 %, 1/168) with wash-out kinetics increasing in size on follow-up MRI. Again MRI-guided biopsy revealed a DCIS [11].

A high malignancy rate of 21 % (14/68) was seen in a series of suspicious small masses (<5 mm) [34]. All lesions remained undetected by MRI-directed ultrasound,

Fig. 14.2 Example of a BI-RADS 3 mass lesion in a 43-year-old woman. Initial examination appears on the *left side* (denoted by 1), final follow-up examination after 24 months on the *right side* (denoted by 2). The lesion initially [1] presented with non-circumscribed margins, and was rather homogeneous with slow initial (**a**) and persistent delayed (**b**) enhancement. A non-circumscribed dark T2w correlate (**c**) disturbs the benign impression, while the ADC map (**d**) showed high ADC values of 1.6×10^{-3} mm²/s. Due to the ambiguous, but predominantly benign findings, a BI-RADS 3 rating was assigned. Follow-up examination [2] gave a stable impression; however, lesion contrast was higher due to a modernized protocol, revealing heterogeneous internal enhancement. The lowest ADC value inside the lesion was 1.4×10^{-3} mm²/s, and the lesion was subsequently downgraded to BI-RADS 2. Due to cosmetic reasons, the patient underwent plastic surgery of both breasts and the lesion was removed after wire localization. Histopathology revealed a fibroadenoma with regressive changes

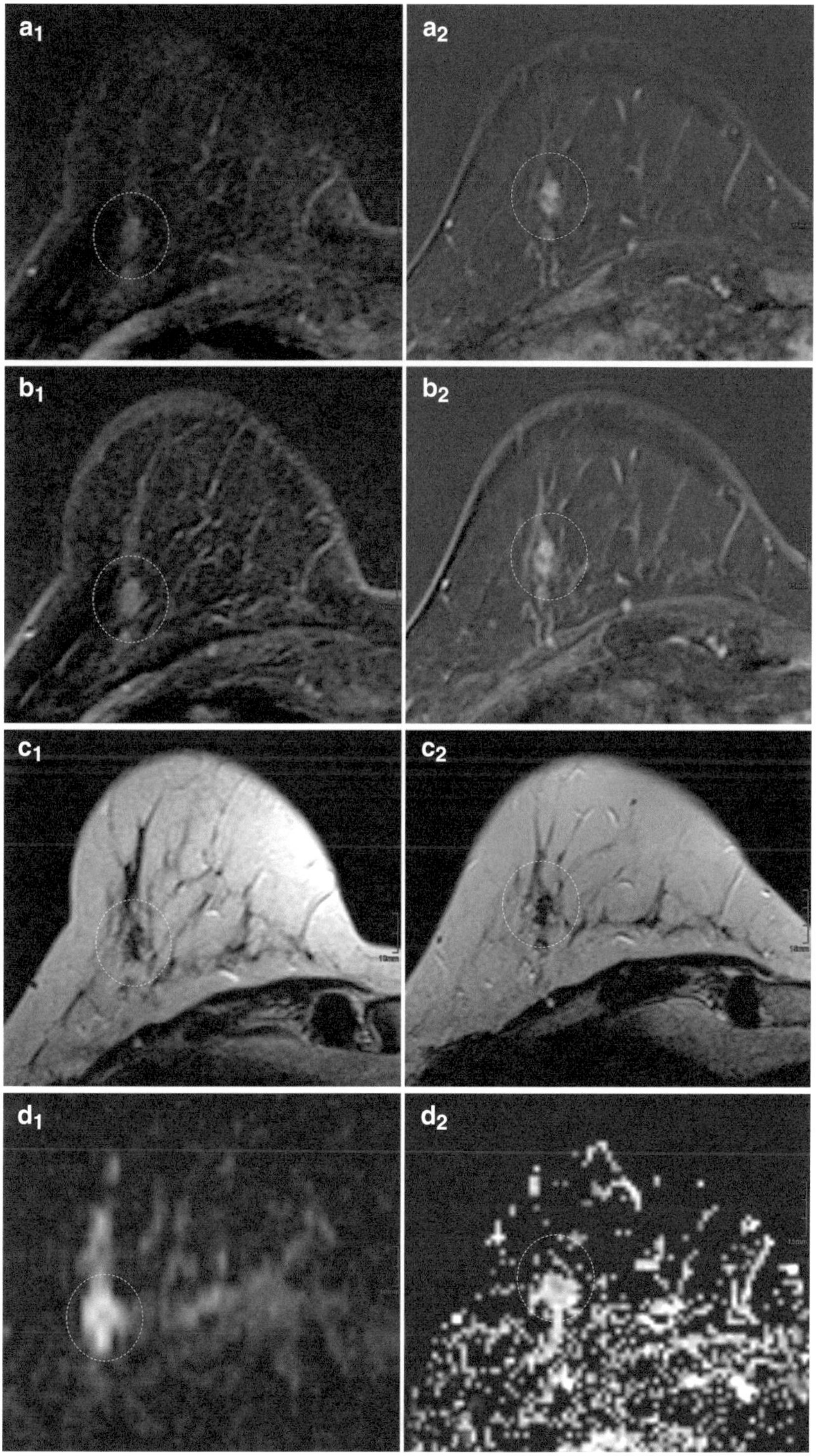
a1
a2
b1
b2
c1
c2
d1
d2

appeared to be suspicious (BI-RADS 4 equivalent) and thus underwent MR-guided biopsy. A final diagnosis of malignancy was associated with recently diagnosed breast cancer and in this case, malignant foci were usually found in the same quadrant [34].

Data suggest that the absence of a high T2 signal and increased size are the most predictive features for malignancy [32, 35]. Importantly, foci presenting with persistent enhancement kinetics are usually benign and might be safely classified as BI-RADS 2 [11, 32, 36]. Finally, the distribution of foci is essential: multiple diffuse bilateral foci should not be considered probably benign but rather benign (BI-RADS 2), as they represent a variation of normal background parenchymal enhancement [1]. Such findings are regularly seen in perimenopausal women. A focus with wash-out harbors a significant risk of malignancy and should thus be categorized BI-RADS 4 instead of BI-RADS 3 [32, 34]. An example of a BI-RADS 3 focus is given in Fig. 14.3.

14.2.4 BI-RADS 3 Non Mass Enhancement on MRI

As opposed to mass lesions, non-mass enhancement (NME) or non-mass lesions are not space-occupying. NME categorized BI-RADS 3 have the highest probability of malignancy in all BI-RADS 3 lesions. The literature reports on 19 out of 467 BI-RADS 3 NME that were finally malignant (4 %) [5, 11–13, 16–19]. Again, no dedicated feature combinations that should lead to a BI-RADS 3 categorization in NME can be extracted from the literature. NME lesions are evaluated by their distribution, enhancement pattern and enhancement kinetics. Diagnostic BI-RADS criteria in non-mass lesions are limited [28, 29]. However, studies have demonstrated that linear and segmental NME have been most predictive for malignancy [15, 37].

Data on BI-RADS 3 NME on MRI are limited. One study reported that BI-RADS 3 may be assigned if the NME is either focal or regional in distribution and homogeneous enhancement and benign enhancment kinetics (persistent type I or plateau type II curves) [18]. Regional, multiple regions, and diffuse distribution patterns have demonstrated the lowest frequency of malignancy [15]. Another study revealed that eight (8.4 %, 8/95) BI-RADS 3 NME were malignant. All of these NME were heterogeneous or clumped or showed wash-out kinetics [19]. Thus, BI-RADS 3 NME on MRI may be appropriately assigned for focal/regional homogeneous or slightly heterogeneous NME that does not show any suspicious features on baseline MRI (Fig. 14.4). Especially the presence of clumped and segmental or linear enhancement in non-mass lesions should be a reason to categorize these lesions as BI-RADS 4 [19, 22, 37].

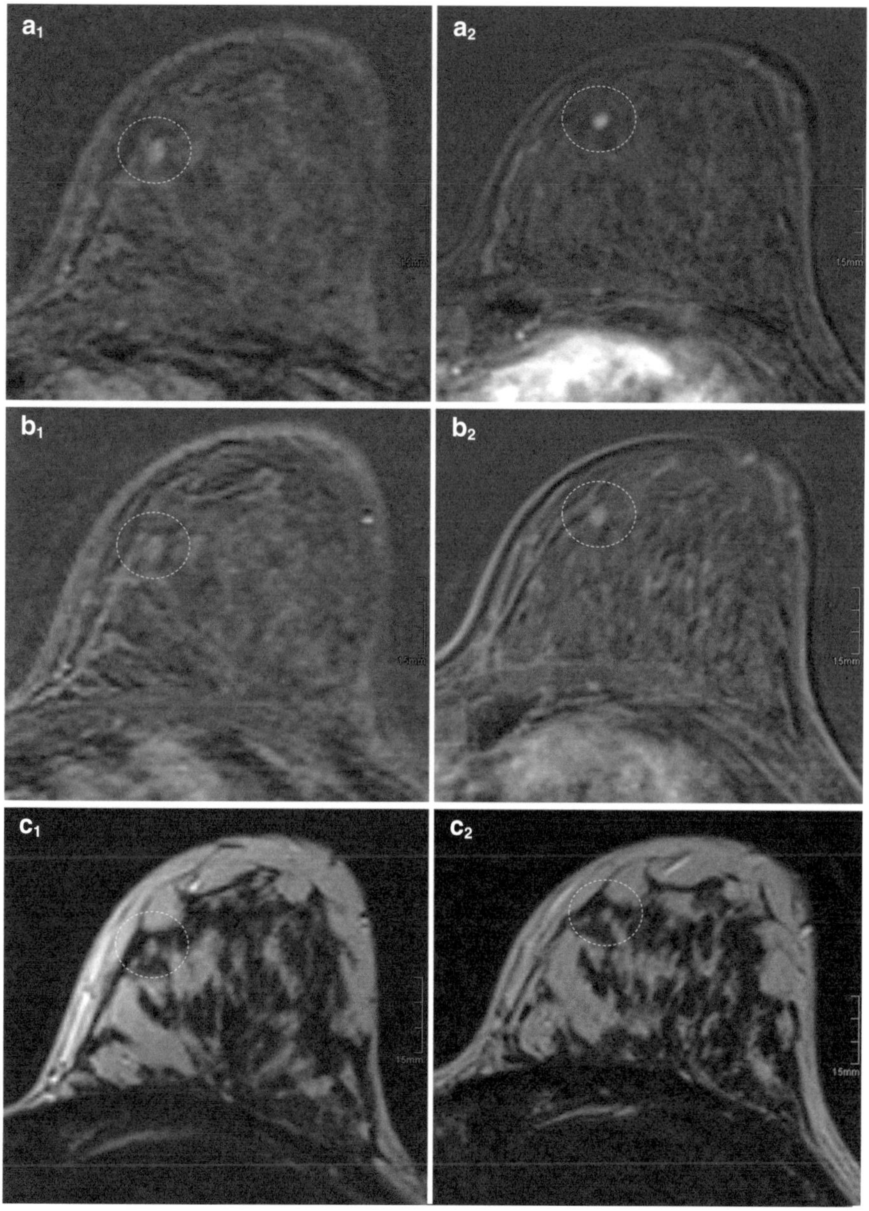

Fig. 14.3 BI-RADS 3 focus in a 41-year-old patient. On the baseline scan (*left hand*, 1), the focus demonstrated an intermediate initial (**a**) enhancement followed by washout (**b**). T2w (**c**) showed a hyperintense correlate with circumscribed margins. The follow-up examination after 12 months (*right hand*, 2) did not show any change in morphology and kinetics. Note the modernized dynamic enhanced protocol, allowing a better depiction of lesion characteristics

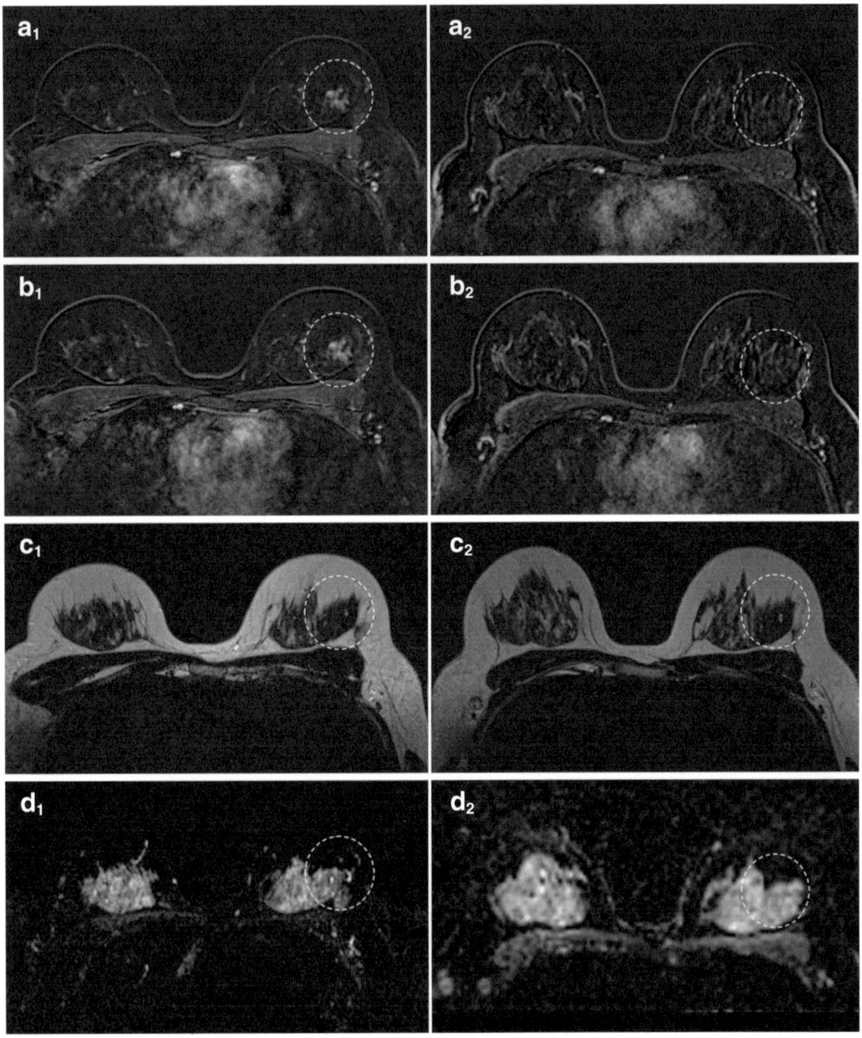

Fig. 14.4 Example of a BI-RADS 3 non-mass lesion (*dashed circle*): a 44-year-old woman who presented with an incidental regional heterogeneous non-mass enhancement with intermediate initial enhancement (**a**$_1$) and a persistent signal increase in the delayed phase (**b**$_1$). Non-specific dark T2w correlate with small cysts (**c**$_1$); ADC map correlate resembles normal breast parenchyma (d1). Follow-up examination after 6 months (*right side*, 2) reveals no residual enhancement

14.2.5 Variations of Background Parenchymal Enhancement

The MRI BI-RADS lexicon term "background parenchymal enhancement" (BPE) is a generalized term for all physiologic enhancements in the breast [1]. Such enhancements comprise regional as well as focal enhancements if they are bilateral and symmetric. In clinical practice, symmetry is not perfect: breasts show slight differences in size, as well as the amount of fibroglandular tissue, cysts, and BPE. Asymmetric focal or patchy BPE often correspond to an ipsilaterally increased amount of cysts and should thus easily be identified. In addition to individual side differences, asymmetric background enhancement can be caused by prior invasive procedures (vacuum-assisted biopsy, open surgery), inflammations and post-radiotherapeutic changes. Radiotherapy has a varying effect immediately after radiation dose delivery but does finally lead to a complete loss of any BPE on the treated side, possibly aggravating a BPE consisting of multiple foci on the contralateral side. If the BPE is clearly asymmetric, and not associated with features of malignancy or pathological findings on conventional imaging, this finding may be called BI-RADS 3 and MRI follow-up may appropriately be initiated.

14.3 Summary/Conclusion

Probably benign (BI-RADS 3) lesions on MRI are an empirically assigned category that lack specific criteria that could be used for an objective diagnosis. That said, rates of BI-RADS 3 ratings will shift towards BI-RADS 2 with reader experience. The rate of malignancy in BI-RADS 3 lesions is below 2 % in the majority of studies. Malignant BI-RADS 3 lesions may be diagnosed by immediate MR-directed ultrasound or a single MRI follow-up in six to 12 months (if a lesion is not visible by MR-directed ultrasound or MR-directed ultrasound was not performed), supporting the recommendation of these two management approaches.

References

1. American College of Radiology. Breast imaging reporting and data system (BI-RADS). 5th ed. Reston: American College of Radiology; 2013.
2. Sickles EA. Probably benign breast lesions: when should follow-up be recommended and what is the optimal follow-up protocol? Radiology. 1999;213(1):11–4.
3. American College of Radiology. American College of Radiology. ACR practice guideline for the performance of contrast-enhanced Magnetic Resonance Imaging (MRI) of the breast. [Internet]. [cited 2016 Feb 1]. http://www.acr.org/~/media/2A0EB28EB59041E2825179AFB72EF624.pdf.
4. Kuhl CK, Schmutzler RK, Leutner CC, Kempe A, Wardelmann E, Hocke A, et al. Breast MR imaging screening in 192 women proved or suspected to be carriers of a breast cancer susceptibility gene: preliminary results. Radiology. 2000;215(1):267–79.
5. Liberman L, Morris EA, Benton CL, Abramson AF, Dershaw DD. Probably benign lesions at breast magnetic resonance imaging: preliminary experience in high-risk women. Cancer. 2003;98(2):377–88.
6. Hartman A-R, Daniel BL, Kurian AW, Mills MA, Nowels KW, Dirbas FM, et al. Breast magnetic resonance image screening and ductal lavage in women at high genetic risk for breast carcinoma. Cancer. 2004;100(3):479–89.

7. Kriege M, Brekelmans CTM, Boetes C, Besnard PE, Zonderland HM, Obdeijn IM, et al. Efficacy of MRI and mammography for breast-cancer screening in women with a familial or genetic predisposition. N Engl J Med. 2004;351(5):427–37.
8. Sadowski EA, Kelcz F. Frequency of malignancy in lesions classified as probably benign after dynamic contrast-enhanced breast MRI examination. J Magn Reson Imaging JMRI. 2005;21(5):556–64.
9. Kuhl CK, Schrading S, Leutner CC, Morakkabati-Spitz N, Wardelmann E, Fimmers R, et al. Mammography, breast ultrasound, and magnetic resonance imaging for surveillance of women at high familial risk for breast cancer. J Clin Oncol Off J Am Soc Clin Oncol. 2005;23(33):8469–76.
10. Eby PR, Demartini WB, Peacock S, Rosen EL, Lauro B, Lehman CD. Cancer yield of probably benign breast MR examinations. J Magn Reson Imaging JMRI. 2007;26(4):950–5.
11. Eby PR, DeMartini WB, Gutierrez RL, Saini MH, Peacock S, Lehman CD. Characteristics of probably benign breast MRI lesions. AJR Am J Roentgenol. 2009;193(3):861–7.
12. Weinstein SP, Hanna LG, Gatsonis C, Schnall MD, Rosen MA, Lehman CD. Frequency of malignancy seen in probably benign lesions at contrast-enhanced breast MR imaging: findings from ACRIN 6667. Radiology. 2010;255(3):731–7.
13. Hauth E, Umutlu L, Kümmel S, Kimmig R, Forsting M. Follow-up of probably benign lesions (BI-RADS 3 category) in breast MR imaging. Breast J. 2010;16(3):297–304.
14. Marshall AL, Domchek SM, Weinstein SP. Follow-up frequency and compliance in women with probably benign findings on breast magnetic resonance imaging. Acad Radiol. 2012;19(4):406–11.
15. Mahoney MC, Gatsonis C, Hanna L, DeMartini WB, Lehman C. Positive predictive value of BI-RADS MR imaging. Radiology. 2012;264(1):51–8.
16. Lourenco AP, Chung MTM, Mainiero MB. Probably benign breast MRI lesions: frequency, lesion type, and rate of malignancy. J Magn Reson Imaging JMRI. 2014;39(4):789–94.
17. Bahrs SD, Baur A, Hattermann V, Hahn M, Vogel U, Claussen CD, et al. BI-RADS® 3 lesions at contrast-enhanced breast MRI: is an initial short-interval follow-up necessary? Acta Radiol Stockh Swed. 1987. 2014;55(3):260–5.
18. Spick C, Szolar DHM, Baltzer PA, Tillich M, Reittner P, Preidler KW, et al. Rate of malignancy in MRI-detected probably benign (BI-RADS 3) lesions. AJR Am J Roentgenol. 2014;202(3):684–9.
19. Grimm LJ, Anderson AL, Baker JA, Johnson KS, Walsh R, Yoon SC, et al. Frequency of malignancy and imaging characteristics of probably benign lesions seen at breast MRI. AJR Am J Roentgenol. 2015;205(2):442–7.
20. Guillaume R, Taieb S, Ceugnart L, Deken-Delannoy V, Faye N. BIRADS 3 MRI lesions: was the initial score appropriate and what is the value of the blooming sign as an additional parameter to better characterize these lesions? Eur J Radiol. 2016;85(2):337–45.
21. Spick C, Baltzer PAT. Diagnostic utility of second-look US for breast lesions identified at MR imaging: systematic review and meta-analysis. Radiology. 2014;273(2):401–9.
22. Kaiser WA. Signs in MR-Mammography [Internet]. Berlin, Heidelberg: Springer Berlin Heidelberg; 2008. [cited 2015 Mar 17]. http://www.springer.com/us/book/9783540732921.
23. Schrading S, Kuhl CK. Mammographic, US, and MR imaging phenotypes of familial breast cancer. Radiology. 2008;246(1):58–70.
24. Baum F, Fischer U, Vosshenrich R, Grabbe E. Classification of hypervascularized lesions in CE MR imaging of the breast. Eur Radiol. 2002;12(5):1087–92.
25. Marino MA, Clauser P, Woitek R, Wengert GJ, Kapetas P, Bernathova M, et al. A simple scoring system for breast MRI interpretation: does it compensate for reader experience?. Eur Radiol. 2016;26(8):2529–37.
26. Baltzer PAT, Dietzel M, Kaiser WA. A simple and robust classification tree for differentiation between benign and malignant lesions in MR-mammography. Eur Radiol. 2013;23(8):2051–60.
27. Houssami N, Ciatto S, Macaskill P, Lord SJ, Warren RM, Dixon JM, et al. Accuracy and surgical impact of magnetic resonance imaging in breast cancer staging: systematic review and

meta-analysis in detection of multifocal and multicentric cancer. J Clin Oncol Off J Am Soc Clin Oncol. 2008;26(19):3248–58.
28. Baltzer PAT, Benndorf M, Dietzel M, Gajda M, Runnebaum IB, Kaiser WA. False-positive findings at contrast-enhanced breast MRI: a BI-RADS descriptor study. AJR Am J Roentgenol. 2010 Jun;194(6):1658–63.
29. Gutierrez RL, DeMartini WB, Eby PR, Kurland BF, Peacock S, Lehman CD. BI-RADS lesion characteristics predict likelihood of malignancy in breast MRI for masses but not for nonmass-like enhancement. AJR Am J Roentgenol. 2009;193(4):994–1000.
30. Lehman CD, Gatsonis C, Kuhl CK, Hendrick RE, Pisano ED, Hanna L, et al. MRI evaluation of the contralateral breast in women with recently diagnosed breast cancer. N Engl J Med. 2007;356(13):1295–303.
31. Schnall MD, Blume J, Bluemke DA, DeAngelis GA, DeBruhl N, Harms S, et al. Diagnostic architectural and dynamic features at breast MR imaging: multicenter study. Radiology. 2006;238(1):42–53.
32. Dietzel M, Baltzer PA, Vag T, Gröschel T, Gajda M, Camara O, et al. Differential diagnosis of breast lesions 5 mm or less: is there a role for magnetic resonance imaging? J Comput Assist Tomogr. 2010;34(3):456–64.
33. Liberman L, Mason G, Morris EA, Dershaw DD. Does size matter? Positive predictive value of MRI-detected breast lesions as a function of lesion size. AJR Am J Roentgenol. 2006;186(2):426–30.
34. Raza S, Sekar M, Ong EMW, Birdwell RL. Small masses on breast MR: is biopsy necessary? Acad Radiol. 2012;19:412–9.
35. Ha R, Sung J, Lee C, Comstock C, Wynn R, Morris E. Characteristics and outcome of enhancing foci followed on breast MRI with management implications. Clin Radiol. 2014;69(7):715–20.
36. Spick C, Szolar DHM, Tillich M, Reittner P, Preidler KW, Baltzer PA. Benign (BI-RADS 2) lesions in breast MRI. Clin Radiol. 2015;70:395–9.
37. Liberman L, Morris EA, Dershaw DD, Abramson AF, Tan LK. Ductal enhancement on MR imaging of the breast. AJR Am J Roentgenol. 2003 Aug;181(2):519–25.

Chapter 15
Multiparametric Imaging: Cutting-Edge Sequences and Techniques Including Diffusion-Weighted Imaging, Magnetic Resonance Spectroscopy, and PET/CT or PET/MRI

Maria Adele Marino and Katja Pinker-Domenig

Abstract Magnetic resonance imaging (MRI) of the breast is an indispensible tool in breast imaging, with several indications. Dynamic contrast-enhanced MRI (DCE-MRI) provides mainly morphological, and, to some extent, functional information about perfusion and vascularity, resulting in excellent sensitivity and good specificity for breast cancer diagnosis. Multiparametric imaging of the breast aims to quantify and visualize biological, physiological, and pathological processes at the cellular and molecular levels. Multiparametric imaging of the breast can be performed at different field-strengths (1.5–7 T) and comprises established and emerging MRI parameters, such as diffusion-weighted imaging (DWI), MR spectroscopy (MRS), sodium imaging (^{23}Na MRI), chemical exchange saturation transfer (CEST) imaging, blood oxygen level–dependent (BOLD) MRI, nuclear imaging, such as positron emission tomography (PET) with different radiotracers, and combinations of techniques (e.g., PET/CT and PET/MRI).

Several functional parameters with MRI and PET have also been assessed for imaging of breast tumors, and their combined application is defined as multiparametric imaging. Available data suggest that multiparametric imaging using different functional MRI and PET parameters can provide detailed information about the hallmarks of cancer and may provide additional specificity.

M.A. Marino
Division of Molecular and Gender Imaging, Department of Biomedical Imaging and Image-guided Therapy, Medical University of Vienna, Vienna, Austria

Department of Biomedical Sciences and Morphologic and Functional Imaging, Policlinico Universitario G. Martino, University of Messina, Messina, Italy

K. Pinker-Domenig, MD (✉)
Department of Biomedical Imaging and Image-guided Therapy, Division of Molecular and Gender Imaging, Medical University Vienna, Waehringer Guertel 18-20, 1090, Vienna, Austria
e-mail: katja.pinker@meduniwien.ac.at

S.L. Heller, L. Moy (eds.), *Breast Oncology: Techniques, Indications, and Interpretation*, DOI 10.1007/978-3-319-42563-4_15

This chapter aims to provide a comprehensive overview of the current possibilities and emerging techniques in multiparametric imaging of the breast with cutting-edge sequences and techniques.

Keywords Dynamic contrast-enhanced MRI (DCE-MRI) • Diffusion-weighted imaging (DWI) • MR spectroscopy (MRS) • Positron emission tomography/computed tomography (PET/CT) • Sodium imaging • Phosphorus spectroscopy • Chemical exchange saturation transfer (CEST) imaging • Blood oxygen level–dependent (BOLD) MRI • PET/MRI • Multiparametric imaging

15.1 Introduction

Breast cancer is the most common cancer in women and the leading cause of female cancer-deaths [1]. Magnetic resonance imaging (MRI) of the breast is an established non-invasive breast imaging modality with several indications, such as pre-operative staging, the monitoring and assessment of treatment response, the differentiation of scar vs. recurrence, the evaluation of breast implants, the screening of high-risk women, and the assessment of patients with cancers of unknown primary (CUP) syndrome. MRI is also a reliable problem-solving tool to accurately exclude malignancy [2–6]. Dynamic contrast-enhanced MRI (DCE-MRI) is the backbone of any given MRI protocol. DCE-MRI provides mainly morphological, and, to some extent, functional information about perfusion and vascularity, resulting in an excellent sensitivity and good specificity [7–9]. Recently, several functional and metabolic MRI and PET parameters have been assessed for the imaging of breast tumors. The combined application of these techniques is defined as multiparametric imaging. Available data suggest that multiparametric imaging using different functional MRI and PET parameters can provide detailed information about the hallmarks of cancer [10], including neo-angiogenesis, cellularity, tumor microenvironment, metabolite concentration, receptor status, tissue pH, and oxygenation, which cannot be obtained with DCE-MRI only, and thus may provide additional specificity [10–13]. In addition to depicting tumor morphology, multiparametric imaging of the breast aims to quantify and visualize biological, physiological, and pathological processes at the cellular and molecular levels to further elucidate the development and progression of breast cancer and the response to treatment. To date, multiparametric imaging of the breast comprises MRI and nuclear imaging parameters as well as hybrid imaging techniques. This chapter aims to review the current and emerging functional parameters for cutting-edge multiparametric imaging of breast tumors with MRI and nuclear imaging.

We will explore the MRI parameters of DCE-MRI, diffusion-weighted imaging (DWI), and proton magnetic resonance spectroscopy (^{1}H-MRS) at 3 T as well as ultra-high field MRI at 7 T. The potential of multiparametric MRI, using cutting-edge sequences and techniques to improve diagnostic accuracy, will be reviewed. In addition, we will discuss emerging MRI parameters, such as sodium imaging (^{23}Na-MRI), phosphorus MRS (^{31}P MRSI), chemical exchange saturation transfer (CEST) imaging, blood oxygen level–dependent (BOLD), and hyperpolarized MRI. We will further discuss the potential for molecular imaging of breast tumors with nuclear imaging methods, such as breast-specific gamma imaging (BSGI), positron emission tomography (PET)/ computed tomography (CT), PET-mammography (PEM), and PET-MRI. Finally, we will review the use of specific tracers for precision medicine in breast cancer imaging.

15.2 MRI of the Breast

DCE-MRI is an indispensible tool in breast imaging with several indications [2–5]. DCE-MRI is able to depict an increased vascular density, microvascular hyper-permeability, and increased interstitial fluid [14–17], resulting in a characteristic enhancement pattern after the intravenous application of gadolinium chelates. The contrast enhancement of tumors is closely related to their microscopic vascular architecture and thus, DCE-MR is able to depict neo-angiogenesis as a tumor-specific feature [18]. DCE-MRI is the most sensitive method for the detection of breast cancer, with a negative predictive value ranging between 89 and 99 %, but reported variable specificities ranging from 47 to 97 % [3, 16, 19–22]. Several attempts have been made to increase both the sensitivity and specificity of DCE-MRI using higher field-strengths and parallel imaging strategies. Recently, other functional and metabolic imaging techniques, such as diffusion-weighted imaging (DWI) and proton MR spectroscopy (^{1}H-MRS), have been introduced to provide complementary information about the cellularity, the metabolism, and the microenvironment of tumors. Available data indicate that the additional use of these functional MRI parameters, in combination with DCE-MRI, increases specificity in breast cancer diagnosis [23, 24]. The combination of DCE-MRI and other functional MRI parameters is defined as multiparametric MRI.

15.2.1 Quantitative DCE-MRI

A hallmark of cancer development and metastatic potential is tumor angiogenesis, i.e., the development of a dedicated vasculature with abnormal vessel permeability that supports the high metabolic demand for oxygen and nutrients, especially in aggressive tumors [19, 20, 25]. Specific peptide hormones released by cancer cells promote tumor angiogenesis as soon as they exceed 2 mm [25, 26]. DCE-MR is able to depict and characterize this abnormal vasculature and permeability as a tumor-specific feature [18] through the assessment of breast kinetic enhancement features [10]. Most commonly, kinetic enhancement analysis of breast tumors is performed semi-quantitatively using a modest temporal resolution with at least two to three post-contrast T1-weighted acquisitions and with k-space centered at approximately 90–120 s after contrast injection for the first post-contrast images [10]. Using the data obtained at these time-points, time signal intensity curves for a region of interest in a given lesion can be calculated. Kinetic characteristics of lesions are categorized by the steepness of the signal intensity increase in the early phase, after the administration of contrast material (initial phase, within approximately 2 min of contrast injection) and by the behavior of signal intensity in the intermediate and late post-contrast periods (delayed phase, after 2 min or after peak enhancement). To account for differences in baseline tissue T1 relaxation times, the percentage of enhancement in the initial phase, classified as slow, medium, or fast, is calculated as signal intensity increase relative to baseline values (SI_{pre} is baseline signal intensity and SI_{post} is signal intensity following contrast agent injection at different time points) [27–29]. The delayed phase refers to the signal intensity changes that occur immediately after the early signal intensity increase and can be further described as persistent, plateau, or wash-out [19]. The rate of contrast agent uptake and washout depends on several factors, such as perfusion, capillary permeability, blood volume, contrast media distribution volume, and other aspects of local anatomy and physiology. Malignant breast tumors are usually characterized by a dense, highly permeable vasculature, a relatively rapid blood flow, and a high degree of micro-heterogeneity. After contrast agent injection, malignant breast tumors tend to enhance more rapidly and intensely than normal tissue or benign lesions. Therefore, malignant lesions often present with "wash-out curves" and benign lesions with "persistent curves" [27, 30]. Plateau curves (type II) are seen in both malignant and benign lesions. Considerable overlap of semi-quantitative kinetic curve types among benign and malignant lesions is often the cause of pitfalls or a challenging diagnosis [27, 30–34].

High-resolution MRI techniques enable a quantitative evaluation of contrast enhancement kinetics through pharmacokinetic modeling. Pharmacokinetic models quantify the contrast agent exchange between the intravascular and the interstitial space, providing measures of tumor blood flow, microvasculature, and capillary permeability. The Tofts Two-Compartment model [35, 36] is the most commonly used approach and measures the exchange between the breast tissue plasma and the plasma space. Contrast agent concentrations for each compartment vary with time after bolus injection and quantitative metrics can be measured with this model using the following relationship: K^{trans} (min^{-1}) is the volume transfer constant and reflects the rate of transfer of contrast agent from the plasma to the tissue. K_{ep} (min^{-1}) is the transfer rate constant and reflects the reflux of contrast agent from the extravascular extracellular space to the plasma compartment. $V_{e(\%)}$ represents the leakage of fractional volume from the extravascular extracellular space into the plasma compartment.

Several studies have shown that pharmacokinetic parameters such as k_{trans} and k_{ep} have the potential to improve discrimination of benign from malignant breast tumors and even can be used to differentiate breast cancer subtypes.

Huang et al. [37] investigated pharmacokinetic parameters in suspicious lesions on standard clinical breast MRI. The authors demonstrated that a potential cutoff could be used such that, in lesions with lower K_{trans} values, biopsy could be obviated, and thus, false-positive MR examinations could be decreased. Li et al. [38] assessed morphological and quantitative DCE-MRI for breast cancer diagnosis and found that K^{trans} and k_{ep} values were significantly higher in invasive ductal carcinoma and DCIS than in borderline and benign lesions or healthy breast tissue.

Another promising application for quantitative DCE MRI is the assessment of the response to neoadjuvant chemotherapy (NAC) in breast cancer patients. It has been demonstrated that MRI is superior to clinical assessment and conventional imaging in measuring response to treatment and in predicting pathologic complete response (pCR) [39]. MRI has the unique ability to provide a volumetric evaluation of tumor size as well as a quantitative assessment of enhancement that is reflective of the intra-tumoral microvascularization. In a recent meta-analysis, Marinovich et al. [40] showed that the measurement of alterations in tumor perfusion in response to preoperative therapy, using K^{trans}, is a powerful predictor of response to NAC and outperforms standard tumor size measurements.

Nevertheless, quantitative DCE–MRI with pharmacokinetic modeling remains challenging. To derive quantitative parameters, knowledge of the pre-contrast T1 relaxation times of the tumor or tissue and the arterial input function (AIF, i.e., the concentration of contrast agent as it changes over time within the arterial blood) is necessary. The measurement of both parameters comes with unique challenges and introduces the potential for error. Pre-contrast T1 mapping requires either the acquisition of an additional series with varying flip angles or an inversion recovery sequence, which adds to examination times. In addition, flip-angle approaches are prone to inaccuracies due to B1 inhomogeneity especially at high field strengths [10, 19, 41]. Most models require that the AIF be measured directly for each subject, which can be challenging to perform and usually requires acquisition tradeoffs in either coverage and/or spatial resolution to achieve the very high temporal resolution necessary to accurately sample the rapidly changing AIF. AIF readings can also be sensitive to patient motion between dynamic acquisitions [37, 42]. The most common approach to circumvent individual calculations of AIF is the use of an average AIF, i.e., the shutter-speed approach, calculated from a larger population for whom the injection site, dose, and rate were kept constant. Another alternative method was proposed by Yankeelov et al., who estimated the AIF using a reference region model and found that this approach correlated well with direct AIF measurement [43]. Novel high spatial and temporal DCE-MRI potentially can provide high temporal resolution sampling of contrast enhancement curves without the undesirable tradeoffs in spatial resolution and coverage, and therefore, might improve the feasibility of quantitative DCE-MRI in clinical breast imaging [21, 44, 45].

In contrast to semi-quantitative enhancement curve assessment, pharmacokinetic modeling should have the advantage of providing objective quantitative measures of the underlying physiology that are not affected by differences in scan parameters. However, due to different modeling algorithms, several challenges and various potential solutions, there are significant differences in quantitative measurements, and thus, the results of individual studies cannot be readily generalized and further data derived with standardized techniques are warranted to fully explore the true potential of quantitative DCE-MRI [46].

15.2.2 *High-Resolution High-Field and Ultra-High-Field DCE-MRI*

Both lesion morphology and enhancement kinetics are necessary for the optimal diagnosis of breast lesions [8, 16, 19, 20, 22, 47, 48]. Several studies by Kuhl et al. [22] and Goto et al. [49] imply that a high spatial resolution improves diagnostic confidence and accuracy with MRI. High-spatial-resolution images must be acquired within a short time span to enable the optimal contrast-enhancement in the arterial phase between the enhancing lesions and the adjacent breast parenchyma. In addition, a high temporal resolution is pivotal for the accurate assessment of lesion enhancement kinetics, as it adds important information for the differentiation between malignant and benign lesions [8, 49, 50]. Due to reasons related to the signal-to-noise ratio (SNR), the maximum achievable spatial resolution at 1.5 T is limited [22, 51]. Methods to overcome these limitations include the application of parallel imaging techniques and the utilization of higher field-strengths (≥3 T), thus resolving the 'temporal versus spatial dilemma' faced by breast MRI protocols at 1.5 T. Several studies have demonstrated increased sensitivity and specificity in breast imaging at 3 T [21, 52, 53], and breast MRI has steadily moved to 3 T. Recently, ultra-high-field MR scanners operating at a field-strength of 7 T have become available. Ultra-high-field MRI at 7 T offers a significantly increased intrinsic SNR [9], which can be translated into even higher temporal and spatial resolution imaging [54, 55] or functional and metabolic imaging [55, 56]. Initial studies investigating unilateral DCE-MRI of the breast at 7 T, in healthy volunteers and a few patients, have demonstrated the feasibility of this technique and encouraged the implementation of further advanced bilateral coil concepts to fully explore the diagnostic potential of DCE-MRI at 7 T [54, 55, 57, 58]. In the first clinical study, Pinker et al. evaluated the application of bilateral DCE MR at 7 T [24] in patients with breast tumors. DCE-MRI at 7 T had a sensitivity of 100 % and a specificity of 90 %, resulting in a diagnostic accuracy of 96.6 %. Overall image quality was excellent in the majority of cases and artifacts did not hamper examinations. The authors concluded that bilateral, high-resolution DCE-MRI of the breast at 7 T is clinically applicable and enables a breast cancer diagnosis with a high diagnostic accuracy and excellent inter-rater agreement and image quality (Fig. 15.1). Gruber et al. [9] compared the image quality, contrast enhancement behavior, and diagnostic value of bilateral high spatial and temporal resolution DCE-MRI at 7 T with 3 T in the same patient group. They found that 7 T DCE-MRI provides simultaneous high temporal and spatial resolution that is significantly improved compared with lower field strengths, resulting in a sensitivity of 100 % and a specificity of 91.67 % for breast cancer diagnosis.

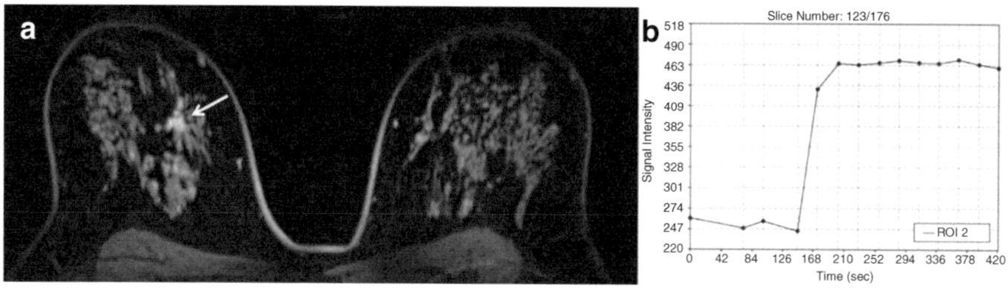

Fig. 15.1 7 T DCE. *Invasive ductal carcinoma G2 in a 50-year-old woman at 1 o'clock in the right breast.* (**a**) At DCE MRI of the breast at 7 T the irregular-shaped mass with spiculated margins (*white arrow*) demonstrates heterogeneous initial strong enhancement followed by a plateau (**b**), and was classified as BI-RADS© 5 (highly suggestive of malignancy)

15.2.3 Diffusion-Weighted Imaging

DWI is a non-contrast MRI parameter, which measures the random movement of water molecules, i.e., Brownian movement, and depicts the diffusivity of the examined tissues. DWI provides a strong surrogate marker for tissue microstructure, membrane integrity, and cell density, and can be quantified by calculating the apparent diffusion coefficient (ADC) [59]. Changes in tissue water diffusion properties can be helpful for the detection and characterization of pathological processes in any part of the body [59, 60]. New developments in imaging techniques (e.g., parallel imaging) and hardware (stronger gradient systems and multi-channel coils) have overcome previous limitations (susceptibility and respiratory motion artifacts) and DWI has been implemented in oncologic imaging in multiple organs. In general, malignant tissue tends to have more restricted diffusion and lower ADC values compared to normal tissue due to the high cellular density and abundance of intra- and intercellular membranes [61].

DWI for breast cancer diagnosis has been evaluated with encouraging results by numerous studies using different ADC thresholds and b-values [62–64]. Bogner et al. compared the diagnostic quality of DWI schemes with respect to ADC accuracy, ADC precision, and DWI contrast-to-noise ratio (CNR) for different types of lesions and breast tissue at 3 T [65]. They concluded that optimal ADC determination and DWI quality at 3 T was found with a combined b-value protocol of 50 and 850 s/mm^2, yielding a diagnostic accuracy of 96 % (Fig. 15.2). In a recent meta-analysis including 26 studies, Dorrius et al. [66] confirmed that ADC values of breast lesions are strongly influenced by the choice of b values. For the most accurate differentiation of benign and malignant lesions, the combination of b = 0 and 1000 s/mm^2 was recommended. Nevertheless, there is a consensus that, in general, breast cancer has lower ADC values compared to healthy breast tissue [43, 62, 67], that the specificity of DWI (75–84 %) is higher than DCE-MRI (67–72 %), and that DWI is a promising imaging biomarker that provides additional functional information to DCE-MRI [68]. DWI also can be easily integrated into a standard MR imaging protocol [11, 13, 69].

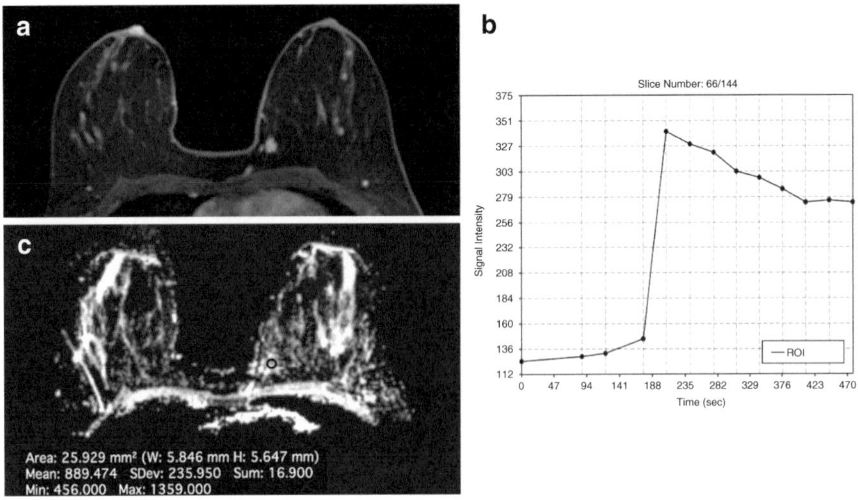

Fig. 15.2 Invasive ductal carcinoma (IDC) medially in the left breast in a 45-year-old woman. (**a**) The irregular shaped and marginated mass lesion demonstrates (**b**) an initial strong heterogeneous contrast enhancement followed by a wash-out, and had decreased (**c**) ADC values (0.889×10^{-3} mm^2/s). DCE-MRI and DWI at 3 T were concordant and both classified the mass lesion as malignant

Several authors recommended cut-off thresholds to discriminate benign and malignant lesions [65, 69–73]. A very low ADC value ($<1.25 \times 10^{-3}$ mm^2/s) is specific for malignancy, whereas high ADC values ($>1.4 \times 10^{-3}$ mm^2/s) are indicative of benignity. Intermediate ADC values are rather unspecific. In a recent study, Spick et al. [74] applied hierarchized ADC thresholds to suspicious breast lesions only visible on DCE MR, and concluded that up to 35 % of MR-guided biopsies could have been omitted when using a high ADC threshold of $>1.4 \times 10^{-3}$ mm^2/s.

In addition to the differentiation of benign and malignant breast tumors, DWI can potentially be used as a non-invasive biomarker for tumor receptor status and tumor grading. Martinicich et al. [75] found that breast cancers characterized by high cellularity or a higher number of mitoses have lower ADC values. Similar observations have been published about triple-negative breast cancers, which are associated with higher ADC values compared to ER+ and HER2/neu-enriched tumors [76–79]. In contrast, mucinous carcinoma usually presents ADC values similar to benign lesions, most likely due to the presence of both low cellularity and mucin-rich compartments [68]. Bickel et al. evaluated whether ADC with DWI at 3 T can be used as an imaging biomarker to differentiate invasive breast cancer from noninvasive ductal carcinoma in situ (DCIS). In that study, in addition to being used as an imaging biomarker for the diagnosis of breast cancer, ADC seemed to be a valuable noninvasive quantitative biomarker to assess breast cancer invasiveness, and thus, has the potential to reduce over-diagnosis and subsequent over-treatment [80]. Another promising application for DWI is the monitoring of breast cancer treatment. ADC values are very sensitive to changes in tumor cellularity and necrosis. The cytotoxic effect of anticancer drugs increases the Brownian movements in damaged tissues and is reflected by an increase in ADC values which occurs earlier than lesion size changes or vascularity, as measured with DCE-MRI, suggesting DWI can provide a valuable early indication of treatment efficacy [81, 82]. Park et al. [83] studied the potential of DWI in the prediction of response to neo-adjuvant chemotherapy in breast cancer patients. Patients with a low pretreatment ADC tended to respond better to chemotherapy. The best pretreatment ADC cutoff with which to differentiate between responders and nonresponders was 1.17×10^{-3} mm^2/s, which yielded a sensitivity of 94 % and a specificity of 71 %. Richards et al. [84] found that pretreatment tumor ADC values differed between intrinsic subtypes and were predictive of pathologic response in triple-negative tumors. However, the literature presents divergent results for the assessment of pre-chemotherapy ADC, and more data to fully elucidate the role of ADC as a potential biomarker for predicting the response to neoadjuvant treatment in the breast is warranted [61, 82, 85, 86].

Several advanced modeling approaches for DWI to extract more biologically relevant information are currently under investigation.

- *Intravoxel incoherent motion (IVIM)*: DWI is also sensitive to perfusion because the flow of blood in randomly oriented capillaries mimics a diffusion process through the IVIM effect [87]. Several studies have investigated IVIM in breast tumors and preliminary data suggests that it can provide valuable information about both tissue microstructure and microvasculature that is beneficial for the diagnosis of breast cancer lesions [88–92].
- *Diffusion-Weighted Kurtosis (DKI)*: In living tissue, DWI is affected by Brownian incoherent motion and micro-perfusion or blood flow showing non Gaussian phenomena [93]. The diffusion-weighted kurtosis (DKI) quantifies the deviation of tissue diffusion from a Gaussian pattern and has demonstrated a substantially higher sensitivity and specificity in cancer detection compared with ADCs [94, 95].
- *Diffusion Tensor Imaging (DTI)*: DTI is considered to be an extension of DWI, which provides information about water motion in six or more directions, and thus, characterizes the motion of water in more detail [96, 97]. DTI provides measurements of two parameters: mean diffusivity (MD) and fractional anisotropy (FA). MD reflects the average anisotropy, whereas FA describes the degree of anisotropy [97, 98]. The diffusion of water molecules in the mammary glandular/ductal system presents an excellent example of restricted movement. There is free diffusion parallel to the walls of the ducts and lobules and a restricted diffusion in the perpendicular directions, leading to an anisotropic diffusion [99]. Based on histopathological data, most breast pathologies result in decreased structuring compared to healthy tissue. Therefore, any changes of this tissue structure by means of benign or malignant tumor growth should be reflected by changes in diffusion anisotropy detectable with DTI [96, 97, 99]. Partidge et al. [100] investigated whether DTI measures of anisotropy in breast tumors are different from those in normal breast tissue and whether this could improve the discrimination between benign and malignant lesions. The authors

demonstrated that diffusion anisotropy is significantly lower in breast cancers than in normal tissue, which may reflect alterations in tissue organization, but that it cannot reliably differentiate between benign and malignant lesions. Baltzer et al. [96] proved that DTI can visualize micro-anatomical differences between benign and malignant breast tumors, as well as normal breast parenchyma. However, FA did not have an incremental value compared to ADC. Although results for the diagnostic accuracy of FA are divergent [96, 97, 101], it seems that DTI has the potential to serve not only as an adjunct method to DCE examination, but also as an alternative method when DCE imaging is contraindicated [96, 99, 100].

15.2.4 Proton MR Spectroscopy

MRS is a non-invasive technique that reflects the chemical composition of tissue by providing spatially localized signal spectra with spectral peaks representing the structure and concentration of different chemical compounds in the region of interest. Based on these signal spectra, which provide information about the varying levels of associated detectable metabolites, MRS is able to differentiate tissue conditions such as normal, benign, malignant, necrotic, or hypoxic. It has been demonstrated that, in breast imaging, the additional application of ^{1}H-MRS aids in the characterization of breast tumors [102, 103]. In breast imaging, the additional value of ^{1}H-MRS is based on the detection of choline (Cho). The Cho peak observed *in vivo* is located at approximately 3.2 ppm and is a composite of several different Cho-containing compounds, such as free choline, phosphocholine, and glycerophosphocholine, and is commonly referred to as total Cho (tCho). Cho is involved in cell membrane turnover and is thus considered an imaging biomarker of cell proliferation. In breast cancer, the elevated Cho signal is thought to result from a combination of increased intracellular phosphocholine concentration and increased cell density in the tumor. At low field-strengths, a choline peak is not regularly identified in normal breast tissue [103, 104], and therefore, its presence helps in the differentiation of benign from malignant lesions [105–107]. ^{1}H-MRS can be performed as single-voxel or multi-voxel MRS. Single-voxel spectroscopy provides a single spatially localized spectrum that represents the average chemical signal from a 3D voxel placed in the lesion detected with DCE-MRI. In multi-voxel MRS using chemical shift, a larger volume is excited, producing a spatially resolved grid of spectra. For a detailed review of acquisition techniques and analysis of breast MRS, refer to a recent review article by Bolan et al. [105]. Assessment of the recorded tCho as an indicator of breast malignancy can be performed either qualitatively—detection of the presence of a tCho peak, semi-quantitatively—measurement of tCho SNR, peak height, or peak integral, or as an absolute quantification—calculation of tCho concentration with water as an internal reference or using an external standard. A detrimental effect of contrast agents on ^{1}H-MRS has been described in both experimental and clinical settings, and therefore, the possibility of altered tCho signal intensities after contrast medium injection have to be considered when calculating absolute tCho quantification [103, 105, 108, 109]. Due to the challenging image acquisition and post-processing, the clinical value of proton ^{1}H-MRS remains controversial. Nevertheless, several studies, mainly performed at 1.5 T and using single-voxel approaches, have demonstrated that ^{1}H-MRS can improve diagnostic accuracy in breast cancer diagnosis [10]. In a recent meta-analysis, which included 19 studies, Baltzer et al. [23] evaluated the diagnostic performance and feasibility of ^{1}H-MRS for differentiating malignant and benign breast lesions. The pooled sensitivity and specificity of ^{1}H-MRS was 73 % and 88 %, respectively. There was a substantial heterogeneity of sensitivity in the studies (42–100 %), whereas specificity showed little variation. The meta-analysis did not show any significant performance advantages of 3 T over 1.5 T field strength or multivoxel over single-voxel techniques, or qualitative over quantitative tCho assessments. However the numbers of studies using 3 T (2/19) and MRSI (3/19) were small. ^{1}H-MRS seems to be limited in the diagnosis of early breast cancer and small breast tumors as well as in non-mass-enhancing lesions.

Recently, Gruber et al. [110] developed a high-spatial-resolution 3D ^{1}H-MRSI protocol at 3 T, designed to cover a large fraction of the breast in a clinically acceptable measurement time of 12–15 min with excellent data quality (Fig. 15.3). In that study, with a Cho SNR threshold level of 2.6, 3D ^{1}H-MRSI provided a sensitivity of 97 % and a specificity of 84 % in breast cancer diagnosis.

^{1}H-MRSI might also be a valuable tool in the assessment of the response to neoadjuvant chemotherapy [102, 111, 112]. Studies indicate that breast tumor tCho levels and the changes in these levels during treatment are reflective of treatment-induced alterations in cell proliferation prior to any changes in tumor size. ^{1}H-MRSI can, therefore, provide an early predictive imaging biomarker of treatment response. Meisamy et al. demonstrated that MRS of the breast was able to detect a change in Cho concentration from baseline (before receiving chemo) within 24 h of administration of the first dose of the regimen. This change had a statistically significant positive correlation with change in final size ($p = 0.001$) [104]. In addition, Shin et al. showed that the tCho of tumors was higher in invasive versus in situ cancers and correlated this with several prognostic factors, including nuclear grade, histologic grade, and estrogen receptor (ER) status [106]. Therefore, it can be expected that the addition of 1H-MRSI of the breast will offer a substantial advantage over contrast-enhanced MRI of the breast alone in the prediction of response to neoadjuvant chemotherapy.

In addition, tCho seems to be indicative not only of an increased proliferation, but also a hallmark of imminent malignant transformation [113, 114]. Recently, Ramadan et al. [115] demonstrated that, in BRCA-1 and BRCA-2 carriers, healthy breast tissue is likely to differ from each other as well as from non-mutation carriers with regard to levels of triglycerides, unsaturated fatty acids, and cholesterol in the absence any other imaging findings. Further studies are warranted, but if these findings may be confirmed there might be relevant clinical implications for the screening of high-risk women.

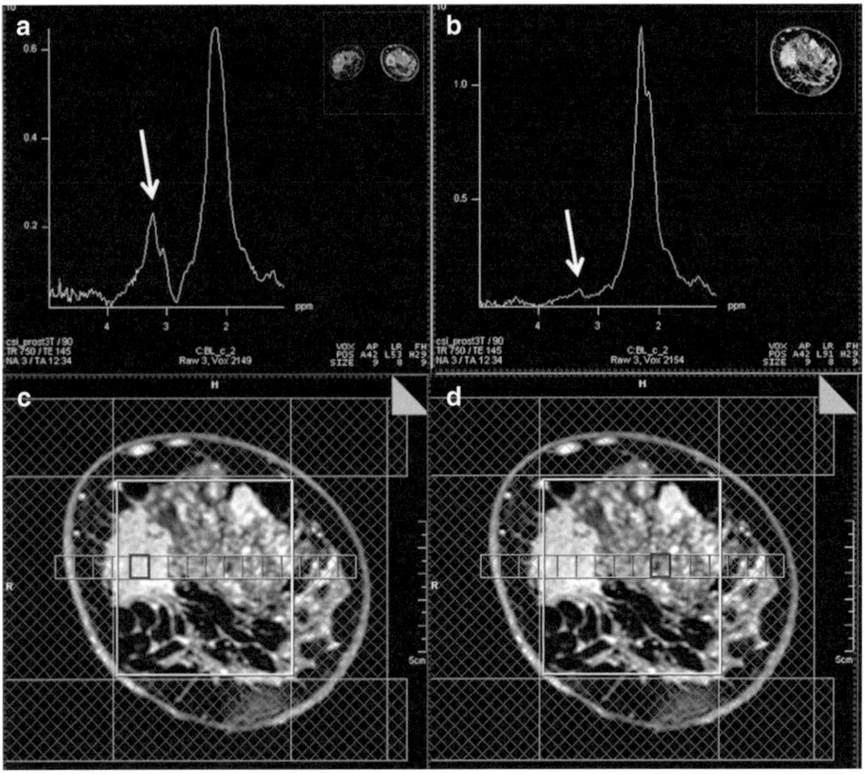

Fig. 15.3 3 T. *Invasive ductal carcinoma G3 in a 47-year-old woman at 9 o'clock in the right breast.* (**a**) The spectrum of the voxel with the highest Cho SNR inside the malignant lesion is displayed. An elevated Cho signal at 3.2 ppm was found and the calculated Cho SNR in this voxel was 10.5 (*white arrow*). (**b**) The DCE MR images are overlaid with the grid used for 3D 1H-MRSI localization. (**c**) Metabolic map of (**d**) adjacent breast tissue without any choline peak (*white arrow*). DCE-MRI demonstrated an irregularly shaped mass lesion with spiculated margins. DCE-MRI and 3D ^{1}H-MRSI at 3 T concordantly classified the lesion as BI-RADS 5 (highly suggestive of malignancy)

15.2.5 Multiparametric MRI

Available data suggests that the addition of functional MRI parameters, in combination with DCE-MRI, may provide additional specificity [23, 24]. Multiparametric MRI of the breast simultaneously and non-invasively acquires multiple imaging biomarkers, and thus, has the potential to significantly improve breast cancer diagnosis, staging, and assessment of treatment response. Several recent studies have assessed multiparametric MRI using DCE-MRI and DWI for breast cancer diagnosis and have demonstrated that an increased diagnostic accuracy in breast cancer diagnosis could be achieved [116, 117]. To solve the dilemma of how to combine the unique information from DCE-MRI and DWI, and to implement multiparametric MRI in the clinical routine, several different approaches have been explored. Pinker et al. [13] developed a reading scheme that adapted ADC thresholds to the

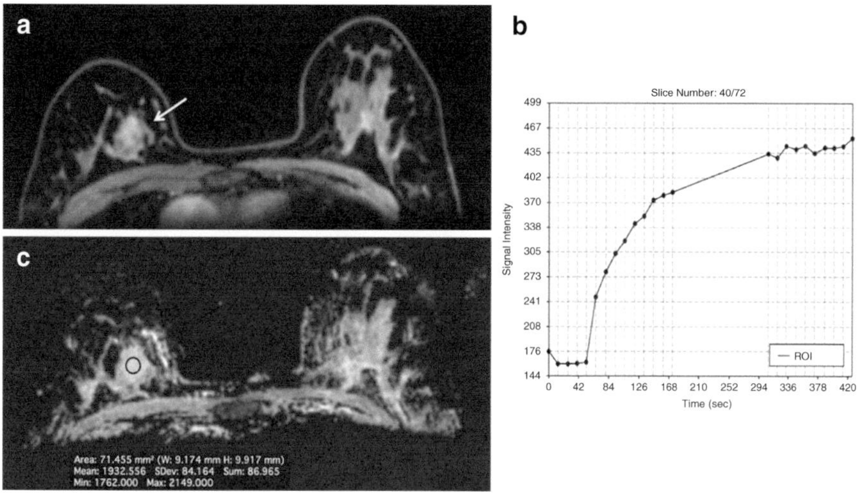

Fig. 15.4 *Fibroadenoma in a 48-year-old woman at 2 o'clock in the right breast.* (**a**) The irregular-shaped and partially irregularly marginated mass (*white arrow*) demonstrated (**b**) an initial fast/persistent (II) heterogeneous contrast enhancement. (**c**) However, on diffusion-weighted imaging (DWI), the ADC values (1.93×10^{-3} mm^2/s) were well above the threshold for malignancy, allowing an accurate classification as a benign finding with the BI-RADS©-adapted reading

assigned BI-RADS® classification. In that study, the sensitivity of the BI-RADS®-adapted reading was not significantly different from the high sensitivity of DCE-MRI ($p = 0.4$), whereas the BI-RADS®-adapted reading maximized specificity to 89.4 %, which was significantly higher compared to DCE-MRI alone ($p < 0.001$). The authors concluded that BI-RADS®-adapted reading, combining DCE-MRI and DWI, improves diagnostic accuracy and is fast and easy to use in routine clinical practice (Fig. 15.4). In a different approach, Baltzer et al. [118] investigated the improvements in specificity of breast MRI by integrating ADC values with DCE-MRI using a simple sum score. The additional integration of ADC scores achieved an improved specificity (92.4 %) compared to DCE-MR-only reading (specificity of 81.8 %), with no false-negative results. Pinker et al. compared the diagnostic accuracy of DCE-MRI as a single parameter to multiparametric MRI with two (DCE-MRI and DWI) and three (DCE-MRI, DWI and 1H-MRSI) parameters in breast cancer diagnosis. Multiparametric MRI with three parameters yielded significantly higher AUCs (0.936) compared to DCE-MRI alone (0.814) ($p < 0.001$). Multiparametric MRI with just two parameters at 3 T did not yield higher AUCs (0.808) than DCE-MRI alone (0.814). Multiparametric MRI with three parameters resulted in elimination of false-negative lesions and significantly reduced the false-positives ($p = 0.002$) (Figs. 15.5 and 15.6). The authors concluded that multiparametric MRI with three parameters increases the diagnostic accuracy of breast cancer, compared to DCE-MRI alone and MP MRI with two parameters, and should be considered for future implementation in breast cancer care [11].

Recently, the concept of multiparametric imaging has been extended to ultra-high-field MRI. Pinker et al. evaluated the clinical application of multiparametric

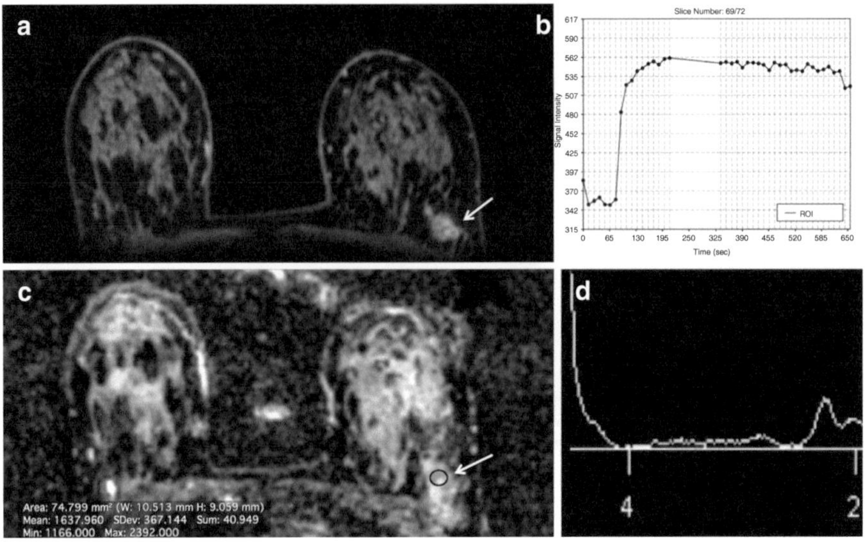

Fig. 15.5 *Fibroadenoma in a 48-year-old woman at the 2 o'clock position of the right breast.* (**a–d**) The slightly irregular, partly indistinct mass (*arrow*) with a heterogeneous initial strong enhancement and plateau curve is classified by DCE-MRI of the breast as BI-RADS© 4 (suspicious abnormality)

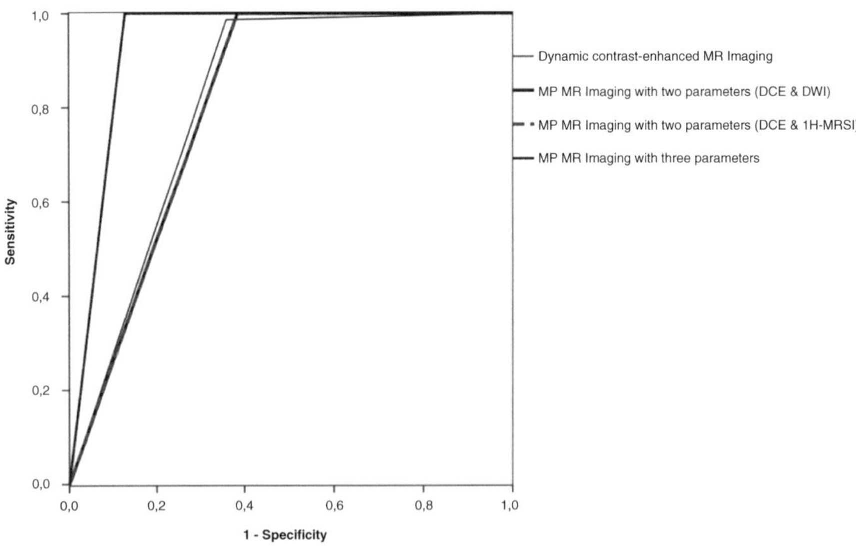

Fig. 15.6 ROC curves illustrate the higher diagnostic value (i.e., higher sensitivity, specificity, and larger area under the curve) that is reached for multiparametric MRI with three parameters, compared to DCE-MRI of the breast and multiparametric MRI with two parameters

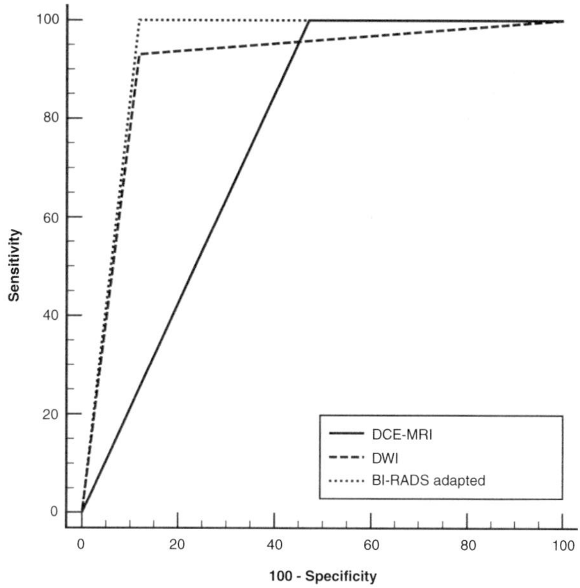

Fig. 15.7 ROC curves illustrate the higher diagnostic value that is reached for multiparametric MRI compared to DCE-MR and DW imaging of the breast at 7 T

MRI using DCE-MRI and DWI at 7 T and its impact on diagnostic accuracy in breast cancer diagnosis [12]. Multiparametric MRI, combining high-resolution DCE-MRI and DWI at 7 T, yielded a sensitivity and specificity of 100 % and 88.2 %, respectively, with an AUC of 0.941, which was significantly greater than DCE-MRI ($p = 0.003$), with a sensitivity and specificity of 100 % and 53.2 %, respectively, with an AUC of 0.765, and greater than DWI, with a sensitivity and specificity of 93.1 % and 88.2 %, respectively, with an AUC of 0.907 (Fig. 15.7). In that study, multiparametric MRI of the breast at 7 T accurately detected all cancers, reduced false-positives from eight with DCE-MRI to two (Fig. 15.8), and thus, could have obviated unnecessary breast biopsies ($p = 0.031$). In a very recent study, Schmitz et al. investigated multiparametric MRI with three parameters, i.e., DCE-MRI, DWI, and phosphorus spectroscopy (31P MRSI) at 7 T for the characterization of breast cancer [119]. The authors concluded that multiparametric 7 T breast MRI with three parameters is feasible in the clinical setting and shows an association between ADC and tumor grade, and between 31P MRSI and mitotic count.

15.3 Emerging MRI Parameters

15.3.1 Sodium Imaging (^{23}Na MRI)

Sodium (^{23}Na) MRI has been introduced as a novel MRI parameter for the detection and therapy monitoring of breast cancer. ^{23}Na MRI provides information about the physiological and biochemical state of tissue, and the sodium concentration is

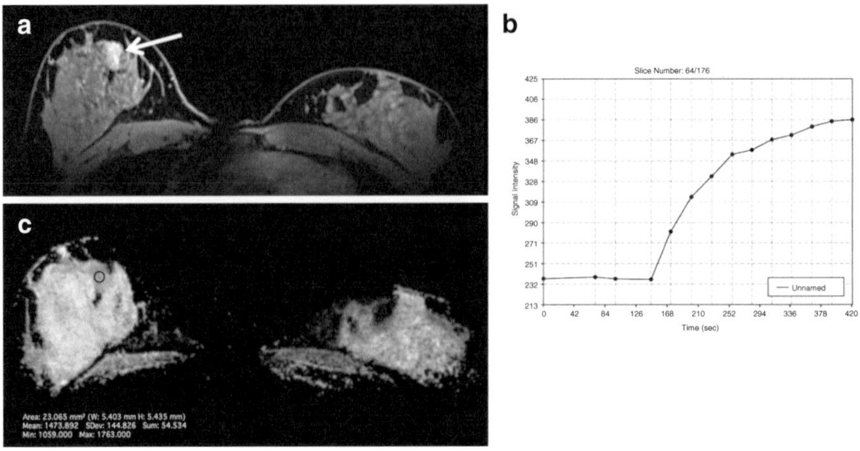

Fig. 15.8 7 T DCE-MR. *Fibroadenoma in a 60-year-old woman at 3 o'clock in the right breast.* (**a**) The irregular-shaped and partially irregularly marginated mass (*white arrow*), demonstrated (**b**) an initial medium/persistent (II) heterogeneous contrast enhancement on DCE-MRI of the breast at 7 T. (**c**) However, on diffusion-weighted imaging (DWI), the ADC values (1.47×10^{-3} mm^2/s) were well above the threshold for malignancy, allowing an accurate classification as a benign finding with the BI-RADS©-adapted reading

a sensitive indicator of cellular metabolic integrity and ion homeostasis [120, 121]. In normal cells, a low intracellular sodium concentration is maintained by the Na^+/K^+ ATPase pump, which actively pumps sodium out of the cell against a concentration gradient formed by the higher extracellular sodium concentration. ^{23}Na MRI is able to detect increased sodium levels secondary to failure of the Na^+/K^+-ATPase pump due to the breakdown of cell membranes, as observed in malignancy. Ouwerkerk et al. investigated the potential of ^{23}Na MRI for the differentiation of benign and malignant breast lesions at 1.5 T [122]. The authors demonstrated that an increased total sodium concentration in breast tumors is a sensitive cellular-level indicator associated with malignancy, and has the potential to increase the specificity of MRI of the breast. However, at field-strengths of 1.5 and 3 T, ^{23}Na MRI is limited. Recently, Zaric et al. investigated quantitative ^{23}Na MRI at 7 T compared to DWI. These authors demonstrated that quantitative ^{23}Na MRI at 7 T can be accomplished with a good resolution and image quality within clinically acceptable measurement times in patients with breast tumors. Quantitative ^{23}Na MRI allowed good discrimination of benign and malignant breast lesions ($p = 0.002$), similar to DWI ($p = 0.002$). ^{23}Na MRI reliably provides complementary information about pathophysiologic changes in neoplasms and has the potential to improve the detection, characterization, and treatment monitoring of breast lesions (Fig. 15.9) [123].

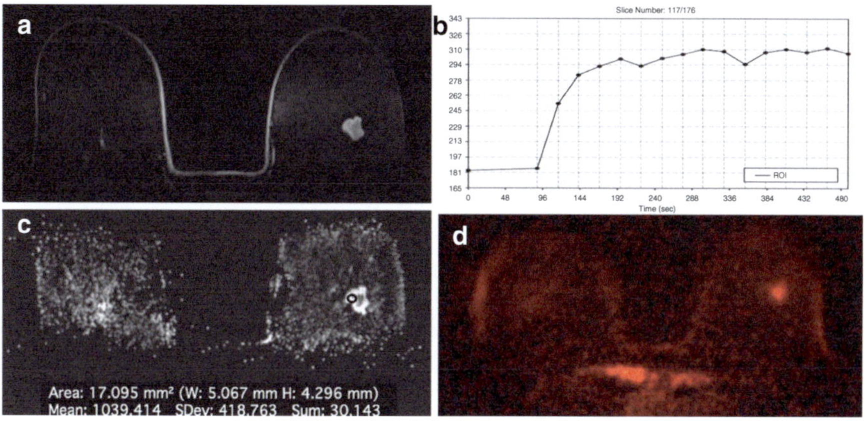

Fig. 15.9 *Invasive ductal carcinoma G1 in a 71-year-old woman at 2 o'clock in the right breast.* (**a**) The irregular shaped and partly irregularly marginated mass lesion demonstrates (**b**) homogeneous initial strong enhancement followed by a plateau. (**c**) The mass demonstrates low ADC values (1.038 × 10^{-3} mm^2/s) and (**d**) shows a high signal intensity on ^{23}Na MRI, indicative of malignancy

15.3.2 Phosphorus Spectroscopy (^{31}P MRS)

Phosphorus spectroscopy (^{31}P MRS) measures the bioenergetics of tissue and membrane phospholipid metabolism. The signals of phospholipid precursors and catabolites can be used as imaging biomarkers for tumor progression and response to therapy [124, 125]. It has been demonstrated in several *in vitro* and *in vivo* ^{31}P MRS studies that elevated levels of phosphocholine (PC)/phosphoethanolamine (PE) are detectable in several cancers. Barzilai et al. showed a significant decrease in the PE/PC ratio in malignant breast tumors compared to benign lesions [126], as well as changes in PE/PC ratios in response to therapy. At field-strengths of 1.5 and 3 T, the application of ^{31}P MRSI is limited to relatively large and primarily superficial tumors [125]. Recently, the feasibility of ^{31}P MRS at 7 T has been demonstrated in healthy volunteers and patients with breast cancer, with excellent quality of (^{31}P)-MR spectra. Patients with breast cancer show higher levels of PE and PC than healthy volunteers. ^{31}P MRS provides a direct method for the *in vivo* detection and quantification of endogenous biomarkers, such as phospholipid metabolism, phosphate energy metabolism, and intracellular pH, and allows monitoring *in vivo* metabolism during neoadjuvant chemotherapy. It can be expected that ^{31}P MRS could used as specific tool for breast cancer diagnosis, tumor staging, and monitoring response to therapy [56, 127].

15.3.3 Chemical Exchange Saturation Transfer (CEST) Imaging

Chemical exchange saturation transfer (CEST) is an MRI parameter that enables visualization of chemical exchange processes between protons bound to solutes and surrounding bulk water molecules [128, 129]. It has been demonstrated that endogenous CEST can discriminate tumor from healthy breast tissue based on the information about protons associated with mobile proteins through the amide proton transfer (APT) effect, and also has been implicated as a prognosticator of response to therapy [130]. Recently, ATP CEST MRI at 3 T has been investigated for its potential in breast cancer diagnosis, with promising results. Schmitt et al. demonstrated lesion detection and differentiation was equally possible with DCE-MRI and ATP CEST-MRI through the CEST contrast generated by endogenous solute molecules. The results of this initial feasibility study hint at a significant potential for ATP CEST-MRI in breast imaging. Recently, animal studies have investigated CEST contrasts other than ATP, exploiting the entire CEST spectrum. Desmond et al. found that imaging of the amide, amine, and aliphatic signal (aaaCEST) allows non-invasive differentiation of areas of apoptosis and/or necrosis from actively progressing tumor [131, 132]. In addition, similar to [^{18}F]Fluorodeoxyglucose positron emission tomography ([^{18}F]FDG), dynamic CEST imaging after the administration of glucose (glucoCEST) has been shown to enable the non-invasive evaluation of the kinetics of glycolysis, which is typically increased in malignant lesions. Initial results indicate that glucoCEST might serve as a potential substitute for PET/CT or PET/MRI in the clinic for the detection of tumors and metastases, distinguishing between malignant and benign tumors and monitoring tumor response to therapy, without the need for radio-labeled isotopes [131, 133–135]. Nevertheless, further studies will be necessary to explore the true potential of CEST imaging in breast cancer.

15.3.4 Blood Oxygen Level–Dependent MRI

Blood oxygen level–dependent (BOLD) MRI or intrinsic susceptibility-weighted imaging is a noninvasive method for the indirect measurement of tumor perfusion and hypoxia. Hypoxia is a feature of most solid tumors, including breast cancer, and is associated with tumor progression, angiogenesis, treatment resistance, local recurrence, and metastasis. BOLD MRI non-invasively detects increased levels of paramagnetic deoxyhemoglobin. Deoxyhemoglobin causes susceptibility variations in the magnetic field, which, in turn, decrease the transverse relaxation rate R2 * (= 1/T2 *) of water in blood and the tissue surrounding blood vessels. An increase in the deoxyhemoglobin concentration, i.e., hypoxia, causes a decrease in the signal intensity on the T2 * image and a faster R2 * [136]. Improvement in tissue oxygenation has the opposite effect. Therefore deoxyhemoglobin acts as an intrinsic BOLD contrast agent for imaging tissue hypoxia [10, 137]. Initial results indicate that BOLD MRI is a simple and non-invasive technique yielding hypoxia information on breast cancer [91, 138, 139], and can be used to assess response to neoadjuvant treatment [140]. Tumor hypoxia might, therefore, have the potential to serve as an imaging biomarker of breast cancer prognosis as well as treatment response [141]. To date, tumor hypoxia is assessed on biopsy-derived tumor tissue samples, with the main limitations being the invasiveness, non-representative sampling (the tumor can be quite heterogeneous and biopsies can be non-representative of the whole tumor), and the necessity to perform multiple evaluations to follow changes in tumor oxygenation after treatment [141]. These limitations highlight the importance of developing imaging biomarkers that can reliably detect tumor hypoxia for tumor grading and non-invasive monitoring spatio-longitudinally during treatment. However, to date, BOLD MRI in breast imaging is in the experimental/translational stage and data is, as yet, scarce. Further studies will be necessary to elucidate the clinical value of BOLD MRI for breast cancer diagnosis and treatment response assessment.

15.3.5 Hyperpolarized MRI (HP MRI)

Hyperpolarized MRI (HP MRI) is one of the most recent advances in molecular imaging. HP MRI allows a rapid, radiation-free, non-invasive investigation of tumor metabolism by exploiting exogenous contrast agents that have been "hyperpolarized." Conventional MR imaging depends on nuclear spins that have been polarized on the order of a few parts per million, whereas, in HP MRI, nuclear spins reach near-unity polarization, resulting in an extensive increase in signal intensity [142, 143]. HP MRI nuclear spins are polarized in an amorphous solid state at ~1.2 K through coupling of the nuclear spins with unpaired electrons that are added to the sample via an organic free radical. In the solid state, the high electron spin polarization is, in part, transferred to the nuclear spins by microwave irradiation and then the sample is rapidly dissolved for injection. Recently, ^{13}C-labeled substrates have been polarized to obtain enhancements of the ^{13}C nuclear MR signals, e.g., >50,000-fold at 3 T in the substrate as well as subsequent metabolic products [144]. The enhancement that is achieved is lost in time as a function of the spin-lattice relaxation time of the nucleus (T1). The HP ^{13}C probes can be injected into living organisms and their metabolism can be observed in real-time by chemical shift imaging. Currently, (^{13}C) pyruvate is the most widely used probe for HP MR studies since it polarizes well, has a long T_1 relaxation time, and is rapidly taken up by the cell and metabolized at the juncture of glycolysis, TCA, amino acid biosynthesis, and other critical pathways. Multiple animal studies have confirmed that the real-time measurement of the relative transformation of pyruvate into lactate and alanine, using HP MRI, allows a differentiation of benign and malignant tissue [145–147]. In addition to the distinction of cancerous and normal cells [146, 148, 149], HP MRSI using ^{13}C pyruvate has been demonstrated to have potential in the assessment of cancer progression [150, 151]. Recently, other novel probes for redox (^{13}C dehydroascorbate), necrosis (^{13}C fumarate), and glutamine metabolism (^{13}C glutamine) have been developed to interrogate other metabolic pathways, with promising results [152]. To date, there is no specific clinical application for HP MRI in breast cancer. Nevertheless, several pre-clinical and initial studies in cancer, including breast cancer [153], indicated that this technique may be applicable for the detection of breast cancer and assessment of treatment response in the future.

15.4 Nuclear Imaging of the Breast

15.4.1 Gamma Camera Imaging: ^{99}mtc-Sestamibi Scintimammography (SM) and Breast-Specific Gamma Imaging (BSGI)

^{99m}Tc-sestamibi scintigraphic mammography (^{99}mTc-MIBI-SM) was introduced in the '90s and can be used as an alternative diagnostic imaging modality in patients with dense breasts. In ^{99}mTc-MIBI-SM, the radiotracer 99mTc-MIBI is injected intravenously and accumulates in tissues with increased perfusion, permeability, and metabolic activity, such as breast cancer. Several studies have investigated the application of 99mTc-MIBI for the assessment of breast tumors, using both planar and single-photon emission computed tomographic radionuclide imaging with a general-purpose gamma camera, and have reported sensitivities ranging from 84 to 93 % [154]. However, ^{99}mTc-MIBI-SM has a relatively low spatial resolution, which impedes the depiction of small cancers and is limited in the detection of low-grade breast tumors [155–157]. To overcome these limitations, ^{99}mTc-MIBI-SM Breast-Specific Gamma Imaging (BSGI) has been developed [158–163]. In a meta-analysis, Sun et al. reviewed the role of BSGI as an adjunct modality to mammography [164] and reported a pooled sensitivity and specificity of 95 % and 80 %, respectively. In patients with normal mammography findings, 4 % were diagnosed with breast cancer by BSGI, and, in those with a suspicious imaging finding on mammography or biopsy-proven breast cancer, 6 % were diagnosed with multifocal disease by BSGI. The authors concluded that BSGI can serve as a valuable adjunct modality to mammography for detecting breast cancer.

15.4.2 Positron Emission Tomography (PET)/Computed Tomography (CT), and PET Mammography (PEM)

Positron emission tomography (PET) is a non-invasive diagnostic nuclear medicine imaging method that enables the assessment of physiological processes using radiotracers. The most commonly used radiotracer is [^{18}F]Fluorodeoxyglucose ([^{18}F]

FDG). [^{18}F]FDG PET allows an assessment of tissue glycolysis, which is typically increased in neoplastic processes, such as breast cancer [165–167]. However, [^{18}F]FDG uptake is variable based on the organ of origin, tumor type, and grade, and a critical mass of tumor cells is necessary for visualization. In addition, [^{18}F]FDG uptake is not tumor-specific and some benign conditions, such as inflammatory processes, can also be [^{18}F]FDG-avid. As [^{18}F]FDG PET alone provides limited anatomical information and has a low spatial resolution that frequently results in difficulties in lesion localization and in the assessment of potential tumor infiltration into adjacent organs, hybrid imaging systems, such as PET/CT, were developed and established in the clinical routine. Numerous studies have investigated [^{18}F]FDG PET and [^{18}F]FDG PET/CT, in the supine position, for breast imaging [165–170]. ^{18}FDG-PET/(CT) is helpful in the staging of locally advanced metastatic or recurrent breast cancer, as well as in evaluating the response of locally advanced and metastatic breast cancer to treatment. Available data indicate that ([^{18}F]FDG PET/CT is valuable in the evaluation of advanced axillary disease and nodal spread in locally advanced breast cancer [165–171]. Whole-body supine [^{18}F]FDG PET/CT has been evaluated for the detection and staging of primary breast cancer with reported sensitivities and specificities of 88 % and 80 %, respectively. However, due to its limited ability in the detection of small lesions and low grade cancers, it is currently not recommended for local staging of known or suspected primary breast malignancies [172, 173]. In a recent study, Magometschnigg et al. compared the diagnostic accuracy of [^{18}F]FDG PET/CT with DCE-MRI at 3 T in suspicious breast lesions, evaluated the influence of tumor size on diagnostic accuracy, and explored the use of SUV_{MAX} thresholds to differentiate malignant and benign breast lesions [173]. In that study, the patients were scanned in the prone position, with a state-of-the-art combined PET/CT system, which might explain the achieved higher sensitivity and diagnostic accuracy. Both [^{18}F]FDG PET/CT and DCE-MRI demonstrate an equal diagnostic accuracy for breast cancer diagnosis of 93 % (Fig. 15.10). Neither sensitivity ($p = 0.125$), specificity ($p = 0.344$), or diagnostic accuracy ($p = 1$) were significantly different. In lesions <10 mm, diagnostic accuracy deteriorated to 91 % for both [^{18}F]FDG PET/CT and DCE-MRI. In lesions <10 mm, CE-MRI at 3 T is more sensitive, but less specific than [^{18}F]FDG PET/CT. Quantitative assessment using an SUV_{MAX} threshold for the differentiation of benign and malignant lesions is not helpful in breast cancer diagnosis.

The authors concluded that [^{18}F]FDG PET/CT can be considered an alternative imaging modality in patients who are not candidates for DCE-MRI.

To overcome the limitations of whole-body [^{18}F]FDG PET/CT in breast imaging, dedicated breast PET systems have been developed. Positron Emission Mammography (PEM) is a high-resolution, breast-specific device that enables co-registration of mammographic and emission [^{18}F]FDG images of the breast by means of two flat detectors integrated into the system on either side of the breast. The more recently developed breast-specific MAMography with MolecularImaging (MAMMI)-PET utilizes a small ring of detectors, which yields an improved contrast and signal-to-noise ratio (SNR). Other alternatives to conventional PEM design are the Clear-PEM system or the Shimadzu, which acquire tomographic breast

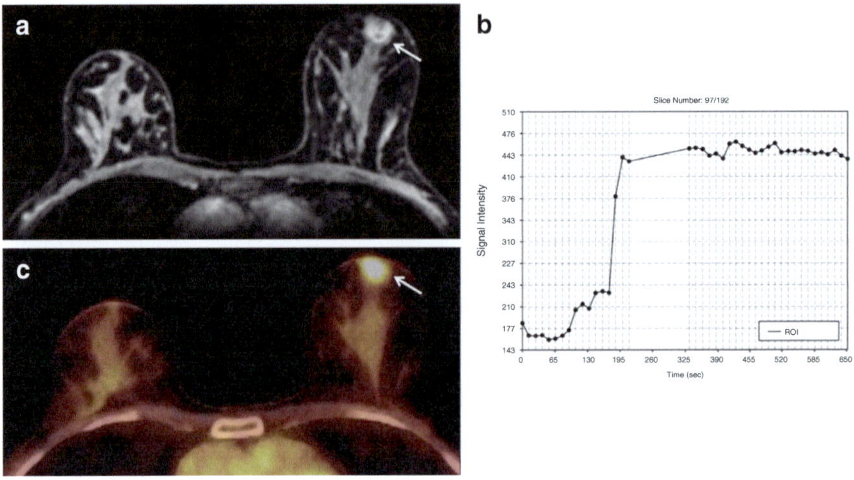

Fig. 15.10 *Invasive ductal carcinoma G2 in a 46-year-old woman, retroareolar in the right breast.* (**a**) The round, irregularly marginated mass lesion (*white arrow*) shows (**b**) a heterogeneous initial strong enhancement followed by a plateau, and was classified by CE-MRI as BI-RADS© 5 (suspicious finding). (**c**) On ^{18}F-FDG PET/CT, the lesion was strongly ^{18}F-FDG-avid, with an SUV_{MAX} of 4.4. The lesion was a true-positive finding on both modalities

images. Dedicated breast PET systems have been shown to have both a high sensitivity and specificity in detecting breast malignancy (<1 cm). Kalles et al. reviewed the role of [^{18}F]FDG PEM in breast cancer imaging, and concluded that [^{18}F]FDG PEM can successfully complement conventional imaging in breast cancer detection by providing information about tumor biology. The current data suggest that PEM might not be far from being included in the first-line modalities for breast cancer screening [174].

15.5 Molecular Imaging with PET/MRI

In their multi-step development, cancers have acquired several biological capabilities, such as sustaining proliferative signaling, evading growth suppressors, resisting cell death, enabling replicative immortality, inducing angiogenesis,s and activating invasion and metastasis [175–179]. To elucidate these hallmarks of cancer, imaging techniques have to be equally sophisticated and multilayered. Both MP MRI and PET of the breast can visualize different processes involved in cancer development and progression, thus providing morphologic, functional, metabolic, and molecular information about breast tumors. To overcome the individual limitations of morphologic and functional imaging techniques, hybrid imaging systems have been developed and introduced into the clinical routine. Initial studies investigating fused [^{18}F]FDG PET and DCE-MRI for breast cancer diagnosis demonstrated that fused [^{18}F]FDG PET/MRI provides accurate morphological and functional data and has the potential to emerge as an all-encompassing alternative to conventional multi-technique tumor staging [180–183]. However, in these studies, the functional information provided by [^{18}F]FDG PET was merely combined with the morphologic and limited functional information of DCE-MRI. Pinker et al. investigated multiparametric PET/MRI using DCE-MRI, DWI, ^{1}H-MRSI, and ^{18}FDG for the assessment of breast tumors at 3 T [184]. The authors demonstrated that MP [^{18}F] FDG PET/MRI provided an improved differentiation of benign and malignant breast tumors when several MRI and PET parameters are combined. In addition, the authors concluded that MP [^{18}F]FDG PET/MRI may lead to a reduction of unnecessary breast biopsies of up to 50 % (Fig. 15.11). In a recent feasibility study, Pinker et al. investigated combined PET/MRI of breast tumors in eight patients with DCE-MRI, DWI, the radiotracer [^{18}F]FDG, and the hypoxia tracer [^{18}F]FMISO (refer to Sect. 15.5.1) at 3 T (Fig. 15.12), and correlated MRI and PET parameters with pathological features, grading, proliferation-rate (ki67), immuno-histochemistry, and the clinical endpoints metastasis and death. Preliminary results showed several moderate to excellent correlations between quantitative imaging markers, grading, receptor status, and proliferation rate (Fig. 15.13) [185]. Multiparametric criteria provided independent information. DCE-MRI, [^{18}F]FDG- and [^{18}F]FMISO-avidity strongly correlated with the presence of metastasis [$r = 0.75$ ($p < 0.01$), 0.63 ($p = 0.212$), and 0.58 ($p = 0.093$)] and death [$r = 0.60$ ($p = 0.09$), 0.62 ($p = 0.08$), 0.56 ($p = 0.11$)]. Multiparametric [^{18}F]FDG /[^{18}F]FMISO PET/MRI provides quantitative prognostic information in breast cancer patients, and thus, might have the potential to enable tailored therapy through improved risk stratification.

15.5.1 Specific Radiotracers

To date, nuclear and hybrid imaging in breast cancer is mainly performed using the radiotracer [^{18}F]FDG. Although [^{18}F]FDG is a very sensitive radiotracer, it is limited with regard to specificity, as there is a significant overlap in uptake behavior for benign and malignant conditions. Recently, more specific radiotracers to target processes involved in cancer development and progression have been developed and introduced into breast imaging:

[^{18}F]Fluoromisonidazole ([^{18}F]FMISO) for the assessment of tumor hypoxia; radioactive-labeled Annexin V for the assessment of tumor-neoangiogenesis; [^{18}F] Fluoro-L-thymidine ([^{18}F]FLT) for the assessment of nucleic acid metabolism; and [^{18}F]Fluoroestradiol ([^{18}F]FES) and radiolabeled trastzumab for the assessment of tumor receptor status.

- Tumor hypoxia

[^{18}F]FMISO has a high affinity to hypoxic cells with active nitroreductase enzymes and accumulates in activated tumor cells, but not necrotic cells. Therefore, [^{18}F]FMISO has the potential to serve as an imaging biomarker for tumor grading and assessment of treatment response. Cheng et al. [186] investigated whether [^{18}F]

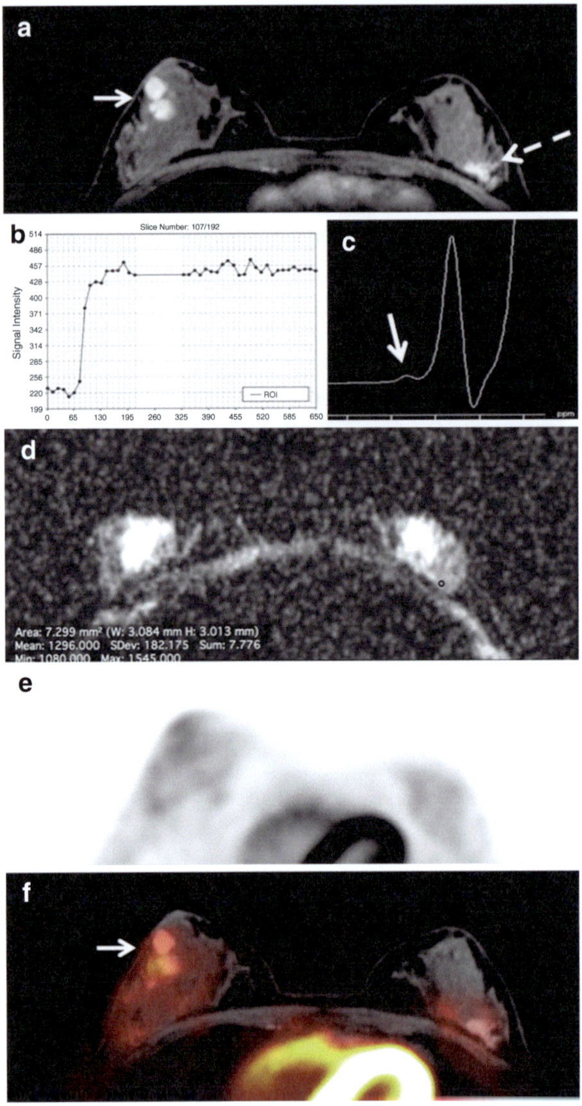

Fig. 15.11 PET/MRI. *Fibroadenomatous hyperplasia in a 22-year-old woman in the upper outer quadrant of the left breast.* (**a**) The irregular shaped and partly irregularly marginated mass lesion (*white dashed arrow*) demonstrates (**b**) homogeneous initial strong enhancement followed by a plateau. (**c**) However, the ADC values are not below the cut-off for malignancy (1.275×10^{-3} mm^2/s). (**d**) There is no Cho peak depicted at 3.23 ppm in 3D ^{1}H-MRSI (*arrow*) and (**e**) the lesion is not [^{18}F]FDG-avid. The lesion is false-positive on DCE-MRI, but true-negative on (**f**) multiparametric PET/MRI. Note two classic, mildly metabolically active fibroadenomas in the right breast, retroareolar (*white arrow*)

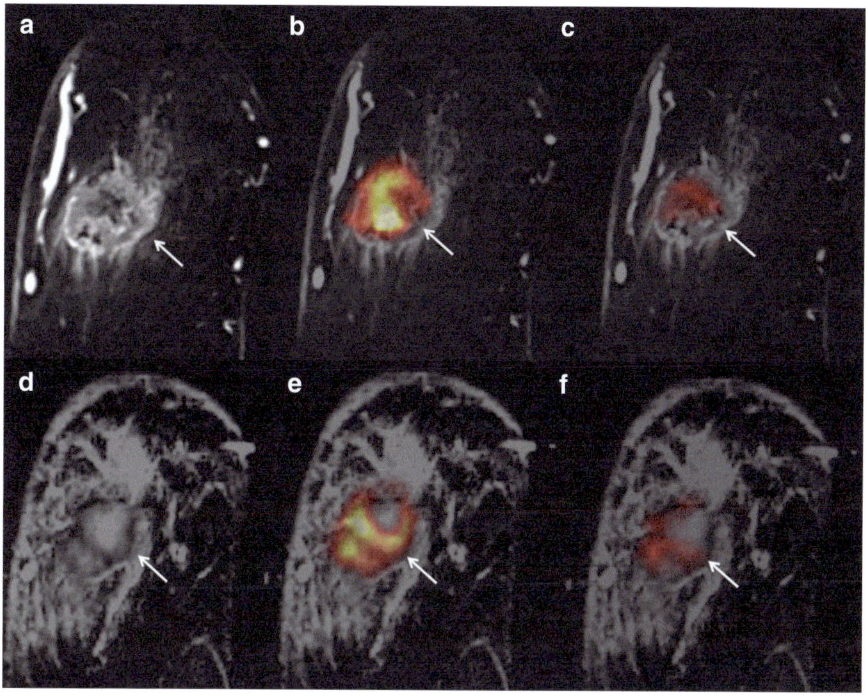

Fig. 15.12 *Invasive ductal carcinoma G3 in a 55-year-old woman at 9 o'clock in the left breast. Upper row*: DCE and fused [^{18}F]FDG and [^{18}F]FMISO PET/MRI. *Lower row*: ADC and fused [^{18}F] FDG and [^{18}F]FMISO PET/MRI. (**a**) The indistinct irregular mass lesion (*white arrow*) with heterogeneous enhancement shows decreased (**d**) ADC values in the enhancing areas. The lesion is (**b**, **e**) highly [^{18}F]FDG-avid and (**c**, **f**) several tumor areas show [^{18}F]FMISO-avidity indicative of tumor hypoxia

FMISO PET/CT can predict primary resistance to endocrine therapy in estrogen-receptor-positive breast cancer, and found a significantly positive correlation between baseline [^{18}F]FMISO uptake and clinical outcomes after ≥3 months of primary endocrine therapy with letrozole. The data suggest that [^{18}F]FMISO PET/CT may be an effective method for monitoring the response to endocrine therapy, and has the potential for early identification of non-responders.

- Apopotosis

Apoptosis plays an important role in tumorgenesis, progression, and therapy. Apopotosis induces a cascade of enzymatic processes, which eventually lead to cell death. The activation of caspsases enables the externalization of phosphatidylserine (PS), which is usually located on the inside of the cell membrane. The protein Annexin V binds to PS with a high affinity, and therefore, is a marker for apoptosis. To date, Annexin V has been labeled with multiple radiotracers for SPECT and PET imaging [187].

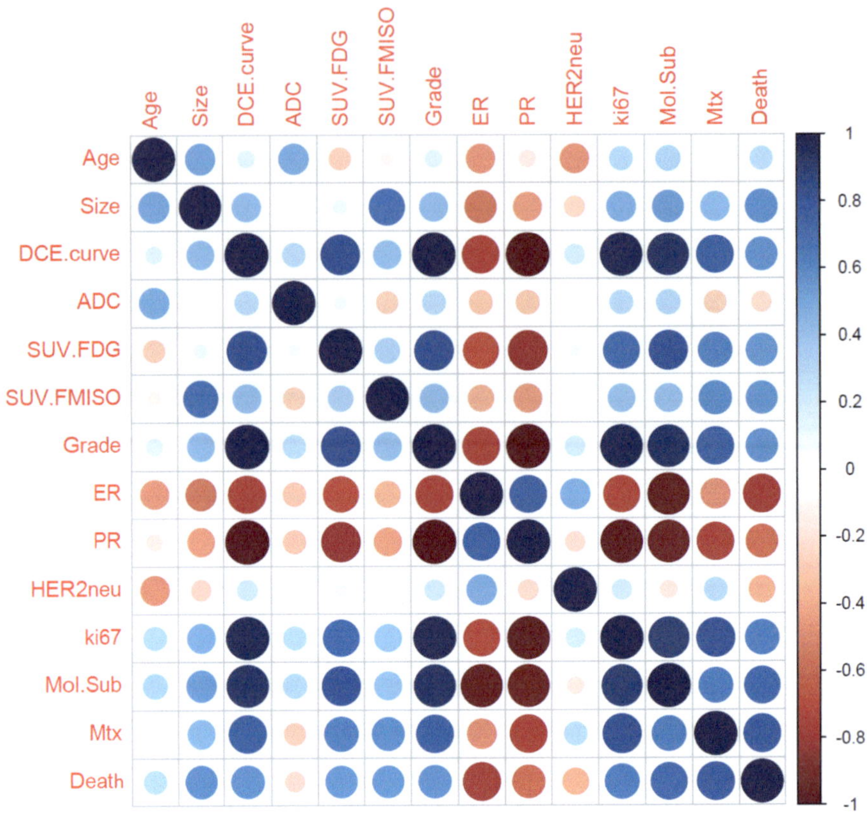

Fig. 15.13 Non-parametric Pearson's correlation coefficient matrix. Correlations are marked in blue if positive and red if negative (cf. legend on the left) *DCE* dynamic contrast enhanced-MRI, *ADC* apparent diffusion coefficient, *SUV* standardized uptake value, *FDG* fluorodeoxyglucose, *FMISO* Fluorine-18 labeled misonidazole, *ER* estrogen receptor, *PR* progesteron receptor, *HER 2 NEU* human epidermal growth factor receptor 2, *Mol.Sub* molecular subtype, *Mtx* metastases

- Proliferation

The radiotracer [^{18}F]FLT accumulates in proliferating cells. The accumulation is regulated by the thymidine salvage pathway and by the activity of thymidine kinase one, and is, therefore, reflective of DNA synthesis. [^{18}F]FLT has demonstrated promising results for the detection of treatment response in preclinical breast cancer mouse models, and is now under investigation in several clinical trials [188].

- Receptor status

[^{18}F]FES PET imaging allows a non-invasive visualization and quantification of estrogen receptor expression of both the primary tumor and metastases [189]. In addition, [^{18}F]FES PET imaging provides valuable information about the response to endocrine therapy, both in the neo-adjuvant and adjuvant setting. In a recent publication by van Kruchten et al., the authors provided a comprehensive overview of the role of [^{18}F]FES PET/CT in breast cancer [190], and concluded that [^{18}F]FES PET/CT has the potential to significantly influence patient management.

Radiolabeled trastuzumab allows the non-invasive visualization and quantification of human epidermal growth factor receptor 2 (HER2) status. In initial studies, Smith-Jones et al. demonstrated the non-invasive measurement of HER2 expression and therapy-induced changes, using a ^{68}Gallium-labeled fragment of trastuzumab in an animal model [191, 192]. In recent clinical PET/CT studies with ^{64}Copper (^{64}Cu)-DOTA-labeled trastuzumab, it was demonstrated that ^{64}Cu-DOTA-trastuzumab PET/CT enables the detection of the primary tumor, as well metastases, with excellent sensitivity, and therefore, has the potential to further improve HER2-targeted therapies [193, 194].

It can be expected that, in the future, specific radiotracers will play a major role in the detection, characterization, staging, and therapy monitoring as part of precision medicine in breast cancer [195–198].

15.6 Conclusion

Within the last few years, multiparametric imaging has entered the field of breast imaging. Multiparametric imaging of the breast comprises established and advanced MRI parameters, such as DWI and MRS, nuclear imaging with PET, PEM, and BSGI, and, more recently, combinations of techniques (e.g., PET/CT and PET/MRI). In addition, novel MRI parameters, such as ^{23}Na-MRI, ^{31}P MRSI, CEST, BOLD, and hyperpolarized MRI, are rapidly evolving and specific radiotracers are being investigated. Multiparametric imaging of the breast is a still-evolving field and more significant advances are imminent. It can be expected that multiparametric imaging of the breast, using cutting-edge sequences and targeted radiotracers, simultaneously at different levels, will provide information, noninvasively, about the hallmarks of cancer. Therefore, multiparametric imaging of the breast has the potential to significantly enhance our understanding of tumor molecular biology and to enable the development of novel personalized approaches in the management of breast cancers thereby significantly impacting not only cancer research, but also clinical practice.

References

1. DeSantis CE, Bray F, Ferlay J, et al. International variation in female breast cancer incidence and mortality rates. Cancer Epidemiol Biomarkers Prev. 2015. doi:10.1158/1055-9965.EPI-15-0535.
2. Spick C, Szolar DHM, Preidler KW, et al. Breast MRI used as a problem-solving tool reliably excludes malignancy. Eur J Radiol. 2015;84:61–4. doi:10.1016/j.ejrad.2014.10.005.

3. Sardanelli F, Boetes C, Borisch B, et al. Magnetic resonance imaging of the breast: recommendations from the EUSOMA working group. Eur J Cancer. 2010;46:1296–316. doi:10.1016/j.ejca.2010.02.015.
4. for the European Society of Breast Imaging (EUSOBI), Sardanelli F, Helbich TH. Mammography: EUSOBI recommendations for women's information. Insights Imaging. 2012;3:7–10. doi:10.1007/s13244-011-0127-y.
5. Mann RM, Balleyguier C, Baltzer PA, et al. Breast MRI: EUSOBI recommendations for women's information. Eur Radiol. 2015. doi:10.1007/s00330-015-3807-z.
6. Lin D, Moy L, Axelrod D, Smith J. Utilization of magnetic resonance imaging in breast cancer screening. Curr Oncol. 2015;22:e332–5. doi:10.3747/co.22.2882.
7. Pinker K, Bogner W, Baltzer P, et al. Clinical application of bilateral high temporal and spatial resolution dynamic contrast-enhanced magnetic resonance imaging of the breast at 7 T. Eur Radiol. 2014;24:913–20. doi:10.1007/s00330-013-3075-8.
8. Kuhl CK, Schild HH, Morakkabati N. Dynamic bilateral contrast-enhanced MR imaging of the breast: trade-off between spatial and temporal resolution. Radiology. 2005;236:789–800. doi:10.1148/radiol.2363040811.
9. Gruber S, Pinker K, Zaric O, et al. Dynamic contrast-enhanced magnetic resonance imaging of breast tumors at 3 and 7 T: a comparison. Invest Radiol. 2014;49:354–62. doi:10.1097/RLI.0000000000000034.
10. Rahbar H, Partridge SC. Multiparametric MR imaging of breast cancer. Magn Reson Imaging Clin N Am. 2016;24:223–38. doi:10.1016/j.mric.2015.08.012.
11. Pinker K, Bogner W, Baltzer P, et al. Improved diagnostic accuracy with multiparametric magnetic resonance imaging of the breast using dynamic contrast-enhanced magnetic resonance imaging, diffusion-weighted imaging, and 3-dimensional proton magnetic resonance spectroscopic imaging. Invest Radiol. 2014;49:421–30. doi:10.1097/RLI.0000000000000029.
12. Pinker K, Baltzer P, Bogner W, et al. Multiparametric MR imaging with high-resolution dynamic contrast-enhanced and diffusion-weighted imaging at 7 T improves the assessment of breast tumors: a feasibility study. Radiology. 2015;276:360–70. doi:10.1148/radiol.15141905.
13. Pinker K, Bickel H, Helbich TH, et al. Combined contrast-enhanced magnetic resonance and diffusion-weighted imaging reading adapted to the "Breast Imaging Reporting and Data System" for multiparametric 3-T imaging of breast lesions. Eur Radiol. 2013;23:1791–802. doi:10.1007/s00330-013-2771-8.
14. Boné B, Szabó BK, Perbeck LG, et al. Can contrast-enhanced MR imaging predict survival in breast cancer? Acta Radiol. 2003;44:373–8.
15. Buckley DL, Drew PJ, Mussurakis S, et al. Microvessel density of invasive breast cancer assessed by dynamic Gd-DTPA enhanced MRI. J Magn Reson Imaging. 1997;7:461–4.
16. Helbich TH. Contrast-enhanced magnetic resonance imaging of the breast. Eur J Radiol. 2000;34:208–19.
17. Wilmes LJ, Pallavicini MG, Fleming LM, et al. AG-013736, a novel inhibitor of VEGF receptor tyrosine kinases, inhibits breast cancer growth and decreases vascular permeability as detected by dynamic contrast-enhanced magnetic resonance imaging. Magn Reson Imaging. 2007;25:319–27. doi:10.1016/j.mri.2006.09.041.
18. Kaiser CG, Reich C, Dietzel M, et al. DCE-MRI of the breast in a stand-alone setting outside a complementary strategy – results of the TK-study. Eur Radiol. 2015;25:1793–800. doi:10.1007/s00330-014-3580-4.
19. Kuhl C. The current status of breast MR imaging. Part I. Choice of technique, image interpretation, diagnostic accuracy, and transfer to clinical practice. Radiology. 2007;244:356–78. doi:10.1148/radiol.2442051620.
20. Kuhl CK. Current status of breast MR imaging. Part 2. Clinical applications. Radiology. 2007;244:672–91. doi:10.1148/radiol.2443051661.
21. Pinker K, Grabner G, Bogner W, et al. A combined high temporal and high spatial resolution 3 Tesla MR imaging protocol for the assessment of breast lesions: initial results. Invest Radiol. 2009;44:553–8. doi:10.1097/RLI.0b013e3181b4c127.

22. Kuhl CK. Breast MR imaging at 3 T. Magn Reson Imaging Clin N Am. 2007;15:315–20, vi. doi:10.1016/j.mric.2007.08.003.
23. Baltzer PAT, Dietzel M. Breast lesions: diagnosis by using proton MR spectroscopy at 1.5 and 3.0 T – systematic review and meta-analysis. Radiology. 2013;267:735–46. doi:10.1148/radiol.13121856.
24. Chen X, Li W, Zhang Y, et al. Meta-analysis of quantitative diffusion-weighted MR imaging in the differential diagnosis of breast lesions. BMC Cancer. 2010;10:693. doi:10.1186/1471-2407-10-693.
25. Folkman J. Seminars in medicine of the Beth Israel Hospital, Boston. Clinical applications of research on angiogenesis. N Engl J Med. 1995;333:1757–63. doi:10.1056/NEJM199512283332608.
26. Folkman J. Tumor angiogenesis: therapeutic implications. N Engl J Med. 1971;285:1182–6. doi:10.1056/NEJM197111182852108.
27. Kaiser WA, Zeitler E. MR imaging of the breast: fast imaging sequences with and without Gd-DTPA. Preliminary Observations Radiol. 1989;170:681–6. doi:10.1148/radiology.170.3.2916021.
28. Helbich TH, Becherer A, Trattnig S, et al. Differentiation of benign and malignant breast lesions: MR imaging versus Tc-99 m sestamibi scintimammography. Radiology. 1997;202:421–9. doi:10.1148/radiology.202.2.9015068.
29. Heywang-Köbrunner SH, Viehweg P, Heinig A, Küchler C. Contrast-enhanced MRI of the breast: accuracy, value, controversies, solutions. Eur J Radiol. 1997;24:94–108.
30. Kuhl CK, Mielcareck P, Klaschik S, et al. Dynamic breast MR imaging: are signal intensity time course data useful for differential diagnosis of enhancing lesions? Radiology. 1999;211:101–10. doi:10.1148/radiology.211.1.r99ap38101.
31. Malich A, Fischer DR, Wurdinger S, et al. Potential MRI interpretation model: differentiation of benign from malignant breast masses. AJR Am J Roentgenol. 2005;185:964–70. doi:10.2214/AJR.04.1073.
32. Kaiser WA. Breast magnetic resonance imaging: principles and techniques. Semin Roentgenol. 2007;42:228–35. doi:10.1053/j.ro.2007.07.003.
33. Fischer DR, Wurdinger S, Boettcher J, et al. Further signs in the evaluation of magnetic resonance mammography: a retrospective study. Invest Radiol. 2005;40:430–5.
34. Berg WA, Gutierrez L, NessAiver MS, et al. Diagnostic accuracy of mammography, clinical examination, US, and MR imaging in preoperative assessment of breast cancer. Radiology. 2004;233:830–49. doi:10.1148/radiol.2333031484.
35. Tofts PS, Kermode AG. Measurement of the blood-brain barrier permeability and leakage space using dynamic MR imaging. 1. Fundamental concepts. Magn Reson Med. 1991;17:357–67.
36. Tofts PS, Berkowitz B, Schnall MD. Quantitative analysis of dynamic Gd-DTPA enhancement in breast tumors using a permeability model. Magn Reson Med. 1995;33:564–8.
37. Huang W, Tudorica LA, Li X, et al. Discrimination of benign and malignant breast lesions by using shutter-speed dynamic contrast-enhanced MR imaging. Radiology. 2011;261:394–403. doi:10.1148/radiol.11102413.
38. Li L, Wang K, Sun X, et al. Parameters of dynamic contrast-enhanced MRI as imaging markers for angiogenesis and proliferation in human breast cancer. Med Sci Monit. 2015;21:376–82. doi:10.12659/MSM.892534.
39. Hylton NM, Blume JD, Bernreuter WK, et al. Locally advanced breast cancer: MR imaging for prediction of response to neoadjuvant chemotherapy – results from ACRIN 6657/I-SPY TRIAL. Radiology. 2012;263:663–72. doi:10.1148/radiol.12110748.
40. Marinovich ML, Macaskill P, Irwig L, et al. Meta-analysis of agreement between MRI and pathologic breast tumour size after neoadjuvant chemotherapy. Br J Cancer. 2013;109:1528–36. doi:10.1038/bjc.2013.473.
41. Kuhl CK, Kooijman H, Gieseke J, Schild HH. Effect of B1 inhomogeneity on breast MR imaging at 3.0 T. Radiology. 2007;244:929–30. doi:10.1148/radiol.2443070266.

42. Tofts PS, Brix G, Buckley DL, et al. Estimating kinetic parameters from dynamic contrast-enhanced T(1)-weighted MRI of a diffusable tracer: standardized quantities and symbols. J Magn Reson Imaging. 1999;10:223–32.
43. Yankeelov TE, Luci JJ, Lepage M, et al. Quantitative pharmacokinetic analysis of DCE-MRI data without an arterial input function: a reference region model. Magn Reson Imaging. 2005;23:519–29. doi:10.1016/j.mri.2005.02.013.
44. Mann RM, Mus RD, van Zelst J, et al. A novel approach to contrast-enhanced breast magnetic resonance imaging for screening: high-resolution ultrafast dynamic imaging. Invest Radiol. 2014;49:579–85. doi:10.1097/RLI.0000000000000057.
45. Tudorica LA, Oh KY, Roy N, et al. A feasible high spatiotemporal resolution breast DCE-MRI protocol for clinical settings. Magn Reson Imaging. 2012;30:1257–67. doi:10.1016/j.mri.2012.04.009.
46. Huang W, Li X, Chen Y, et al. Variations of dynamic contrast-enhanced magnetic resonance imaging in evaluation of breast cancer therapy response: a multicenter data analysis challenge. Transl Oncol. 2014;7:153–66.
47. Kinkel K, Helbich TH, Esserman LJ, et al. Dynamic high-spatial-resolution MR imaging of suspicious breast lesions: diagnostic criteria and interobserver variability. AJR Am J Roentgenol. 2000;175:35–43. doi:10.2214/ajr.175.1.1750035.
48. Turnbull LW. Dynamic contrast-enhanced MRI in the diagnosis and management of breast cancer. NMR Biomed. 2009;22:28–39. doi:10.1002/nbm.1273.
49. Goto M, Ito H, Akazawa K, et al. Diagnosis of breast tumors by contrast-enhanced MR imaging: comparison between the diagnostic performance of dynamic enhancement patterns and morphologic features. J Magn Reson Imaging. 2007;25:104–12. doi:10.1002/jmri.20812.
50. Veltman J, Stoutjesdijk M, Mann R, et al. Contrast-enhanced magnetic resonance imaging of the breast: the value of pharmacokinetic parameters derived from fast dynamic imaging during initial enhancement in classifying lesions. Eur Radiol. 2008;18:1123–33. doi:10.1007/s00330-008-0870-8.
51. Kuhl CK, Jost P, Morakkabati N, et al. Contrast-enhanced MR imaging of the breast at 3.0 and 1.5 T in the same patients: initial experience. Radiology. 2006;239:666–76. doi:10.1148/radiol.2392050509.
52. Lourenco AP, Donegan L, Khalil H, Mainiero MB. Improving outcomes of screening breast MRI with practice evolution: initial clinical experience with 3 T compared to 1.5 T. J Magn Reson Imaging. 2014;39:535–9. doi:10.1002/jmri.24198.
53. Pinker-Domenig K, Bogner W, Gruber S, et al. High resolution MRI of the breast at 3 T: which BI-RADS® descriptors are most strongly associated with the diagnosis of breast cancer? Eur Radiol. 2012;22:322–30. doi:10.1007/s00330-011-2256-6.
54. van de Bank BL, Voogt IJ, Italiaander M, et al. Ultra high spatial and temporal resolution breast imaging at 7 T. NMR Biomed. 2013;26:367–75. doi:10.1002/nbm.2868.
55. Korteweg MA, Veldhuis WB, Visser F, et al. Feasibility of 7 Tesla breast magnetic resonance imaging determination of intrinsic sensitivity and high-resolution magnetic resonance imaging, diffusion-weighted imaging, and (1)H-magnetic resonance spectroscopy of breast cancer patients receiving neoadjuvant therapy. Invest Radiol. 2011;46:370–6. doi:10.1097/RLI.0b013e31820df706.
56. Klomp DWJ, van de Bank BL, Raaijmakers A, et al. 31P MRSI and 1H MRS at 7 T: initial results in human breast cancer. NMR Biomed. 2011;24:1337–42. doi:10.1002/nbm.1696.
57. Stehouwer BL, Klomp DWJ, Korteweg MA, et al. 7 T versus 3 T contrast-enhanced breast magnetic resonance imaging of invasive ductulolobular carcinoma: first clinical experience. Magn Reson Imaging. 2013;31:613–7. doi:10.1016/j.mri.2012.09.005.
58. Brown R, Storey P, Geppert C, et al. Breast MRI at 7 Tesla with a bilateral coil and T1-weighted acquisition with robust fat suppression: image evaluation and comparison with 3 Tesla. Eur Radiol. 2013;23:2969–78. doi:10.1007/s00330-013-2972-1.
59. Baltzer PA, Renz DM, Herrmann K-H, et al. (2009) Diffusion-weighted imaging (DWI) in MR mammography (MRM): clinical comparison of echo planar imaging (EPI) and half-Fourier single-shot turbo spin echo (HASTE) diffusion techniques. Eur Radiol 19:1612–1620. doi: 10.1007/s00330-009-1326-5

60. Baltzer PAT, Benndorf M, Dietzel M, et al. Sensitivity and specificity of unenhanced MR mammography (DWI combined with T2-weighted TSE imaging, ueMRM) for the differentiation of mass lesions. Eur Radiol. 2010;20:1101–10. doi:10.1007/s00330-009-1654-5.
61. Woodhams R, Kakita S, Hata H, et al. Identification of residual breast carcinoma following neoadjuvant chemotherapy: diffusion-weighted imaging – comparison with contrast-enhanced MR imaging and pathologic findings. Radiology. 2010;254:357–66. doi:10.1148/radiol.2542090405.
62. Marini C, Iacconi C, Giannelli M, et al. Quantitative diffusion-weighted MR imaging in the differential diagnosis of breast lesion. Eur Radiol. 2007;17:2646–55. doi:10.1007/s00330-007-0621-2.
63. Thomassin-Naggara I, De Bazelaire C, Chopier J, et al. Diffusion-weighted MR imaging of the breast: advantages and pitfalls. Eur J Radiol. 2013;82:435–43. doi:10.1016/j.ejrad.2012.03.002.
64. Cho GY, Moy L, Kim SG, et al. Comparison of contrast enhancement and diffusion-weighted magnetic resonance imaging in healthy and cancerous breast tissue. Eur J Radiol. 2015;84:1888–93. doi:10.1016/j.ejrad.2015.06.023.
65. Bogner W, Gruber S, Pinker K, et al. Diffusion-weighted MR for differentiation of breast lesions at 3.0 T: how does selection of diffusion protocols affect diagnosis? Radiology. 2009;253:341–51. doi:10.1148/radiol.2532081718.
66. Dorrius MD, Dijkstra H, Oudkerk M, Sijens PE. Effect of b value and pre-admission of contrast on diagnostic accuracy of 1.5-T breast DWI: a systematic review and meta-analysis. Eur Radiol. 2014;24:2835–47. doi:10.1007/s00330-014-3338-z.
67. Guo Y, Cai Y-Q, Cai Z-L, et al. Differentiation of clinically benign and malignant breast lesions using diffusion-weighted imaging. J Magn Reson Imaging. 2002;16:172–8. doi:10.1002/jmri.10140.
68. Woodhams R, Ramadan S, Stanwell P, et al. Diffusion-weighted imaging of the breast: principles and clinical applications. Radiographics. 2011;31:1059–84. doi:10.1148/rg.314105160.
69. Bogner W, Pinker-Domenig K, Bickel H, et al. Readout-segmented echo-planar imaging improves the diagnostic performance of diffusion-weighted MR breast examinations at 3.0 T. Radiology. 2012;263:64–76. doi:10.1148/radiol.12111494.
70. Tsushima Y, Takahashi-Taketomi A, Endo K. Magnetic resonance (MR) differential diagnosis of breast tumors using apparent diffusion coefficient (ADC) on 1.5-T. J Magn Reson Imaging. 2009;30:249–55. doi:10.1002/jmri.21854.
71. Costantini M, Belli P, Rinaldi P, et al. Diffusion-weighted imaging in breast cancer: relationship between apparent diffusion coefficient and tumour aggressiveness. Clin Radiol. 2010;65:1005–12. doi:10.1016/j.crad.2010.07.008.
72. Hatakenaka M, Soeda H, Yabuuchi H, et al. Apparent diffusion coefficients of breast tumors: clinical application. Magn Reson Med Sci. 2008;7:23–9.
73. Woodhams R, Matsunaga K, Iwabuchi K, et al. Diffusion-weighted imaging of malignant breast tumors: the usefulness of apparent diffusion coefficient (ADC) value and ADC map for the detection of malignant breast tumors and evaluation of cancer extension. J Comput Assist Tomogr. 2005;29:644–9.
74. Spick C, Pinker-Domenig K, Rudas M, et al. MRI-only lesions: application of diffusion-weighted imaging obviates unnecessary MR-guided breast biopsies. Eur Radiol. 2014;24:1204–10. doi:10.1007/s00330-014-3153-6.
75. Martincich L, Deantoni V, Bertotto I, et al. Correlations between diffusion-weighted imaging and breast cancer biomarkers. Eur Radiol. 2012;22:1519–28. doi:10.1007/s00330-012-2403-8.
76. Uematsu T, Kasami M, Yuen S. Triple-negative breast cancer: correlation between MR imaging and pathologic findings. Radiology. 2009;250:638–47. doi:10.1148/radiol.2503081054.
77. Foulkes WD, Smith IE, Reis-Filho JS. Triple-negative breast cancer. N Engl J Med. 2010;363:1938–48. doi:10.1056/NEJMra1001389.
78. Dogan BE, Gonzalez-Angulo AM, Gilcrease M, et al. Multimodality imaging of triple receptor-negative tumors with mammography, ultrasound, and MRI. AJR Am J Roentgenol. 2010;194:1160–6. doi:10.2214/AJR.09.2355.

79. Kawashima H. Imaging findings of triple-negative breast cancer. Breast Cancer. 2011;18:145. doi:10.1007/s12282-010-0247-0.
80. Bickel H, Pinker-Domenig K, Bogner W, et al. Quantitative apparent diffusion coefficient as a noninvasive imaging biomarker for the differentiation of invasive breast cancer and ductal carcinoma in situ. Invest Radiol. 2015;50:95–100. doi:10.1097/RLI.0000000000000104.
81. Padhani AR, Liu G, Koh DM, et al. Diffusion-weighted magnetic resonance imaging as a cancer biomarker: consensus and recommendations. Neoplasia. 2009;11:102–25.
82. Pickles MD, Gibbs P, Lowry M, Turnbull LW. Diffusion changes precede size reduction in neoadjuvant treatment of breast cancer. Magn Reson Imaging. 2006;24:843–7. doi:10.1016/j.mri.2005.11.005.
83. Park SH, Moon WK, Cho N, et al. Diffusion-weighted MR imaging: pretreatment prediction of response to neoadjuvant chemotherapy in patients with breast cancer. Radiology. 2010;257:56–63. doi:10.1148/radiol.10092021.
84. Richard R, Thomassin I, Chapellier M, et al. Diffusion-weighted MRI in pretreatment prediction of response to neoadjuvant chemotherapy in patients with breast cancer. Eur Radiol. 2013;23:2420–31. doi:10.1007/s00330-013-2850-x.
85. Sharma U, Danishad KKA, Seenu V, Jagannathan NR. Longitudinal study of the assessment by MRI and diffusion-weighted imaging of tumor response in patients with locally advanced breast cancer undergoing neoadjuvant chemotherapy. NMR Biomed. 2009;22:104–13. doi:10.1002/nbm.1245.
86. Iacconi C, Giannelli M, Marini C, et al. The role of mean diffusivity (MD) as a predictive index of the response to chemotherapy in locally advanced breast cancer: a preliminary study. Eur Radiol. 2010;20:303–8. doi:10.1007/s00330-009-1550-z.
87. Le Bihan D, Breton E, Lallemand D, et al. Separation of diffusion and perfusion in intravoxel incoherent motion MR imaging. Radiology. 1988;168:497–505. doi:10.1148/radiology.168.2.3393671.
88. Cho GY, Moy L, Kim SG, et al. Evaluation of breast cancer using intravoxel incoherent motion (IVIM) histogram analysis: comparison with malignant status, histological subtype, and molecular prognostic factors. Eur Radiol. 2015. doi:10.1007/s00330-015-4087-3.
89. Bokacheva L, Kaplan JB, Giri DD, et al. Intravoxel incoherent motion diffusion-weighted MRI at 3.0 T differentiates malignant breast lesions from benign lesions and breast parenchyma. J Magn Reson Imaging. 2014;40:813–23. doi:10.1002/jmri.24462.
90. Iima M, Yano K, Kataoka M, et al. Quantitative non-Gaussian diffusion and intravoxel incoherent motion magnetic resonance imaging: differentiation of malignant and benign breast lesions. Invest Radiol. 2015;50:205–11. doi:10.1097/RLI.0000000000000094.
91. Liu C, Liang C, Liu Z, et al. Intravoxel incoherent motion (IVIM) in evaluation of breast lesions: comparison with conventional DWI. Eur J Radiol. 2013;82:e782–9. doi:10.1016/j.ejrad.2013.08.006.
92. Cho GY, Moy L, Zhang JL, et al. Comparison of fitting methods and b-value sampling strategies for intravoxel incoherent motion in breast cancer. Magn Reson Med. 2015;74:1077–85. doi:10.1002/mrm.25484.
93. Jensen JH, Helpern JA, Ramani A, et al. Diffusional kurtosis imaging: the quantification of non-gaussian water diffusion by means of magnetic resonance imaging. Magn Reson Med. 2005;53:1432–40. doi:10.1002/mrm.20508.
94. Nogueira L, Brandão S, Matos E, et al. Application of the diffusion kurtosis model for the study of breast lesions. Eur Radiol. 2014;24:1197–203. doi:10.1007/s00330-014-3146-5.
95. Sun K, Chen X, Chai W, et al. Breast cancer: diffusion kurtosis MR imaging-diagnostic accuracy and correlation with clinical-pathologic factors. Radiology. 2015;277:46–55. doi:10.1148/radiol.15141625.
96. Baltzer PAT, Schäfer A, Dietzel M, et al. Diffusion tensor magnetic resonance imaging of the breast: a pilot study. Eur Radiol. 2011;21:1–10. doi:10.1007/s00330-010-1901-9.

97. Cakir O, Arslan A, Inan N, et al. Comparison of the diagnostic performances of diffusion parameters in diffusion weighted imaging and diffusion tensor imaging of breast lesions. Eur J Radiol. 2013;82:e801–6. doi:10.1016/j.ejrad.2013.09.001.
98. Le Bihan D, Mangin JF, Poupon C, et al. Diffusion tensor imaging: concepts and applications. J Magn Reson Imaging. 2001;13:534–46.
99. Eyal E, Shapiro-Feinberg M, Furman-Haran E, et al. Parametric diffusion tensor imaging of the breast. Invest Radiol. 2012;47:284–91. doi:10.1097/RLI.0b013e3182438e5d.
100. Partridge SC, Ziadloo A, Murthy R, et al. Diffusion tensor MRI: preliminary anisotropy measures and mapping of breast tumors. J Magn Reson Imaging. 2010;31:339–47. doi:10.1002/jmri.22045.
101. Partridge SC, DeMartini WB, Kurland BF, et al. Quantitative diffusion-weighted imaging as an adjunct to conventional breast MRI for improved positive predictive value. AJR Am J Roentgenol. 2009;193:1716–22. doi:10.2214/AJR.08.2139.
102. Jagannathan NR, Kumar M, Seenu V, et al. Evaluation of total choline from in-vivo volume localized proton MR spectroscopy and its response to neoadjuvant chemotherapy in locally advanced breast cancer. Br J Cancer. 2001;84:1016–22. doi:10.1054/bjoc.2000.1711.
103. Baik H-M, Su M-Y, Yu H, et al. Quantification of choline-containing compounds in malignant breast tumors by 1H MR spectroscopy using water as an internal reference at 1.5 T. MAGMA. 2006;19:96–104. doi:10.1007/s10334-006-0032-4.
104. Meisamy S, Bolan PJ, Baker EH, et al. Adding in vivo quantitative 1H MR spectroscopy to improve diagnostic accuracy of breast MR imaging: preliminary results of observer performance study at 4.0 T. Radiology. 2005;236:465–75. doi:10.1148/radiol.2362040836.
105. Bolan PJ. Magnetic resonance spectroscopy of the breast: current status. Magn Reson Imaging Clin N Am. 2013;21:625–39. doi:10.1016/j.mric.2013.04.008.
106. Shin HJ, Baek H-M, Cha JH, Kim HH. Evaluation of breast cancer using proton MR spectroscopy: total choline peak integral and signal-to-noise ratio as prognostic indicators. AJR Am J Roentgenol. 2012;198:W488–97. doi:10.2214/AJR.11.7292.
107. Roebuck JR, Cecil KM, Schnall MD, Lenkinski RE. Human breast lesions: characterization with proton MR spectroscopy. Radiology. 1998;209:269–75. doi:10.1148/radiology.209.1.9769842.
108. Lenkinski RE, Wang X, Elian M, Goldberg SN. Interaction of gadolinium-based MR contrast agents with choline: implications for MR spectroscopy (MRS) of the breast. Magn Reson Med. 2009;61:1286–92. doi:10.1002/mrm.21937.
109. Baltzer PAT, Dietzel M, Kaiser WA. MR-spectroscopy at 1.5 tesla and 3 tesla. Useful? A systematic review and meta-analysis. Eur J Radiol. 2012;81 Suppl 1:S6–9. doi:10.1016/S0720-048X(12)70003-7.
110. Gruber S, Debski B-K, Pinker K, et al. Three-dimensional proton MR spectroscopic imaging at 3 T for the differentiation of benign and malignant breast lesions. Radiology. 2011;261:752–61. doi:10.1148/radiol.11102096.
111. Danishad KKA, Sharma U, Sah RG, et al. Assessment of therapeutic response of locally advanced breast cancer (LABC) patients undergoing neoadjuvant chemotherapy (NACT) monitored using sequential magnetic resonance spectroscopic imaging (MRSI). NMR Biomed. 2010;23:233–41. doi:10.1002/nbm.1436.
112. Sharma U, Baek HM, Su MY, Jagannathan NR. In vivo 1H MRS in the assessment of the therapeutic response of breast cancer patients. NMR Biomed. 2011;24:700–11. doi:10.1002/nbm.1654.
113. Glunde K, Bhujwalla ZM, Ronen SM. Choline metabolism in malignant transformation. Nat Rev Cancer. 2011;11:835–48. doi:10.1038/nrc3162.
114. Aboagye EO, Bhujwalla ZM. Malignant transformation alters membrane choline phospholipid metabolism of human mammary epithelial cells. Cancer Res. 1999;59:80–4.
115. Ramadan S, Arm J, Silcock J, et al. Lipid and metabolite deregulation in the breast tissue of women carrying BRCA1 and BRCA2 genetic mutations. Radiology. 2015;275:675–82. doi:10.1148/radiol.15140967.

116. Kul S, Cansu A, Alhan E, et al. Contribution of diffusion-weighted imaging to dynamic contrast-enhanced MRI in the characterization of breast tumors. AJR Am J Roentgenol. 2011;196:210–7. doi:10.2214/AJR.10.4258.
117. Ei Khouli RH, Jacobs MA, Mezban SD, et al. Diffusion-weighted imaging improves the diagnostic accuracy of conventional 3.0-T breast MR imaging. Radiology. 2010;256:64–73. doi:10.1148/radiol.10091367.
118. Baltzer A, Dietzel M, Kaiser CG, Baltzer PA. Combined reading of contrast enhanced and diffusion weighted magnetic resonance imaging by using a simple sum score. Eur Radiol. 2015. doi:10.1007/s00330-015-3886-x.
119. Schmitz AMT, Veldhuis WB, Menke-Pluijmers MBE, et al. Multiparametric MRI with dynamic contrast enhancement, diffusion-weighted imaging, and 31-phosphorus spectroscopy at 7 T for characterization of breast cancer. Invest Radiol. 2015;50:766–71. doi:10.1097/RLI.0000000000000183.
120. Madelin G, Regatte RR. Biomedical applications of sodium MRI in vivo. J Magn Reson Imaging. 2013;38:511–29. doi:10.1002/jmri.24168.
121. Ouwerkerk R. Sodium MRI. Methods Mol Biol. 2011;711:175–201. doi:10.1007/978-1-61737-992-5_8.
122. Ouwerkerk R, Jacobs MA, Macura KJ, et al. Elevated tissue sodium concentration in malignant breast lesions detected with non-invasive 23Na MRI. Breast Cancer Res Treat. 2007;106:151–60. doi:10.1007/s10549-006-9485-4.
123. Zaric O, Pinker K, Zbyn S, Strasser S, Robinson S, Minarikova L, Gruber S, Farr A, Singer C, TH H, Trattnig S, Bogner W. Quantitative sodium MR imaging at 7 tesla – initial results and comparison with diffusion-weighted imaging in patients with breast tumors. Radiology. 2016;280(1):39–48.
124. Ackerstaff E, Glunde K, Bhujwalla ZM. Choline phospholipid metabolism: a target in cancer cells? J Cell Biochem. 2003;90:525–33. doi:10.1002/jcb.10659.
125. Arias-Mendoza F, Payne GS, Zakian KL, et al. In vivo 31P MR spectral patterns and reproducibility in cancer patients studied in a multi-institutional trial. NMR Biomed. 2006;19:504–12. doi:10.1002/nbm.1057.
126. Barzilai A, Horowitz A, Geier A, Degani H. Phosphate metabolites and steroid hormone receptors of benign and malignant breast tumors. A Nuclear Magnetic Resonance study. Cancer. 1991;67:2919–25.
127. Wijnen JP, van der Kemp WJM, Luttje MP, et al. Quantitative 31P magnetic resonance spectroscopy of the human breast at 7 T. Magn Reson Med. 2012;68:339–48. doi:10.1002/mrm.23249.
128. Ward KM, Aletras AH, Balaban RS. A new class of contrast agents for MRI based on proton chemical exchange dependent saturation transfer (CEST). J Magn Reson. 2000;143:79–87. doi:10.1006/jmre.1999.1956.
129. Schmitt B, Trattnig S, Schlemmer H-P. CEST-imaging: a new contrast in MR-mammography by means of chemical exchange saturation transfer. Eur J Radiol. 2012;81 Suppl 1:S144–6. doi:10.1016/S0720-048X(12)70060-8.
130. Klomp DWJ, Dula AN, Arlinghaus LR, et al. Amide proton transfer imaging of the human breast at 7 T: development and reproducibility. NMR Biomed. 2013;26:1271–7. doi:10.1002/nbm.2947.
131. Rivlin M, Horev J, Tsarfaty I, Navon G. Molecular imaging of tumors and metastases using chemical exchange saturation transfer (CEST) MRI. Sci Rep. 2013;3:3045. doi:10.1038/srep03045.
132. Desmond KL, Moosvi F, Stanisz GJ. Mapping of amide, amine, and aliphatic peaks in the CEST spectra of murine xenografts at 7 T. Magn Reson Med. 2014;71:1841–53. doi:10.1002/mrm.24822.
133. Chan KWY, McMahon MT, Kato Y, et al. Natural D-glucose as a biodegradable MRI contrast agent for detecting cancer. Magn Reson Med. 2012;68:1764–73. doi:10.1002/mrm.24520.
134. Walker-Samuel S, Ramasawmy R, Torrealdea F, et al. In vivo imaging of glucose uptake and metabolism in tumors. Nat Med. 2013;19:1067–72. doi:10.1038/nm.3252.

135. Nasrallah FA, Pagès G, Kuchel PW, et al. Imaging brain deoxyglucose uptake and metabolism by glucoCEST MRI. J Cereb Blood Flow Metab. 2013;33:1270–8. doi:10.1038/jcbfm.2013.79.
136. Robinson SP, Howe FA, Rodrigues LM, et al. Magnetic resonance imaging techniques for monitoring changes in tumor oxygenation and blood flow. Semin Radiat Oncol. 1998;8:197–207.
137. O'Flynn EAM, DeSouza NM. Functional magnetic resonance: biomarkers of response in breast cancer. Breast Cancer Res. 2011;13:204. doi:10.1186/bcr2815.
138. Rakow-Penner R, Daniel B, Glover GH. Detecting blood oxygen level-dependent (BOLD) contrast in the breast. J Magn Reson Imaging. 2010;32:120–9. doi:10.1002/jmri.22227.
139. Li SP, Taylor NJ, Makris A, et al. Primary human breast adenocarcinoma: imaging and histologic correlates of intrinsic susceptibility-weighted MR imaging before and during chemotherapy. Radiology. 2010;257:643–52. doi:10.1148/radiol.10100421.
140. Jiang L, Weatherall PT, McColl RW, et al. Blood oxygenation level-dependent (BOLD) contrast magnetic resonance imaging (MRI) for prediction of breast cancer chemotherapy response: a pilot study. J Magn Reson Imaging. 2013;37:1083–92. doi:10.1002/jmri.23891.
141. Tatum JL, Kelloff GJ, Gillies RJ, et al. Hypoxia: importance in tumor biology, noninvasive measurement by imaging, and value of its measurement in the management of cancer therapy. Int J Radiat Biol. 2006;82:699–757. doi:10.1080/09553000601002324.
142. Ardenkjaer-Larsen JH, Fridlund B, Gram A, et al. Increase in signal-to-noise ratio of >10,000 times in liquid-state NMR. Proc Natl Acad Sci U S A. 2003;100:10158–63. doi:10.1073/pnas.1733835100.
143. Brindle KM, Bohndiek SE, Gallagher FA, Kettunen MI. Tumor imaging using hyperpolarized 13C magnetic resonance spectroscopy. Magn Reson Med. 2011;66:505–19. doi:10.1002/mrm.22999.
144. Jóhannesson H, Macholl S, Ardenkjaer-Larsen JH. Dynamic nuclear polarization of [1-13C] pyruvic acid at 4.6 tesla. J Magn Reson. 2009;197:167–75. doi:10.1016/j.jmr.2008.12.016.
145. Golman K, Ardenkjaer-Larsen JH, Petersson JS, et al. Molecular imaging with endogenous substances. Proc Natl Acad Sci U S A. 2003;100:10435–9. doi:10.1073/pnas.1733836100.
146. Golman K, Zandt RI, Lerche M, et al. Metabolic imaging by hyperpolarized 13C magnetic resonance imaging for in vivo tumor diagnosis. Cancer Res. 2006;66:10855–60. doi:10.1158/0008-5472.CAN-06-2564.
147. Park I, Larson PEZ, Zierhut ML, et al. Hyperpolarized 13C magnetic resonance metabolic imaging: application to brain tumors. Neuro Oncol. 2010;12:133–44. doi:10.1093/neuonc/nop043.
148. Chen AP, Albers MJ, Cunningham CH, et al. Hyperpolarized C-13 spectroscopic imaging of the TRAMP mouse at 3 T-initial experience. Magn Reson Med. 2007;58:1099–106. doi:10.1002/mrm.21256.
149. Kurhanewicz J, Bok R, Nelson SJ, Vigneron DB. Current and potential applications of clinical 13C MR spectroscopy. J Nucl Med. 2008;49:341–4. doi:10.2967/jnumed.107.045112.
150. Albers MJ, Bok R, Chen AP, et al. Hyperpolarized 13C lactate, pyruvate, and alanine: noninvasive biomarkers for prostate cancer detection and grading. Cancer Res. 2008;68:8607–15. doi:10.1158/0008-5472.CAN-08-0749.
151. Zierhut ML, Yen Y-F, Chen AP, et al. Kinetic modeling of hyperpolarized 13C1-pyruvate metabolism in normal rats and TRAMP mice. J Magn Reson. 2010;202:85–92. doi:10.1016/j.jmr.2009.10.003.
152. Keshari KR, Sai V, Wang ZJ, et al. Hyperpolarized [1-13C]dehydroascorbate MR spectroscopy in a murine model of prostate cancer: comparison with 18F-FDG PET. J Nucl Med. 2013;54:922–8. doi:10.2967/jnumed.112.115402.
153. Asghar Butt S, Søgaard LV, Ardenkjaer-Larsen JH, et al. Monitoring mammary tumor progression and effect of tamoxifen treatment in MMTV-PymT using MRI and magnetic resonance spectroscopy with hyperpolarized [1-(13) C]pyruvate. Magn Reson Med. 2014. doi:10.1002/mrm.25095.
154. Taillefer R. Clinical applications of 99mTc-sestamibi scintimammography. Semin Nucl Med. 2005;35:100–15. doi:10.1053/j.semnuclmed.2004.11.002.

155. Scopinaro F, Schillaci O, Ussof W, et al. A three center study on the diagnostic accuracy of 99mTc-MIBI scintimammography. Anticancer Res. 1997;17:1631–4.
156. Arslan N, Oztürk E, Ilgan S, et al. 99Tcm-MIBI scintimammography in the evaluation of breast lesions and axillary involvement: a comparison with mammography and histopathological diagnosis. Nucl Med Commun. 1999;20:317–25.
157. Maffioli L, Agresti R, Chiti A, et al. Prone scintimammography in patients with non-palpable breast lesions. Anticancer Res. 1996;16:1269–73.
158. Brem RF, Rapelyea JA, Zisman G, et al. Occult breast cancer: scintimammography with high-resolution breast-specific gamma camera in women at high risk for breast cancer. Radiology. 2005;237:274–80. doi:10.1148/radiol.2371040758.
159. Brem RF, Shahan C, Rapleyea JA, et al. Detection of occult foci of breast cancer using breast-specific gamma imaging in women with one mammographic or clinically suspicious breast lesion. Acad Radiol. 2010;17:735–43. doi:10.1016/j.acra.2010.01.017.
160. Coover LR, Caravaglia G, Kuhn P. Scintimammography with dedicated breast camera detects and localizes occult carcinoma. J Nucl Med. 2004;45:553–8.
161. Rhodes DJ, O'Connor MK, Phillips SW, et al. Molecular breast imaging: a new technique using technetium Tc 99 m scintimammography to detect small tumors of the breast. Mayo Clin Proc. 2005;80:24–30. doi:10.1016/S0025-6196(11)62953-4.
162. Brem RF, Floerke AC, Rapelyea JA, et al. Breast-specific gamma imaging as an adjunct imaging modality for the diagnosis of breast cancer. Radiology. 2008;247:651–7. doi:10.1148/radiol.2473061678.
163. Brem RF, Fishman M, Rapelyea JA. Detection of ductal carcinoma in situ with mammography, breast specific gamma imaging, and magnetic resonance imaging: a comparative study. Acad Radiol. 2007;14:945–50. doi:10.1016/j.acra.2007.04.004.
164. Sun Y, Wei W, Yang H-W, Liu J-L. Clinical usefulness of breast-specific gamma imaging as an adjunct modality to mammography for diagnosis of breast cancer: a systemic review and meta-analysis. Eur J Nucl Med Mol Imaging. 2013;40:450–63. doi:10.1007/s00259-012-2279-5.
165. Avril N, Adler LP. F-18 fluorodeoxyglucose-positron emission tomography imaging for primary breast cancer and loco-regional staging. Radiol Clin North Am. 2007;45:645–57, vi. doi:10.1016/j.rcl.2007.05.004.
166. Quon A, Gambhir SS. FDG-PET and beyond: molecular breast cancer imaging. J Clin Oncol. 2005;23:1664–73. doi:10.1200/JCO.2005.11.024.
167. Avril N, Rosé CA, Schelling M, et al. Breast imaging with positron emission tomography and fluorine-18 fluorodeoxyglucose: use and limitations. J Clin Oncol. 2000;18:3495–502.
168. Kumar R, Lal N, Alavi A. 18F-FDG PET in detecting primary breast cancer. J Nucl Med. 2007;48:1751 . doi:10.2967/jnumed.107.043265.author reply 1752
169. Tatsumi M, Cohade C, Mourtzikos KA, et al. Initial experience with FDG-PET/CT in the evaluation of breast cancer. Eur J Nucl Med Mol Imaging. 2006;33:254–62. doi:10.1007/s00259-005-1835-7.
170. Escalona S, Blasco JA, Reza MM, et al. A systematic review of FDG-PET in breast cancer. Med Oncol. 2010;27:114–29. doi:10.1007/s12032-009-9182-3.
171. Rosen EL, Eubank WB, Mankoff DA. FDG PET, PET/CT, and breast cancer imaging. Radiographics. 2007;27 Suppl 1:S215–29. doi:10.1148/rg.27si075517.
172. Samson DJ, Flamm CR, Pisano ED, Aronson N. Should FDG PET be used to decide whether a patient with an abnormal mammogram or breast finding at physical examination should undergo biopsy? Acad Radiol. 2002;9:773–83.
173. Magometschnigg HF, Baltzer PA, Fueger B, et al. Diagnostic accuracy of (18)F-FDG PET/CT compared with that of contrast-enhanced MRI of the breast at 3 T. Eur J Nucl Med Mol Imaging. 2015;42:1656–65. doi:10.1007/s00259-015-3099-1.
174. Kalles V, Zografos GC, Provatopoulou X, et al. The current status of positron emission mammography in breast cancer diagnosis. Breast Cancer. 2013;20:123–30. doi:10.1007/s12282-012-0433-3.

175. Hanahan D, Weinberg RA. Hallmarks of cancer: the next generation. Cell. 2011;144:646–74. doi:10.1016/j.cell.2011.02.013.
176. Hanahan D, Weinberg RA. The hallmarks of cancer. Cell. 2000;100:57–70.
177. Tennant DA, Durán RV, Gottlieb E. Targeting metabolic transformation for cancer therapy. Nat Rev Cancer. 2010;10:267–77. doi:10.1038/nrc2817.
178. Tennant DA, Durán RV, Boulahbel H, Gottlieb E. Metabolic transformation in cancer. Carcinogenesis. 2009;30:1269–80. doi:10.1093/carcin/bgp070.
179. Trosko JE, Chang C-C, Upham BL, Tai M-H. Ignored hallmarks of carcinogenesis: stem cells and cell-cell communication. Ann N Y Acad Sci. 2004;1028:192–201. doi:10.1196/annals.1322.023.
180. Moy L, Ponzo F, Noz ME, et al. Improving specificity of breast MRI using prone PET and fused MRI and PET 3D volume datasets. J Nucl Med. 2007;48:528–37.
181. Domingues RC, Carneiro MP, Lopes FCR, et al. Whole-body MRI and FDG PET fused images for evaluation of patients with cancer. AJR Am J Roentgenol. 2009;192:1012–20. doi:10.2214/AJR.08.1498.
182. Moy L, Noz ME, Maguire GQ, et al. Role of fusion of prone FDG-PET and magnetic resonance imaging of the breasts in the evaluation of breast cancer. Breast J. 2010;16:369–76. doi:10.1111/j.1524-4741.2010.00927.x.
183. Moy L, Noz ME, Maguire GQ, et al. Prone mammoPET acquisition improves the ability to fuse MRI and PET breast scans. Clin Nucl Med. 2007;32:194–8. doi:10.1097/01.rlu.0000255055.10177.80.
184. Pinker K, Bickel H, Magometschnigg H et al Molecular imaging of breast tumours with PET-MRI – proof of concept. In: ISMRM 2011, editor. (European Journal of Cancer, Montreal); 2011.
185. Pinker-Domenig K, Baltzer PA, Andrzejewski P, Magometschnigg H, Georg D, Karanikas G, Wadsak W, Kapetas P, Helbich TH. World molecular imaging congress 2015 scientific presentation dual tracer PET/MRI of breast tumors: insights into tumor biology.
186. Cheng J, Lei L, Xu J, et al. 18F-fluoromisonidazole PET/CT: a potential tool for predicting primary endocrine therapy resistance in breast cancer. J Nucl Med. 2013;54:333–40. doi:10.2967/jnumed.112.111963.
187. Blankenberg FG. In vivo detection of apoptosis. J Nucl Med. 2008;49 Suppl 2:81S–95. doi:10.2967/jnumed.107.045898.
188. Whisenant JG, Peterson TE, Fluckiger JU, et al. Reproducibility of static and dynamic (18)F-FDG, (18)F-FLT, and (18)F-FMISO MicroPET studies in a murine model of HER2+ breast cancer. Mol Imaging Biol. 2013;15:87–96. doi:10.1007/s11307-012-0564-0.
189. Yang Z, Sun Y, Zhang Y, et al. Can fluorine-18 fluoroestradiol positron emission tomography-computed tomography demonstrate the heterogeneity of breast cancer in vivo? Clin Breast Cancer. 2013;13:359–63. doi:10.1016/j.clbc.2013.02.012.
190. van Kruchten M, de Vries EGE, Brown M, et al. PET imaging of oestrogen receptors in patients with breast cancer. Lancet Oncol. 2013;14:e465–75. doi:10.1016/S1470-2045(13)70292-4.
191. Smith-Jones PM, Solit DB, Akhurst T, et al. Imaging the pharmacodynamics of HER2 degradation in response to Hsp90 inhibitors. Nat Biotechnol. 2004;22:701–6. doi:10.1038/nbt968.
192. Smith-Jones PM, Solit D, Afroze F, et al. Early tumor response to Hsp90 therapy using HER2 PET: comparison with 18F-FDG PET. J Nucl Med. 2006;47:793–6.
193. Tamura K, Kurihara H, Yonemori K, et al. 64Cu-DOTA-trastuzumab PET imaging in patients with HER2-positive breast cancer. J Nucl Med. 2013;54:1869–75. doi:10.2967/jnumed.112.118612.
194. Mortimer JE, Bading JR, Colcher DM, et al. Functional imaging of human epidermal growth factor receptor 2-positive metastatic breast cancer using (64)Cu-DOTA-trastuzumab PET. J Nucl Med. 2014;55:23–9. doi:10.2967/jnumed.113.122630.
195. Imbriaco M, Caprio MG, Limite G, et al. Dual-time-point 18F-FDG PET/CT versus dynamic breast MRI of suspicious breast lesions. AJR Am J Roentgenol. 2008;191:1323–30. doi:10.2214/AJR.07.3439.

196. van de Wiele C, Lahorte C, Vermeersch H, et al. Quantitative tumor apoptosis imaging using technetium-99 m-HYNIC annexin V single photon emission computed tomography. J Clin Oncol. 2003;21:3483–7. doi:10.1200/JCO.2003.12.096.
197. Vera P, Bohn P, Edet-Sanson A, et al. Simultaneous positron emission tomography (PET) assessment of metabolism with ^{18}F-fluoro-2-deoxy-d-glucose (FDG), proliferation with ^{18}F-fluoro-thymidine (FLT), and hypoxia with ^{18}fluoro-misonidazole (F-miso) before and during radiotherapy in patients with non-small-cell lung cancer (NSCLC): a pilot study. Radiother Oncol. 2011;98:109–16. doi:10.1016/j.radonc.2010.10.011.
198. Rajendran JG, Wilson DC, Conrad EU, et al. [(18)F]FMISO and [(18)F]FDG PET imaging in soft tissue sarcomas: correlation of hypoxia, metabolism and VEGF expression. Eur J Nucl Med Mol Imaging. 2003;30:695–704. doi:10.1007/s00259-002-1096-7.

Chapter 16
Abbreviated Breast MRI

Victoria Mango and Linda Moy

Abstract Breast MRI demonstrates high sensitivity for breast cancer detection, beyond that of mammography and ultrasound. Numerous factors limit the widespread application of MRI as a screening modality for all women, including time-consuming protocols which may occupy the MRI system for 30–60 min, and which are costly, difficult for patients and limit clinical accessibility. Recently researchers have questioned which MR sequences are truly necessary in the screening setting to achieve the desired sensitivity of a screening examination. The definition of an abbreviated MR protocol varies from study to study and research is ongoing to optimize such a protocol. Possibilities include limiting the exam to one post-contrast sequence, utilizing T2-weighted or diffusion weighted imaging (DWI) or employing time-resolved angiography with stochastic trajectories (TWIST) sequences. Decreased image acquisition and reading time in the screening MRI setting could potentially decrease cost and increase women's access to screening breast MRI without sacrificing diagnostic accuracy and cancer yield.

Keywords Breast MRI • Abbreviated protocol • Breast cancer • Supplemental screening • Breast density • Screening costs • MR protocol optimization • Interpretation times • DWI • TWIST

Breast MRI demonstrates high sensitivity for breast cancer detection, beyond that of mammography and ultrasound [1–3]. According to the American Cancer Society, screening breast MRI should be used for patients with >20 % lifetime risk of developing breast cancer, BRCA 1 or 2 mutation carriers, and patients with a history of mantle radiation before age 30 [4]. In these high risk groups MRI screening enables breast cancer diagnosis at a lower stage and reduces interval cancers [2, 5–13]. There is indirect evidence that MR screening improves prognosis [12, 13]; however,

V. Mango, MD (✉)
Department of Radiology, Memorial Sloan Kettering Cancer Center, New York, NY, USA
e-mail: mangov@mskcc.org

L. Moy, MD
Department of Radiology, New York University School of Medicine, New York University Langone Medical Center, Laura and Isaac Perlmutter Cancer Center, New York, NY, USA

S.L. Heller, L. Moy (eds.), *Breast Oncology: Techniques, Indications, and Interpretation*, DOI 10.1007/978-3-319-42563-4_16

cost effectiveness of breast MRI has been evaluated by multiple studies with differing conclusions [14–19].

Although most studies focus on women at high risk, patients of mildly elevated risk may benefit from breast MRI screening as well [20]; however, numerous factors limit the widespread application of MRI as a screening modality. Breast MRI is technically demanding and therefore associated with high costs, directly and indirectly [21, 22]. This is partly due to protocols that are time consuming to acquire and read. A full diagnostic protocol may occupy the MRI system for 30–60 min [23, 24]. The length of the exam may also be difficult for patients, particularly those with claustrophobia or musculoskeletal issues that create discomfort or prohibit laying stationary in the prone position for long periods of time. Indirect costs result from false positive findings with subsequent biopsy and follow up exams for BI-RADS 3 findings. Availability of facilities with scanners and radiologists trained in breast MRI limits clinical accessibility [25]. Additionally the need for intravenous contrast increases the cost of the exam and may limit MR use due to patient allergy or renal insufficiency [26].

The reported length of a full diagnostic breast MRI examination varies between institutions; scan time, contrast injection, providing patient instructions and getting the patient on and off the table can occupy up to 60 min of magnet and technologist time. Standard full diagnostic protocols vary slightly but usually include a non-fat saturated T1 sequence, a T2 weighted sequence, pre and several post-contrast sequences with generation of subtraction images and kinetic enhancement curves. Maximum Intensity Projection (MIP) images are often generated from the data set and fuse a stack of images into a single 3-dimensional like image allowing quick overview of the entire volume imaged with increased conspicuity of enhancing lesions. Subtraction images are created by subtracting unenhanced images from contrast-enhanced images on a pixel-by-pixel basis producing a subtracted post-contrast image. While the full diagnostic protocol is informative, in many ways it has been lengthened to maximize specificity in order to best characterize lesions and establish disease extent. Currently this diagnostic protocol is uniformly applied to screening patients as well as to those undergoing extent of disease evaluation and problem solving. However, the goal in screening is to identify the small number of patients amongst a large population who have otherwise undetectable disease; it is therefore possible that the screening population may warrant a different approach [27].

Recently researchers have questioned which MR sequences are truly necessary in the screening setting. If a shorter or abbreviated MRI protocol were to be applied to a screening population patients could be called back for the full diagnostic examination only if necessary. This model would conform to the routine practice in screening and diagnostic mammography in which a small percentage of patients with indeterminate or suspicious findings on the screening exam are recalled for additional diagnostic imaging. Alternatively researchers have suggested that the abbreviated MRI protocol could be a stand alone exam; interpreted without the need for the patient to be recalled for additional imaging. Regardless, a shortened MRI examination could reduce the time to acquire and interpret the exam, leading to decreased costs and improved patient comfort. Such improvements could ultimately enable breast MRI to be available to more women and potentially to function as a routine screening exam.

The definition of an abbreviated MR protocol, both sequences used and imaging plane, varies from study to study and research is ongoing to optimize such a protocol. The various abbreviated protocols investigated in the currently available literature are summarized in Table 16.1. In the seminal prospective study by Kuhl et al., the feasibility of an abbreviated MRI protocol was explored in a high risk screening population. The authors analyzed 606 MRI exams in 443 women, prospectively utilizing an abbreviated protocol consisting of one axial pre-contrast T1 and one single axial post-contrast T1 with subsequent first post-contrast subtraction and MIP images generated [28]. This patient population was at mild to moderately increased risk for breast cancer and had normal/benign mammograms, normal clinical exams and, for those with heterogeneously or extremely dense tissue, a normal/benign ultrasound. The authors found 11 breast cancers (4 DCIS, 7 invasive; all T1N0 intermediate or high grade, median invasive cancer size 0.8 cm) for an additional cancer yield of 18.2 per 1000 (Fig. 16.1). Reading the MIP image alone demonstrated 10/11 (90.9 % sensitivity) cancers with a negative predictive value (NPV) of 99.8 %. When reading the complete abbreviated protocol (MIP, first post-contrast subtracted and optionally their non-subtracted source images), 11/11 cancers were diagnosed with equivalent specificity and positive predictive value compared to the full diagnostic protocol. They found the NPV for the complete abbreviated protocol and full diagnostic protocol were 100 % with 2 year follow up used to validate negative screening MR results. Specificity and PPV of the abbreviated protocol did not differ significantly from the full diagnostic protocol (94.3 % v 93.9 % and 24.4 % v 23.4 %) (Table 16.2).

Achieving such high sensitivity and specificity with limited MR sequences would be ideal in the screening setting. The Kuhl study also demonstrated expected decreased radiologist reading time of the abbreviated protocol, on average 2.8 s for the single MIP image and 28 s for the complete abbreviated protocol which is faster than published screening mammogram reading times of 60–120 s [29, 30] (Table 16.3). Such short reading times could allow for batch reading of MR screening exams similar to the model currently used for mammography. The reported full diagnostic protocol acquisition time was 17 min but only 3 min for the abbreviated protocol. Comparing this time to other breast cancer supplemental screening options is striking given the average ultrasound screening time of 19 min reported in the American College of Radiology Imaging Network breast ultrasound screening trial by Berg et al. [2, 31]. In this trial a doubled cancer yield (14.9 %) was achieved by adding MRI following ultrasound, showing the superiority of MRI over ultrasound for breast cancer detection.

Findings in the Kuhl study are further supported in a study by Mango, et al. which examined an abbreviated protocol consisting of a pre-contrast fat saturated sagittal T1 image and single early post-contrast sagittal T1 image [32]. In this study four experienced breast radiologists reviewed 100 cases of biopsy proven unicentric breast carcinoma including the first post-contrast T1, post processed subtracted first

Table 16.1 Overview of published abbreviated breast MRI protocols

	Scout/localizer	Pre-contrast[a]	Inject	1st post contrast[a]	2nd post contrast[a]	3rd post contrast[a]	4th post contrast[a]	Axial post delayed	Non fat sat T1	T2	DWI
Full diagnostic MRI	x	x	x	x	x	x	x	x	x	x	x
Kuhl et al. abbreviated	x	x (axial, non-fat sat)	x	x (axial, non-fat sat)							
Mango et al. abbreviated	x	x (sag)	x	x (sag)							
Grimm et al. abbreviated 1	x	x (axial)	x	x (axial)						x	
Grimm et al. abbreviated 2	x	x (axial)	x	x (axial)	x					x	
Trimboli et al.	x	x								x	x
Heacock et al. abbreviated 1	x	x (sag)	x	x (sag)							
Heacock et al. abbreviated 2[b]	x	x (sag)	x	x (sag)							
Heacock et al. abbreviated 3	x	x (sag)	x	x (sag)						x(sag)	

Note full diagnostic MRI protocol varies between institutions
[a]images from which additional subtraction series and MIP images may be generated
[b]second abbreviated protocol was distinguished from the first in this study by availability of clinical history and prior imaging

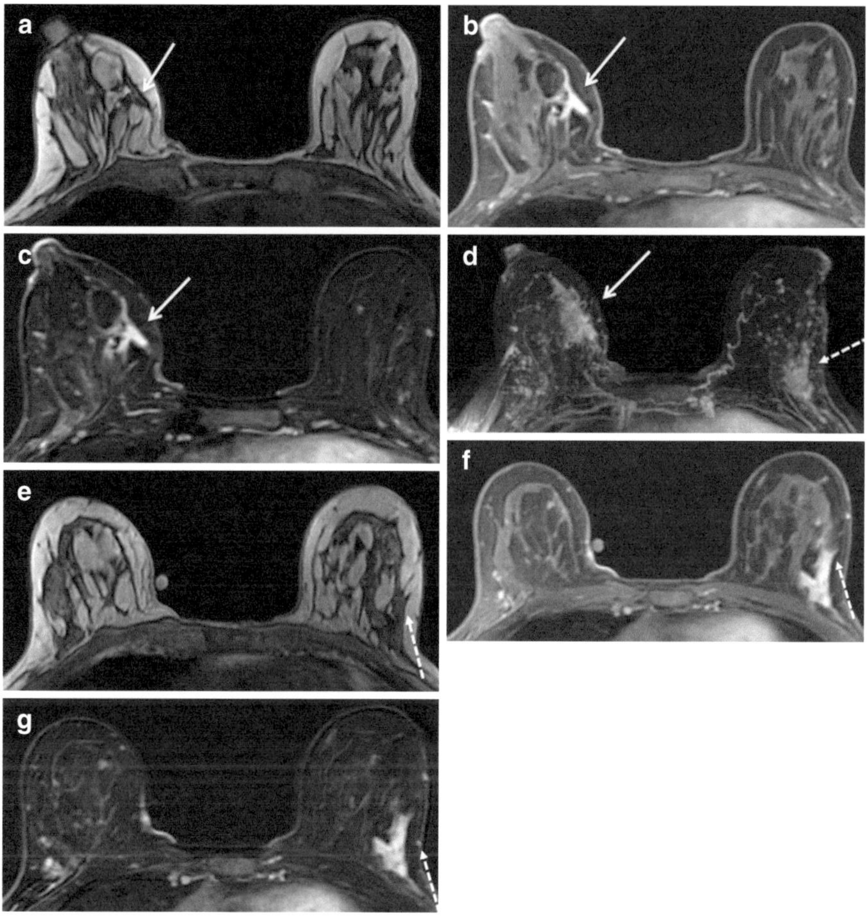

Fig. 16.1 Forty-six-year-old female with a palpable right 3:00, 1.4 cm moderately differentiated invasive ductal carcinoma (*white solid arrow*). Selected sequences provide an example of the abbreviated breast MRI protocol investigated by Kuhl et al. [28]. (**a**) Axial pre-contrast non-fat saturated T1-weighted image (**b**) Axial first post-contrast fat saturated T1-weighted image (**c**) Axial first post-contrast subtracted T1-weighted image and (**d**) Axial MIP image. Note the MIP shows bilateral asymmetric enhancement. The MRI demonstrates suspicious non mass enhancement in the contralateral breast (*white dash arrow*). (**e**) Axial pre-contrast non-fat saturated T1-weighted image (**f**) Axial first post-contrast fat saturated T1-weighted image (**g**) Axial first post-contrast subtracted T1-weighted image. MR biopsy of the left breast yielded fibrocystic change and marked adenosis deemed concordant with imaging findings

post-contrast and subtraction MIP images. As all the patients had cancer, this study addressed cancer visualization but did not simulate a true screening environment. Nonetheless results for cancer localization and detection were promising as all 100 cancers (21 DCIS and 79 invasive cancers; mean cancer size 2.2 cm) were visualized on initial reading of the abbreviated protocol by at least one reader and 92/100 by all four readers (Fig. 16.2). This resulted in a mean sensitivity of 96 % for the

Table 16.2 Comparison of sensitivity, specificity, negative predictive value (NPV) and positive predictive value (PPV) of published abbreviated protocols compared to the full diagnostic MR protocol

	Sensitivity[a]	Specificity	PPV	NPV
MIP (Kuhl et al.)	90.9	NA	NA	99.8
1st post (Kuhl et al.)	100	94.3	24.4	100
Full MR (Kuhl et al.)	100	93.9	23.4	100
MIP (Mango et al.)	93	NA	NA	NA
1st post (Mango et al.)	96	NA	NA	NA
1st post sub (Mango et al.)	96	NA	NA	NA
Abbreviated 1 (Grimm et al.)	86	52	NA	NA
Abbreviated 2 (Grimm et al.)	89	45	NA	NA
Full MR (Grimm et al.)	95	52	NA	NA
Abbreviated (Trimboli et al.)	78	87	74	90
abbreviated 1 (Heacock et al.)	97.8	NA	NA	NA
abbreviated 2 (Heacock et al.)	99.4	NA	NA	NA
abbreviated 3 (Heacock et al.)	99.4	NA	NA	NA

NA not available
[a]Or percentage detected in studies of only cancer cases

Table 16.3 Comparison of time to acquire and read the full diagnostic breast MRI to the abbreviated protocol

	Full protocol scan time	Full protocol radiologist interpretation time	Abbreviated scan time	Abbreviated protocol radiologist interpretation time
Kuhl et al.	17 min	NA	3 min	28 s
Mango et al.	30–40 min	NA	10–15 min[a]	44 s
Grimm et al. (abbreviated 1)	30–45 min	2.95 min		2.98 min
Heacock et al. (abbreviated 1)	35 min	15 min	7 min	14–25.4 s

[a]included time for patient instructions, transition between sequences and getting patient on/off table, other studies report acquisition time only

first post-contrast sequence, 96 % for the first post-contrast subtraction and 93 % for the subtraction MIP sequence, the MIP sequence was statistically significantly inferior. These sequences were interpreted together as one examination and there was no significant difference between sensitivities for the different readers. Both the Kuhl and Mango studies suggest the subtraction MIP sequence alone is not sufficient for detection of all cancers. Kuhl et al. also noted that MIP images did not provide enough information for the reader to provide a BI-RADS assessment if a lesion was present and thus readers in that study simply determined the presence or absence of significant enhancement (i.e. above background parenchymal enhancement) when reading the MIP alone. However, they found just the first post-contrast image was sufficient to provide a BI-RADS assessment.

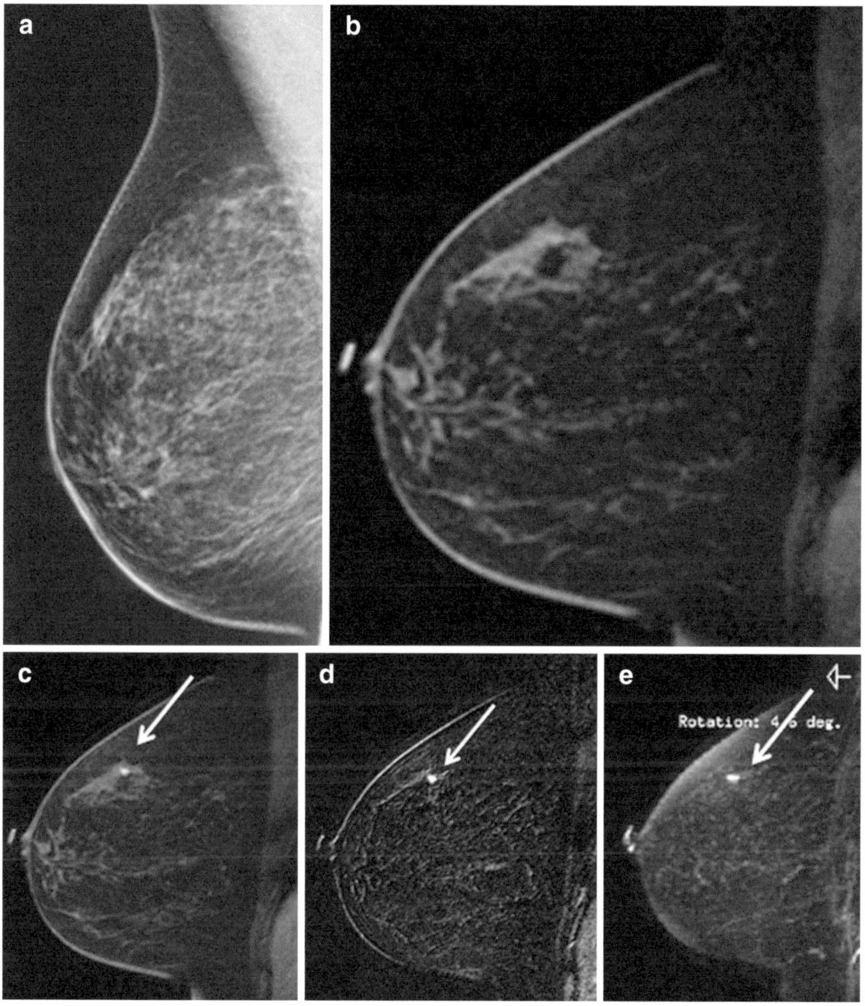

Fig. 16.2 Fifty-four-year-old woman with right 12:00, 0.7 cm invasive ductal carcinoma (*white arrow*). (**a**) Mammogram, MLO image. Cancer mammographically occult. Selected MR sequences provide an example of the abbreviated breast MRI protocol investigated by Mango et al. [32]. (**b**) Sagittal precontrast fat saturated T1-weighted image, cancer not visualized (**c**) Sagittal early post-contrast fat saturated T1-weighted image (**d**) Sagittal postcontrast T1-weighted subtraction image (**e**) Sagittal subtraction MIP

Similar to the Kuhl study, Mango et al. demonstrated decreased image acquisition and radiologist reading times. They estimated the abbreviated imaging protocol to take 10–15 min of magnet time including image acquisition, patient transitions/instructions and contrast injection compared with 30–40 min for the full protocol. Interpretation of the abbreviated protocol averaged 44 s compared with published mean time to read standard breast MRI of 4.7 min [33].

A more recent study by Heacock et al. supports these results and examines utilization of the T2-weighted sequence and history/prior imaging in an abbreviated MR protocol [34]. Their abridged protocol consisted of T1-weighted images (non-contrast, first post-contrast and first post-contrast subtraction sequences) read with and without history/prior imaging available (abbreviated protocols 1 and 2). An additional reading was performed with T2-weighted images also available (abbreviated protocol 3). Total MR acquisition time was 12 min including a reported 5 min for the T2-weighted sequence. Looking at 107 patients with known unifocal breast carcinoma they found all cancers were identified on the T1-weighted sequences by at least one reader with a mean cancer detection rate of 97.8–99.4 %. T2-weighted imaging increased lesion conspicuity but did not improve cancer detection. Given study design the effect of T2-weighted images on specificity could not be evaluated. Mean interpretation times for 3 readers for T1-weighted sequences was 14.0–25.4 s with T2-sequences adding an average of 5.0–9.9 s to the interpretation time. Improved cancer detection rates were seen for all readers with prior imaging and clinical history available.

Studies of such abbreviated protocols highlight limitations when depending on just a few sequences for interpretation. For example, a protocol consisting of a single MIP image may be insufficient for interpretation due to extensive background parenchymal enhancement (BPE) or subtraction errors secondary to patient motion. Kuhl et al. noted 3.6 % of their cases required reading of the complete abbreviated protocol due to these limitations on the MIP [28] (Fig. 16.1). Additionally, lack of the T2 sequence eliminates assessment for lesion T2 hyperintensity which may enable the benign assessment of a finding. Absence of a T1 non-fat saturated image may limit diagnosis of fat necrosis or identification of an intramammary node fatty hilum and result in patients being recalled for the full diagnostic exam [32]. In addition, only obtaining one post-contrast sequence prohibits kinetic analysis of a lesion.

Before abbreviated breast MRI is utilized as a mass population screening tool one must also consider the indirect costs of the abbreviated protocol through BI-RADS 3 follow up or biopsy recommendations. In Kuhl's study the full diagnostic protocol and complete abbreviated protocol performed similarly for cancer detection and had similar false-positive diagnoses; however, the full protocol enabled downgrading of 37.7 % of lesions (20 of 53) to BI-RADS 2 initially characterized as BI-RADS 3 on the complete abbreviated protocol [28]. This supports the impression that the full protocol sequences assist more in lesion characterization than lesion detection. In patients with BI-RADS 3 lesions on the abbreviated MR exam a decision must be made to perform a full diagnostic exam for further lesion characterization versus 2 year abridged MR imaging follow up to assess for stability. A cost benefit analysis is necessary to see if the expense and time of the full diagnostic protocol would be worthwhile in this setting. Interestingly Kuhl et al. also demonstrated that reading the full diagnostic protocol upgraded lesion assessment to BI-RADS 4 in 4 of 53 women, leading to biopsy of a papilloma but no additional cancers. Thus the additional sequences of the full diagnostic protocol did not always improve patient outcomes and may result in additional procedures in a few cases.

These studies have focused on the early postcontrast phase as it is thought early arterial enhancement is best suited for visualization of invasive breast cancers [28]; however, optimal timing needs to be established. A recent study by Grimm et al. looked at the addition of a second post-contrast image and a T2 weighted image to an abbreviated protocol [20]. T2 hyperintensity may increase exam specificity by enabling benign assessment of a finding; however, it adds substantial scan time, reportedly 6 min for the T2 sequence in this study compared with 2 min each for T1 pre and post contrast images [20]. In Grimm's study three fellowship-trained breast imagers evaluated 48 breast MRIs (24 normal, 12 benign and 12 malignant-3 DCIS and 9 invasive cancers) from a high risk screening population comparing two abbreviated protocols to the full diagnostic protocol. The first abbreviated protocol (abbreviated 1) included fat-saturated pre contrast T2-weighted and first post contrast T1-weighted images. Readers had the option to generate a first post contrast subtraction image at the workstation. The second abbreviated protocol (abbreviated 2) included those same images plus a second post contrast T1-weighted sequence that enabled generation of kinetic curves (Fig. 16.3). They observed no statistically significant difference in sensitivity or specificity between the two abbreviated protocols and the full protocol. Lower specificities, 52 % abbreviated 1, 45 % abbreviated 2 and 52 % full protocol, compared to those typically reported in prospective

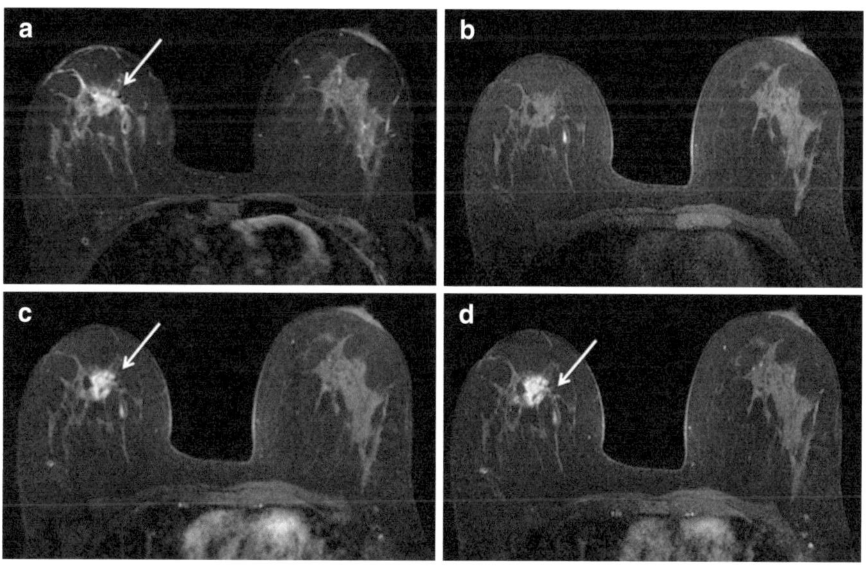

Fig. 16.3 Fifty-three-year-old female with right 12:00, 2.2 cm invasive ductal carcinoma (*white arrow*). Selected sequences provide an example of the abbreviated breast MRI protocol (abbreviated 1) investigated by Grimm et al. [20] (**a**) Axial fat saturated precontrast T2-weighted image (**b**) Axial pre contrast T1-weighted image (**c**) Axial first post-contrast T1-weighted image. Readers had the option to generate a first postcontrast subtraction image at the workstation. The second abbreviated protocol (abbreviated 2) included those same images plus (**d**) a second postcontrast T1-weighted sequence which enabled generation of kinetic curves

breast MR studies [6, 8, 9, 35] were likely because the study population included 25 % biopsy proven benign lesions and readers did not have access to prior studies or correlation with other modalities [20]. Interestingly, the ability to calculate lesion kinetics did not alter specificities given the abbreviated 1 and abbreviated 2 protocols performed similarly. Surprisingly reader interpretation times were not significantly different for the abbreviated 1 and full diagnostic protocol (2.98 vs 2.95 min) and the authors hypothesize that the additional sequences in the full diagnostic protocol are either not routinely used for assessment or alternatively readers spent more time on abbreviated sequences to be confident in their interpretations in the absence of additional sequences [20]; further study into this is necessary.

The sensitivity of breast MRI in these studies of abbreviated protocols is comparable to the sensitivity of the breast MRI full diagnostic protocol reported by other investigators including a meta-analysis of 44 breast MRI studies which calculated a pooled sensitivity of 0.90 and specificity of 0.72 [36] (Table 16.2). In comparison, the sensitivity of screening breast ultrasound is considerably lower than breast MRI and has higher false positive results [2, 31].

Additional efforts to shorten the standard diagnostic breast MRI protocol but maintain dynamic contrast information have come from Mann et al. looking at obtaining such information with time-resolved angiography with stochastic trajectories (TWIST) instead of standard dynamic post-contrast sequences [37]. The TWIST technique captures contrast inflow to lesions (as opposed to the washout phase) allowing calculations for rate of enhancement. This ultrafast sequence heavily undersamples the outer part of k-space and shares data points between successive time points (known as view sharing) to improve spatial resolution [37]. As image contrast is determined by the center of k-space the rate of enhancement can still be accurately measured [37]. Visually this enables successive MIPs presented as a movie of contrast inflow with "light bulb" tumor enhancement before the remainder of the normal breast facilitating lesion detection. This differs from standard breast MRI where vessels on subtraction MIPs are usually venous in origin [37]. Mann et al. interleaved 20 ultrafast TWIST acquisitions during contrast inflow in a regular high-resolution dynamic MRI protocol for a total sequence duration of 102 s. They calculated the maximum slope of the contrast enhancement versus time curve (MS) as a dynamic parameter to differentiate benign and malignant disease. Looking at 199 enhancing lesions (95 benign and 104 malignant) with pathology or 2 year follow up available they compared the MS obtained from the TWIST to the kinetic curves from the conventional dynamic contrast enhanced MRI as defined by the BI-RADS lexicon. They found all lesions were visible on the TWIST and standard series. The TWIST MS allowed discrimination between benign and malignant disease, the steeper the MS the higher the likelihood of malignancy, with maximum slope as a dynamic parameter achieving a higher accuracy in differentiation between benign and malignant disease than traditional BI-RADS curve type analysis [37]. Based on ROC curve analysis, regarding all lesions with an MS higher than 6.4 %/s to be malignant results in 90 % sensitivity and 67 % specificity. Such a technique could allow acquisition of dynamic information in a fraction of the time; however, future studies are warranted to determine utility in a screening setting.

Also assessment of lesion morphology on TWIST images was beyond the scope of their study. Having MS data for lesion characterization may be useful to improve sensitivity and specificity of an abbreviated protocol without significantly lengthening the exam.

Other authors have examined shortening the breast MRI exam by eliminating contrast administration and utilizing diffusion weighted imaging (DWI). DWI provides information about the degree of water molecule diffusion which is inversely correlated with tissue cellularity and cell membrane integrity [38]. Breast cancers have been shown to have high signal and increased conspicuity on DWI [39] (Fig. 16.4). Trimboli et al. looked at an unenhanced protocol in 67 women using axial T1-weighted gradient-echo, T2-weighted STIR, and echo-planar DWI with

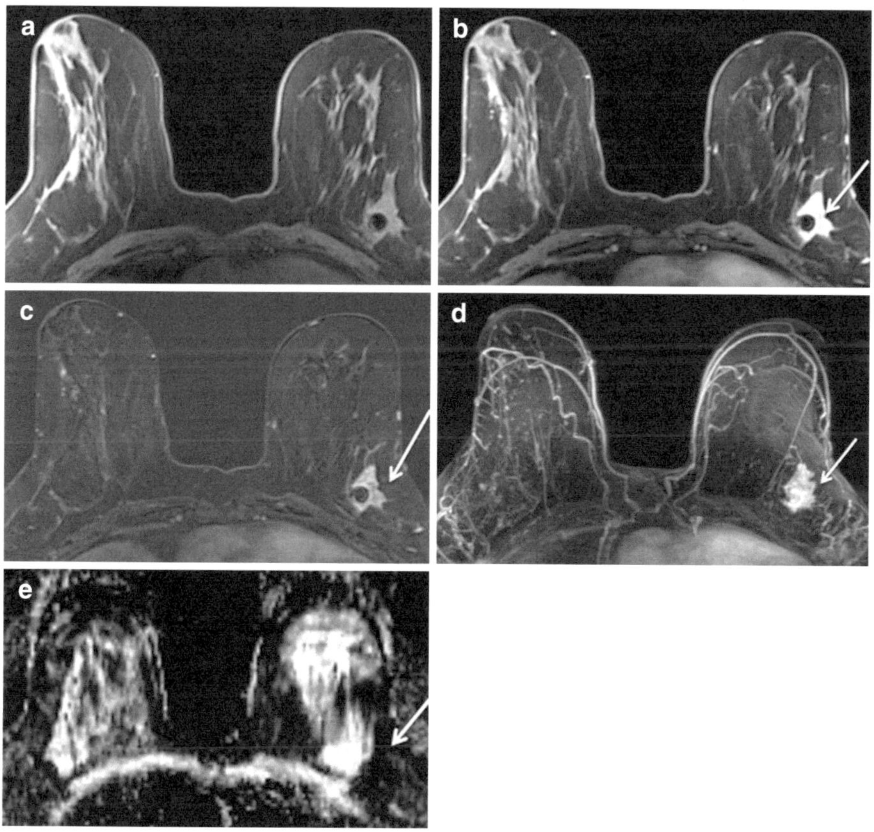

Fig. 16.4 Sixty-seven-year-old female with left 2:00, 3.1 cm invasive ductal carcinoma and DCIS (*white arrow*). MR demonstrates an irregular, heterogeneously enhancing mass with central susceptibility artifact consistent with a biopsy clip marking the site of biopsy-proven malignancy. (**a**) Axial precontrast fat saturated T1-weighted image (**b**) Axial first postcontrast fat saturated T1-weighted image (**c**) Axial first postcontrast subtracted T1-weighted image and (**d**) Axial MIP image. (**e**) DWI showed low ADC values (0.782×10^{-3} mm^2/s) consistent with a malignancy

associated ADC maps which enabled breast cancer detection with a sensitivity of 78 % and specificity of 90 % [26]. It is notable the sensitivity of this technique is less than reported for other abbreviated protocols and detected cancers appear to be larger, with a median size of 1.7 cm, possibly due to decreased resolution; however this was not a screening population. The authors point out the sensitivity is comparable to that of screening mammography in the general population [26] and specificity of their abbreviated protocol is improved in the absence of contrast likely due to lack of enhancing normal tissue or enhancing benign lesions [5, 36]. This study did not demonstrate improved sensitivity despite double reading; however, unlike the other cited studies, the two readers in this study were residents and not experienced breast radiologists, likely limiting results. The lower spatial resolution of DWI limits its use in isolation [39] with the greatest limitation seen in identification of cancers manifesting as nonmasslike enhancement, 60 % (3/5) of non-mass cancers were missed compared with 18 % (5/28) of those with mass enhancement [26]. Also this MR population included symptomatic women and patients undergoing extent of disease evaluation for known breast cancer resulting in a 32 % breast cancer prevalence, much higher than the general population or a high risk screening group [26].

Breast radiologists are currently faced with difficult questions about what modalities to utilize for supplemental screening and which patients should be offered supplemental screening. There is a lack of consensus for such recommendations at a time when these questions are asked with increasing frequency given how many states now mandate patient notification of breast density [40, 41]. Patients with heterogeneously or extremely dense breasts on mammography have an increased risk of developing breast cancer but as an independent risk factor these patients do not meet the 20 % risk threshold to qualify for MR screening under current guidelines [42, 43]. Additionally MRI demonstrates the highest sensitivity for breast carcinoma detection regardless of breast density, thus patients with scattered fibroglandular tissue or fatty breasts may benefit from breast MRI as well [44]. The advantages of screening with MRI over other modalities such as ultrasound include an improved PPV_3, the positive predictive value for malignancy of biopsied lesions detected at screening [41]. Decreased image acquisition and reading time in the screening MR setting could potentially decrease cost and increase women's access to screening breast MRI without sacrificing diagnostic accuracy and cancer yield. Additionally as studies have demonstrated additional small invasive cancers with negative nodes not detected on mammography, ultrasound or physical exam, initial results seem promising to hopefully demonstrate a mortality benefit of abbreviated MRI on future studies.

Limitations of abbreviated breast MR studies to date include performance at high volume centers with most readings done by experienced dedicated breast radiologists which may reduce applicability of the currently available data to the community practice setting. Some hypothesize the radiologists' learning curve associated with increased breast MRI volume would be similar to that undergone by the radiology community at the beginning of screening mammography programs [28]. Most of the currently available studies did not include pure screening populations, limiting our ability to generalize results to these populations and thus caution in applying these results in practice is warranted. In addition it is important to note that MRI acquisition time estimates for the abbreviated protocol may not accurately reflect the entire time the MRI room is occupied given time spent transitioning patients on and off the table, providing patient instructions and contrast injection time. Additionally most studies did not allow readers to utilize important information normally available in a clinical setting such as exam indication, prior MRI studies and correlation with patient's prior mammogram or breast ultrasound potentially improving results in a true practice setting. Finally, another hurdle to the implementation of an abbreviated MRI is cost. Currently, the vast majority of third-party carriers are not reimbursing for this study. Therefore, the cost of the abbreviated MRI exam may fall on the patient. In private communication, (non published data), a practice in Michigan has performed over 671 abbreviated MRI exams that were paid for by one third party carrier.

Future research into the applicability of abbreviated breast MRI screening is needed including refining which sequences should be included to improve specificity and looking at the cost-benefit analysis for average to intermediate risk patients and true screening populations. It remains to be seen if initial results are applicable to general radiologists and to mass population screening. Some authors point out further study is necessary to determine time spent reading individual sequences and to determine the influence of that sequence on the final BI-RADS assessment [20]. In addition, in the context of screening breast MRI at regular intervals one notes that the long-term effect of annual or biannual IV administration of gadolinium for decades is unknown [26].

16.1 Conclusions

Overall the currently available data suggests that abbreviated breast MRI is feasible without sacrificing sensitivity or specificity, compared with the standard full diagnostic MR protocol. Abbreviated-MRI may have the potential to decrease costs associated with the exam and increase patient access to breast MRI. Larger prospective studies are necessary to refine abbreviated protocols in patients with various levels of risk and ultimately as our healthcare system focuses on value based care, demonstrate a patient mortality benefit at an acceptable cost through mass MRI screening with an abbreviated protocol.

References

1. Morris EA, Liberman L, Ballon DJ, Robson M, Abramson AF, Heerdt A, et al. MRI of occult breast carcinoma in a high-risk population. Am J Roentgenol. 2003;181:619–26.
2. Berg WA, Zhang Z, Lehrer D, Jong RA, Pisano ED, Barr RG, et al. Detection of breast cancer with addition of annual screening ultrasound or a single screening MRI to mammography in women with elevated breast cancer risk. JAMA. 2012;307:1394–404.

3. Lehman CD, Isaacs C, Schnall MD. Cancer yield of mammography, MR, and US in high-risk women: prospective multi-institution breast cancer screen study. Radiology. 2007;244(2):381–8.
4. Saslow D, Boetes C, Burke W, et al. American Cancer Society guidelines for breast screening with MRI as an adjunct to mammography. CA Cancer J Clin. 2007;57(2):75–89.
5. Sardanelli F, Podo F, Santoro F, et al. Multi-center surveillance of women at high genetic breast cancer risk using mammography, ultrasonography, and contrast-enhanced magnetic resonance imaging (the high breast cancer risk Italian 1 study): final results. Invest Radiol. 2011;46:94–105.
6. Lehman CD, Gatsonis C, Kuhl CK, et al. MRI evaluation of the contralateral breast in women with recently diagnosed breast cancer. N Engl J Med. 2007;356:1295–303.
7. Warner E, Plewes DB, Hill KA, et al. Surveillance of BRCA 1 and BRCA 2 mutation carriers with magnetic resonance imaging, ultrasound, mammography, and clinical breast examination. JAMA. 2004;292:1317–25.
8. Kriege M, Brekelmans CT, Boetes C, et al. Efficacy of MRI and mammography for breast cancer screening in women with a familial or genetic predisposition. N Engl J Med. 2004;351:427–37.
9. Kuhl CK, Schrading S, Leutner CC, et al. Mammography, breast ultrasound, and magnetic resonance imaging for surveillance of women at high familial risk for breast cancer. J Clin Oncol. 2005;23:8469–76.
10. Leach MO, Boggis CR, Dixon AK, et al. Screening with magnetic resonance imaging and mammography of a UK population at high familial risk of breast cancer: a prospective multicentre cohort study (MARIBS). Lancet. 2005;365:1769–78.
11. Lehman CD, Blume JD, Weatherall P, et al. Screening women at high risk for breast cancer with mammography and magnetic resonance imaging. Cancer. 2005;103:1898–905.
12. Passaperuma K, Warner E, Causer PA, et al. Long-term results of screening with magnetic resonance imaging in women with BRCA mutations. Br J Cancer. 2012;107:24–30.
13. Warner E, Hill K, Causer P, et al. Prospective study of breast cancer incidence in women with a BRCA 1 or BRCA 2 mutation under surveillance with and without magnetic resonance imaging. J Clin Oncol. 2011;29:1664–9.
14. Sickles EA. The use of breast imaging to screen women at high risk for cancer. Radiol Clin North Am. 2010;48:859–78.
15. Ahern CH, Shih YC, Dong W, et al. Cost-effectiveness of alternative strategies for integrating MRI into breast cancer screening for women at high risk. Br J Cancer. 2014;111:1542–51.
16. Feig S. Cost-effectiveness of mammography, MRI, and ultrasonography for breast cancer screening. Radiol Clin North Am. 2010;48:879–91.
17. Moore SG, Shenoy PJ, Fanucchi L, et al. Cost-effectiveness of MRI compared to mammography for breast cancer screening in a high risk population. BMC Health Serv Res. 2009;9:9.
18. Pataky R, Armstrong L, Chia S, et al. Cost-effectiveness of MRI for breast cancer screening in BRCA ½ mutation carriers. BMC Cancer. 2013;13:339.
19. Taneja C, Edelsberg J, Weycker D, et al. Cost-effectiveness of breast cancer screening with contrast-enhanced MRI in high-risk women. J Am Coll Radiol. 2009;6:171–9.
20. Grimm LJ, Soo MS, Yoon S, Kim C, Ghate SV, Johnson KS. Abbreviated screening protocol for breast MRI: a feasibility study. Acad Radiol. 2015;22:1157–62.
21. Lowry KP, Lee JM, Kong CY, et al. Annual screening strategies in BRCA 1 and BRCA 2 gene mutation carriers: a comparative effectiveness analysis. Cancer. 2012;118:2021–30.
22. Cott Chubiz JE, Lee JM, Gilmore ME, et al. Cost-effectiveness of alternating magnetic resonance imaging and digital mammography screening in BRCA 1 and BRCA 2 gene mutation carriers. Cancer. 2013;119:1266–76.
23. Ivanov EN, Pogromsky AY, Van Den Brink JS, et al. Optimization of duty cycles for MRI scanners. Concepts Magn Reson Part B Magn Reson Eng. 2010;37B:180–92.
24. Carpenter AP, Leemis LM, Papir AS, et al. Managing magnetic resonance imaging machines: support tools for scheduling and planning. Health Care Manag Sci. 2011;14:158–73.

25. Wernli KJ, Demartini WB, Ichikawa L, et al. Patterns of breast magnetic imaging use in community practice. JAMA Intern Med. 2014;174:125–32.
26. Trimboli RM, Verardi N, Cartia F, Carbonaro LA, Sardanelli F. Breast cancer detection using double reading of unenhanced MRI including T1-weighted, T2-weighted STIR, and diffusion-weighted imaging: a proof of concept study. Am J Roentgenol. 2014;203:674–81.
27. Wilson JMG, Junger G. Principles and practice of screening for disease. Geneva, Switzerland: World Health Organization; 1968.
28. Kuhl CK, Schrading S, Strobel K, Schild HH, Hilgers RD, Beiling HB. Abbreviated breast magnetic resonance imaging (MRI): first postcontrast subtracted images and maximum-intensity projection- a novel approach to breast cancer screening with MRI. J Clin Oncol. 2014;32:2304–10.
29. Garg AS, Rapelyea JA, Rechtman LR, et al. Full-field digital mammographic interpretation with prior analog versus prior digitized analog mammography: Time for interpretation. Am J Roentgenol. 2011;196:1436–8.
30. Tchou PM, Haygood TM, Atkinson EN, et al. Interpretation time of computer-aided detection at screening mammography. Radiology. 2010;257:40–6.
31. Berg WA, Blume JD, Cormack JB, et al. Combined screening with ultrasound and mammography vs mammography alone in women at elevated risk of breast cancer. JAMA. 2008;299:2151–63.
32. Mango VL, Morris EA, Dershaw DD, Abramson A, Fry C, Moskowitz CS, Hughes M, Kaplan J, Jochelson M. Abbreviated protocol for breast MRI: are multiple sequences needed for cancer detection? Eur J Radiol. 2015;84:65–70.
33. Lehman CD, Blume JD, DeMartini WB, Hylton NM, Herman B, Schnall MD, et al. Accuracy and interpretation time of computer-aided detection among novice and experience breast MRI readers. Am J Roentgenol. 2013;200:W683–9.
34. Heacock L, Melsaether AN, Heller SL, et al. Evaluation of a known breast cancer using an abbreviated breast MRI protocol: correlation of imaging characteristics and pathology with lesion detection and conspicuity. Eur J Radiol. 2016;85(4):815–23.
35. Warner E, Messersmith H, Causer P, et al. Systematic review: using magnetic resonance imaging to screen women at high risk for breast cancer. Ann Intern Med. 2008;148:671–9.
36. Peters NH, Borel Rinkes IH, Zuithoff NP, et al. Meta-analysis of MR imaging in the diagnosis of breast lesions. Radiology. 2008;246:116–24.
37. Mann RM, Mus RD, Zelst JV, Geppert C, Karssemeijer N, Platel B. A novel approach to contrast-enhanced breast magnetic resonance imaging for screening: high-resolution ultrafast dynamic imaging. Invest Radiol. 2014;49(9):579–85.
38. Englander SA, Ulug AM, Brem R, Glickson JD, van Zijl PC. Diffusion imaging of human breast. NMR Biomed. 1997;10:348–52.
39. Woodhams R, Ramadan S, Stanwell P, et al. Diffusion-weighted imaging of the breast: principles and clinical applications. Radiographics. 2011;31:1059–84.
40. Ho JM, Jafferjee N, Covarrubias GM, et al. Dense breasts: a review of reporting legislation and available supplemental screening options. Am J Roentgenol. 2014;203:449–56.
41. Freer PE. Mammographic breast density: impact on breast cancer risk and implications for screening. Radiographics. 2015;35(2):302–15.
42. Harvey JA, Bovbjerg VE. Quantitative assessment of mammographic breast density: relationship with breast cancer risk. Radiology. 2004;230:29–41.
43. Sprague BL, Gangnon RE, Burt V, et al. Prevalence of mammographically dense breasts in the United States. J Natl Cancer Inst. 2014;106:1–6.
44. Riedl CC, Luft N, Bernhart C, et al. Triple-modality screening trial for familial breast cancer underlines the importance of magnetic resonance imaging and questions the role of mammography and ultrasound regardless of patient mutations status, age, and breast density. J Clin Oncol. 2015;33:1128–35.

Chapter 17
Personalized Medicine, Biomarkers of Risk and Breast MRI

Elizabeth J. Sutton, Nina Purvis, Katja Pinker-Domenig, and Elizabeth A. Morris

Abstract Breast cancer is a heterogeneous disease with inter- and intra-tumor genetic variation impacting predictive and prognostic risk. This chapter discusses the use of breast MRI, the most sensitive imaging modality for high-risk screening and pre-operative assessment, to predict breast cancer risk, to define extent of disease and to monitor neoadjuvant chemotherapeutic response at the level of the individual patient. In the current clinical landscape, immunohistochemical surrogates are used to define molecular subtypes and personalized cancer treatment and care. Radiogenomics involves the correlation of genomic information with imaging features. Feature extraction from breast MRI is being pursued on a large scale as a potential non-invasive means of defining molecular subtypes and/or developing phenotypic biomarkers that can be clinically analogous to commercially available genomic assays. Neoadjuvant chemotherapy, treatment administered in operable cancers before surgery, is increasingly used, allowing for breast conservation in women who would traditionally require mastectomy. As breast cancer genetic molecular subtypes are predictive of recurrence free and overall survival, treatment based on breast cancer molecular subtype and breast MRI is critical in evaluating response though improvement in its sensitivity for pathologic complete response. Breast MRI in the neoadjuvant cohort has provided biomarkers of response and insight into the biologic basis of disease. MRI is at the forefront of technology providing prognostic indicators as well as a crucial tool in personalizing medicine.

E.J. Sutton, MDCM (✉) • N. Purvis, MPhys, PhD • E.A. Morris, MD, FACR
Department of Radiology, Memorial Sloan Kettering Cancer Center,
New York, NY 10021, USA
e-mail: suttone@mskcc.org

K. Pinker-Domenig, MD, PhD
Department of Radiology, Memorial Sloan Kettering Cancer Center,
New York, NY 10021, USA

Department of Biomedical Imaging and Image-guided Therapy, Division of Molecular and Gender Imaging, Medical University of Vienna/General Hospital Vienna, Vienna, Austria

S.L. Heller, L. Moy (eds.), *Breast Oncology: Techniques, Indications, and Interpretation*, DOI 10.1007/978-3-319-42563-4_17

Keywords Breast MRI • High-risk screening • Background parenchymal enhancement • Breast cancer molecular subtype • Genetics • Radiogenomics • Radiomics • Neoadjuvant chemotherapy • Biomarkers • Texture features • Personalized medicine • Risk markers • Response assessment • Big data • Tumor segmentation

17.1 Introduction

Breast cancer prevention based on risk-adjusted screening and targeted therapeutics based on genetic molecular subtype both epitomize personalized cancer care. Breast magnetic resonance imaging (MRI) is the most sensitive imaging modality for both high-risk screening and diagnoses. MR images are now being mined for information pertaining to the biologic basis of this disease. This chapter will explore the evolving role of breast MRI in predicting risk as well as in defining biomarkers of breast cancer and its response to treatment.

17.2 Breast Cancer Risk

Despite tremendous advances in the understanding of breast cancer, it remains unknown which individuals will ultimately develop breast malignancy. In addition, the type of breast tissue that fosters a microenvironment conducive to the growth of breast cancer also remains unknown.

We do know that certain genetic mutations and phenotypic syndromes result in a high, greater than or equal to 20 %, lifetime risk of breast cancer and these include the deleterious type 1 or 2 BRCA mutation, Li-Fraumeni syndrome, Cowden syndrome and Bannayan-Riley-Ruvalcaba syndrome as well as all of their respective first-degree relatives. We also know that women with a history of chest irradiation also have a high lifetime risk of breast cancer. Other genomic biomarkers of breast cancer, including a moderately penetrant mutation of the CHEK2 gene, have been identified and will continue to be with variable penetrance [1].

The role of breast MRI continues to evolve in the screening of women with a low or moderate risk of breast cancer, even as current recommendations state that evidence is insufficient for or against its use. Currently, in the United States of America, high-risk breast MRI screening is performed as an adjunct to mammography in the aforementioned women as well as in women with a strong family history and who are defined as high-risk based upon a risk assessment model [2, 3]. High-risk screening with MRI has been associated with a significant increase in overall survival compared to a mammography-only screening [4].

Breast MRI has now been used as a screening tool for almost 20 years. There is a vast amount of information contained within MRI images that can be processed to identify and validate potential biomarkers associated with individual patient risk or an outcome. An imaging biomarker is a broad term for either a feature or prognostic indicator of biologic behavior that is detectable in an image. Biomarkers can either be qualitative or quantitative. Researchers are exploring if breast tissue can be used as a biomarker of risk. We discuss fibroglandular tissue and background parenchymal enhancement as imaging biomarkers of risk below.

17.2.1 Fibroglandular Tissue

The amount of fibroglandular tissue, often referred to as breast density, is strongly associated with increased risk of breast cancer [5, 6]. The underlying reason why women with dense breasts have a higher risk of breast cancer remains unclear [7]. Currently, the amount of fibroglandular tissue on MRI is a qualitative assessment made by the radiologist and even when standardized criteria is used there remains significant inter- and intra-observer agreement variability (the degree is unclear due to the paucity of research in this area). Because of this strong association between the amount of fibroglandular tissue and breast cancer, research into the development of computer-assisted devices for fibroglandular tissue segmentation began in the 1990s [8]. There is continuing research focusing on the development of robust computer algorithms that can automatically segment fibroglandular tissue and provide a quantitative metric of volume and density. Different methods are being evaluated including fuzzy clustering and fuzzy-C-means; however, a detailed review of all techniques is beyond the scope of this chapter [9]. At this time, there is neither any clinically available software program nor agreement regarding the most accurate and robust method of segmentation that can be applied universally across different images and vendor platforms.

17.2.2 Background Parenchymal Enhancement

Background parenchymal enhancement refers to the proportion of normal fibroglandular tissue that enhances [5]. It is physiologically defined as the amount of contrast agent that reaches normal fibroglandular breast tissue and is an indicator of blood perfusion to the normal tissue [10, 11]. As with the amount of fibroglandular tissue, the degree of background parenchymal enhancement is also a significant predictor of breast cancer. Specifically, increased background parenchymal enhancement is associated with an increased risk of breast cancer [7]. Similar to fibroglandular tissue, background parenchymal enhancement is evaluated qualitatively by a radiologist (Fig. 17.1) [10, 11]. Background parenchymal enhancement has also been shown to be affected by factors such as hormonal status, menopausal status, age and hormonal therapies [5].

Computer algorithms are also being developed to provide a quantitative metric of background parenchymal enhancement [12, 13]. From a computing standpoint, this is more complicated then the volumetric assessment of fibroglandular tissue because it involves the evaluation of contrast enhancement, which itself is dependent on a number of different factors. A detailed discussion is beyond the scope of this chapter, but variables include time, type of contrast and dose. Robust and standard quantitative methods are needed but do not currently exist.

There has been current investigation into whether background parenchymal enhancement in the healthy breast can be predictive or prognostic of the breast cancer in the contralateral breast. In a recent study, authors reported that neoadjuvant chemotherapy patients with higher pre-treatment background parenchymal enhancement in the contralateral normal breasts went on to show a significant decrease of background parenchymal enhancement early after neoadjuvant chemotherapy and were more likely to achieve pathologic complete response [14]. Another study evaluated the parenchymal enhancement in the contralateral breast in patients with unilateral breast cancer; the results suggested that parenchymal enhancement was significantly associated with long-term outcome [15].

No studies to date have employed the power of more than a few parameters together to explore background parenchymal enhancement as a predictive biomarker, nor have they tried to quantify it on a voxel-by-voxel basis. Background parenchymal enhancement should be further utilized by exploring its potential as a predictive biomarker through the means of multiparametric MRI and advanced image analysis.

Analysis of information inherent in breast MRI images such as fibroglandular tissue and background parenchymal enhancement may ultimately lead to the development of risk-adjusted screening algorithms. Understanding the impact of these entities for risk has the potential to obviate the current blanket recommendation for a yearly screening mammogram beginning at the age of 40 as recommended by the American College of Radiology [16] and the Society of Breast Imaging [17]. Larger studies are needed to investigate and support this possibility.

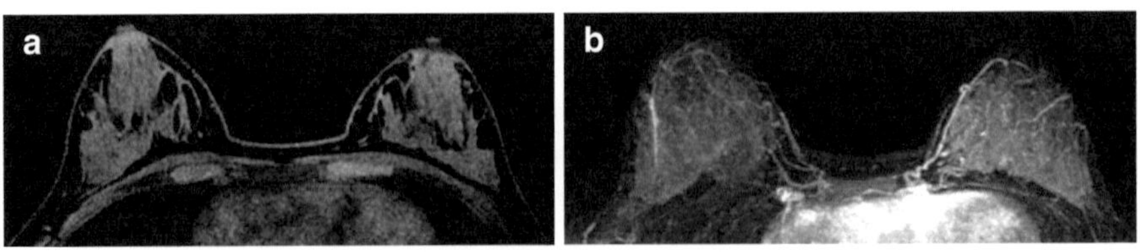

Fig. 17.1 Axial T1 fat-suppressed images before (**a**) and after (**b**) the administration of intravenous contrast in a woman with extremely dense fibroglandular tissue and marked background parenchymal enhancement on the first post-contrast image (**b**)

17.3 Breast Cancer Genetics

Our current understanding of breast cancer genetics continues to evolve rapidly. As researchers increasingly perform next generation DNA and RNA sequencing, our understanding of breast cancers will continue to grow and the currently defined molecular subtypes described below will likely become further subcategorized in the next few years.

Breast cancer is a heterogeneous disease. The discovery of different molecular subtypes based upon genetic variation has markedly impacted the treatment of breast cancer and helped develop the concept of personalized clinical care [18]. These subtypes have been shown to be predictive of disease-free and overall survival [19] and are used to guide targeted therapy. Full genome sequencing of all diagnosed breast cancers is not yet a clinical reality, although it is possible for a price. Therefore, immunohistochemical surrogates, specifically estrogen receptor (ER), progesterone receptor (PR) and human epidermal growth factor receptor 2 (HER2) status, are used to approximate the following molecular subtypes: 1- luminal A (ER positive (+) and/or PR+, HER2 negative (−)), 2- luminal B (ER+ and/or PR+, HER2 +), 3- HER2-over-expressing (ER-, PR- and HER2+) and 4- basal-like/triple negative (ER-, PR- and HER2-) (Fig. 17.2). The luminal A subtype is the most common and is significantly associated with the best disease-free and overall survival compared to luminal B, HER2-overexpressing and basal-like subtypes. HER2-overexpressing and basal-like subtypes have the worst outcome. However, Herceptin has significantly improved the disease free and overall survival of HER-2-overexpressing cancers [19].

In addition, within each molecular subtype, it is becoming increasingly clear that there is genotypic variation between tumors (inter-tumoral heterogeneity). This

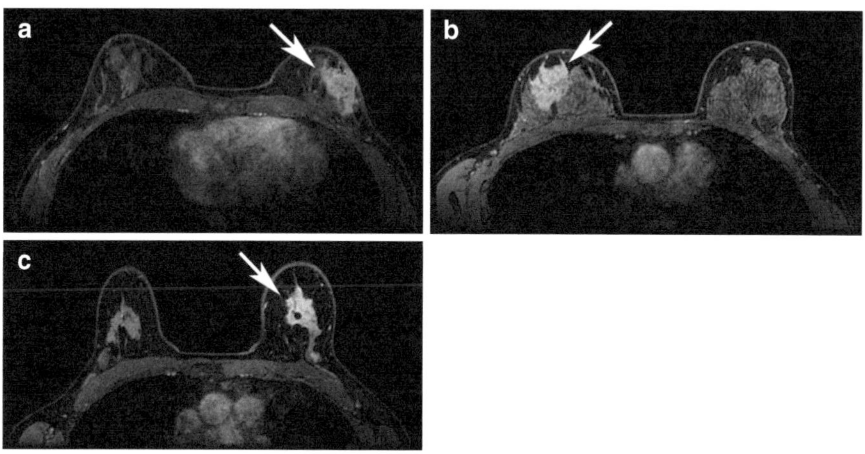

Fig. 17.2 Axial T1 fat-suppressed post-contrast images of (**a**) Estrogen Receptor positive HER2 negative (**b**) HER2 overexpressing and (**c**) Triple negative breast cancers (*arrows*). Research is currently evaluating if the MR imaging phenotype correlates with the molecular subtype

knowledge has resulted in the development and clinical use of predictive and prognostic assays. For example, the American Society of Clinical Oncology has recommended the clinical use of Oncotype Dx (Genomic Health, Redwood City, CA) in early-stage ER+/HER2− invasive breast cancers because it has been shown to be both predictive (likelihood of recurrence) and prognostic (magnitude of chemotherapy benefit). Oncotype Dx is a clinically validated, gene-expression based prognostic and predictive assay that incorporates the mRNA expression of 21 genes, resulting in the so-called Recurrence Score. This Recurrence Score quantifies the magnitude of chemotherapy benefit as well as the 10-year risk of distant recurrence, both increasing with higher Recurrence Scores [20]. This Recurrence Score significantly impacts treatment decisions; women with low recurrence scores can avoid unnecessary chemotherapy [21]. Mammaprint (Agendia) and PAM50 (Prosigna) are other predictive and prognostic genomic assays, which are both clinically available.

Breast MRI is the most sensitive imaging modality for tumor characterization and accurate size measurement at present. There have been major technological advances in MRI which complement the above-described discoveries of the genetic heterogeneity of breast cancer. Advances in MRI include the now clinically available 3-Tesla MRI scanners as well as 8 and 16-channel breast coils. High temporal and spatial resolution imaging is also now a clinical reality. Isotropic MR imaging, which means the voxel is equal in three dimensions allows for multiplanar reconstruction. Clinical indications for breast MRI include pre-operative evaluation to define extent of disease in newly diagnosed breast cancer [5, 22]. Clinically, tumors are still characterized by using the American College of Radiology Breast Imaging-Reporting and Data System (BI-RADS) Lexicon. Besides tumor size measurement, BI-RADS characteristics are qualitative assessments of tumor features or semi-quantitative analyses of contrast enhancement kinetics.

One consequence of technological advances in imaging is that a large volume of data exists. Data mining (also referred to in the literature as data or knowledge discovery) involves computer extraction and analysis of data with the goal of discovering useful information. As it pertains to the field of radiology, this type of computer analytics is referred to as 'radiomics'. Radiomics involves the computer extraction and analysis of quantitative imaging features [23]. One example of this is in the characterization of tumor morphology, texture and enhancement kinetics [24]. This data can be used to build models, which could be used to predict tumor type, behavior or response. Radiomics enables the correlation of imaging phenotypes with genomic information; this is called radiogenomics [25].

Currently the benefit of radiomics and radiogenomics is the identification of tumor imaging biomarkers. As explained earlier in this chapter, an imaging biomarker is a broad term implying either a biologic feature or indicator of biologic behavior that is detectable on an image. Biomarkers are either qualitative or quantitative. A quantifiable imaging biomarker is one that can be objectively measured, which is preferable because it eliminates inter-reader variability and allows change to be assessed on follow-up scans. This is particularly relevant to those patients undergoing treatment. A simple example of a quantifiable imaging biomarker is tumor size. The types of biomarkers that are being researched are broad but include subtle imaging changes, often imperceptible to the eye (features that can be generated by sophisticated computer algorithms) as they pertain to biology, physiology and treatment response, functioning as surrogate markers of tumor behavior and/or endpoints.

Research in this area includes the development of predictive models that correlate breast cancer MRI features with breast cancer molecular subtypes [26–28]. For example, machine-learning-based (support vector machines) models using leave-one-out cross validation have been used to identify significant MR image features associated with three different invasive ductal carcinoma molecular subtypes (ERPR+ (n = 95, 53.4 %); ERPR−/HER2+ (n = 35, 19.6 %); triple negative (n = 48, 27.0 %)). This study developed a predictive model that could distinguish the breast cancer (n = 178) with significant predictive power. When combining the top nine imaging features, the model distinguished the subtypes with an overall accuracy of 71.2 % [26].

Breast cancer MRI features are also being correlated with clinically available genomic assays [29, 30]. MR morphologic and texture-based image features of ER+, PR+ and HER2− invasive ductal carcinomas have been extracted to investigate their association with Oncotype Dx. Ninty-five patients were included with a median Oncotype Dx Recurrence Score of 16 (range: 0–45). Using stepwise multiple linear regression, a model was developed using imaging and pathology information that correlated with the Oncotype Dx recurrence score [30]. Additionally, MR imaging radiomics of 108 breast cancers from The Cancer Imaging Archive (TCIA; (*http://www.cancerimagingarchive.net*)) have been correlated with their respective genomic analyses in The Cancer Genome Atlas (TCGA)—both of which are open-source and open-access information resources [31]. This study also demonstrated significant associations between breast cancer MR radiomics signatures and multigene assay recurrence scores, specifically Mammaprint (Agendia), Oncotype Dx and PAM50 risk of relapse based on subtype (Prosigna) [29].

Currently, researchers are using different computer algorithms to extract MR imaging phenotypes. Large scale datasets are necessary to validate all observations are needed and this will be facilitated by multi-institutional collaboration. This will allow researchers to test their results models on MR images acquired by different vendors, magnet strength and imaging protocols.

17.4 Therapy

As stated above, breast cancer encompasses a heterogeneous group of tumors; this heterogeneity results in very different outcomes. Targeted systemic therapy, based upon a tumor's molecular subtype, epitomizes the concept of precision medicine. Breast cancer systemic recurrence remains a major cause of morbidity and mortality [32]. Historically, chemotherapy was administered after tumor surgical resection and was termed adjuvant chemotherapy. Recently, research has demonstrated equivalent success of adjuvant and neoadjuvant chemotherapy in preventing breast cancer

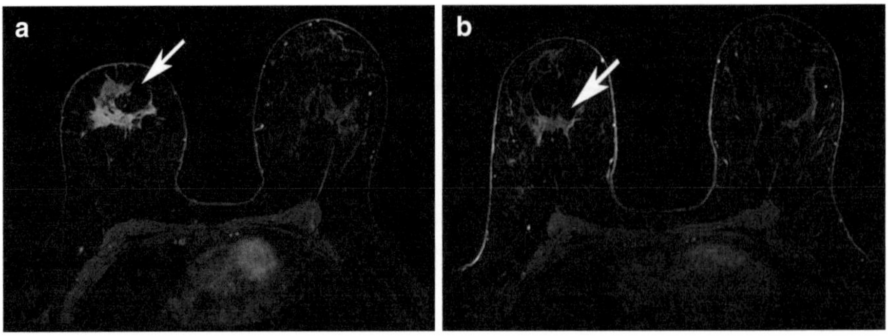

Fig. 17.3 HER2 overexpressing right breast cancer axial T1 fat-suppressed post-contrast image pre (**a**) and post (**b**) neoadjuvant chemotherapy (*arrows*). This case was interpreted as a complete radiologic response because of the absence of any residual enhancement on the post-neoadjuvant chemotherapy images (**b**). Surgical excision confirmed a complete pathologic response

local recurrence. Neoadjuvant chemotherapy (NAC) is used to treat breast cancer pre-operatively and historically it was used for patients with inflammatory or inoperable locally advanced breast cancer. A major shift in breast cancer treatment is currently taking place whereby NAC is being increasingly used because it enables more patients to be treated with breast-conserving surgery whereas traditionally they would have required a mastectomy [32, 33]. NAC is now being increasingly used to establish tumor chemosensitivity in vivo with the goal of a pathologic complete response [34]. Pathologic complete response, an intermediate endpoint, serves as a biomarker for improved disease free and overall survival [34]. The focus in this section will be on the use of NAC since MRI plays a critical role in operable breast cancer. Discussion of all oncologic treatments exceeds the breadth of this chapter.

A study in 2006 reported that approximately 70 % of patients responded to NAC, with pathologic complete response (pCR) in 13–26 % [35]; however, more recent studies suggest the pCR rate is higher [36, 37]. Breast cancer genetics plays a significant role: it has been shown that the likelihood of a tumor responding to NAC is based upon its specific subtype, with triple negative and HER2 over-expressing tumors having a higher likelihood of complete pathologic response (pCR), of up to 38.2 % and 45.4 %, respectively (Fig. 17.3, 17.4, and 17.5) [36, 37]. Currently, no imaging biomarker has been validated to detect a pathologic complete response post NAC preoperatively. Therefore, all patients still undergo breast surgery post NAC.

As our understanding of breast cancer genetic subtypes expands, so too the availability of novel therapies will increase. The National Comprehensive Cancer Network guidelines currently recommend a breast MRI before and after NAC. Clinical breast MRI detects breast cancer by contrast enhancement related to tumor angiogenesis; quantitative guidelines to determine complete pCR are lacking. Better methods are needed to detect complete pCR. The definition of a pCR varies with some groups defining it as the absence of residual invasive breast cancer (ductal carcinoma can be present) while others define it as the absence of residual invasive and in situ breast cancer [38].

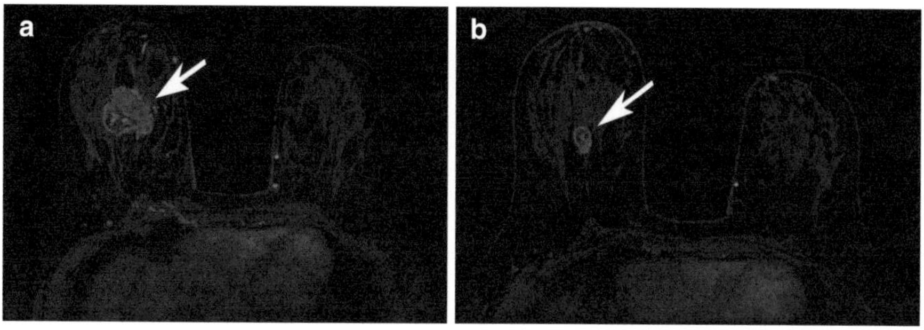

Fig. 17.4 Triple negative right breast right breast cancer axial T1 fat-suppressed post-contrast image pre (**a**) and post (**b**) neoadjuvant chemotherapy (*arrows*). This case was interpreted as a partial radiologic response because there has been a decrease in size of the persistently enhancing mass on the post-neoadjuvant chemotherapy images (**b**). Surgical excision confirmed a partial pathologic response

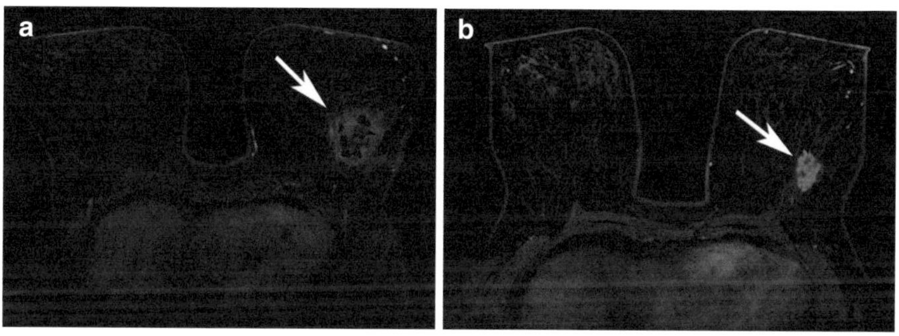

Fig. 17.5 Estrogen receptor positive HER2 negative left breast cancer axial T1 fat-suppressed post-contrast image pre (**a**) and post (**b**) neoadjuvant chemotherapy (*arrows*). This case was interpreted as a partial radiologic response because there has been a decrease in size of the persistently enhancing mass on the post-neoadjuvant chemotherapy images (**b**). Surgical excision confirmed a partial pathologic response

One novel MRI approach to detect complete pCR combines multiparametric breast MRI parameters, enabling a voxel-based analysis of hemodynamics and other changes in tumor physiology including perfusion, diffusion and metabolism [39]. Such techniques may improve overall sensitivity and specificity for evaluation. The literature substantiate the claim that employing multiple MRI parameters in combination has the highest diagnostic accuracy, increasing both sensitivity and specificity (Fig. 17.6) [38, 40]. Post-processing techniques enable volumetric voxel-based analysis of histograms and co-occurrence matrices, generating information that is imperceptible to the eye but improves evaluation of treatment response. A recent study of 48 patients undergoing treatment with NAC found that multiparametric MRI response maps could reliably predict pCR after one cycle of NAC. Specifically, mean voxel signal intensity was lower in those women who went on to have pCR [39].

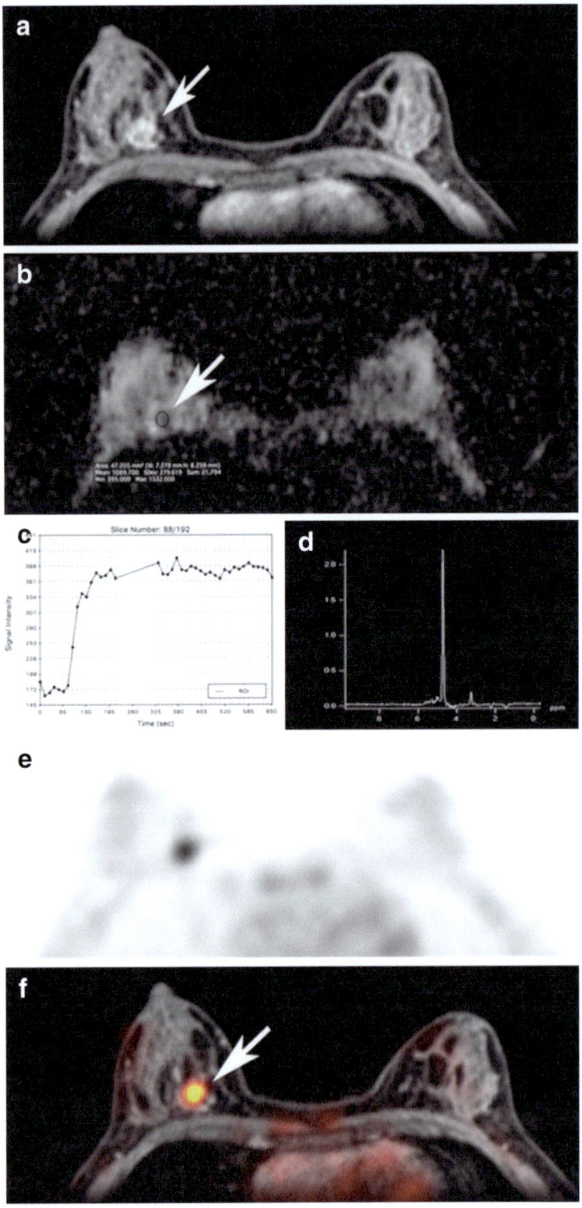

Fig. 17.6 Multiparametric PET-MRI at 3 T with DCE MRI, DWI, 3D ^{1}H-MRSI and the radiotracer [^{18}F]FDG: *Poorly differentiated invasive ductal carcinoma in a 46-year-old woman at 2 o'clock in the right breast.* (**a**) The irregularly shaped and marginated mass showed rapid wash-in enhancement followed by plateau kinetics and was classified as BI-RADS 5 (*arrow*). (**b**) The mass demonstrates decreased ADC values (1.089×10^{-3} mm^2/s) on DWI (*arrow*). (**c**) The mass (*arrow*) has a heterogeneous initial strong enhancement and plateau curve. (**d**) In 3D ^{1}H-MRSI there is a choline peak at 3,2 ppm and (**e**) in [^{18}F]FDG PET, the mass is highly [^{18}F]FDG avid (*arrow*). (**f**) Multiparametric PET-MRI accurately classified the mass as malignant (*arrow*)

Other studies have also demonstrated that diffusion weighted imaging (DWI) is a robust method of distinguishing breast cancers that respond to NAC. Apparent diffusion coefficient (ADC) values can increase post NAC, which is thought to be due to the decrease in tumor cellularity [41, 42]. Further, lower tumor ADC values have been reported to be associated with breast cancers that are more likely to respond to NAC [43]. Intravoxel incoherent motion (IVIM), a method that uses a DWI sequence, can provide microcirculatory perfusion information. Such information can reveal the state of the tumor before NAC and identify changes induced by treatment. T2-weighted imaging can provide information about tumor edema related to breast cancer cell death. T1 and T2 mapping techniques may be used to provide a quantitative assessment of the breast cancer before and after NAC by measuring T1 and T2 relaxation times. High temporal and spatial resolution dynamic contrast enhancement (DCE) will provide information regarding tumor morphology, angiogenesis and tumor vascularity. High temporal resolution DCE has also been shown to provide functional information pertaining to gadolinium uptake curves, improving the ability to detect changes in the pharmacokinetic modeling parameters, especially volume transfer constant (K^{trans}) [44]. The role of high temporal resolution MR imaging in predicting breast cancer NAC response is being investigated. For example, tumor subregion heterogeneity associated with fast washout was found to predict pathologic response to NAC in a group of 35 patients [45].

17.5 Conclusion

Breast MRI has the potential to contribute to our understanding of tumor biology, behavior and treatment response and to help identify risk factors and treatment regimens at the individual level. Quantifiable image biomarkers need to be validated and this can only be done by large-scale institutional collaborations where computer algorithms and data are shared for the greater good.

References

1. Walsh MF, Nathanson KL, Couch FJ, Offit K. Genomic biomarkers for breast cancer risk. Adv Exp Med Biol. 2016;882:1–32.
2. Saslow D, Boetes C, Burke W, et al. American Cancer Society guidelines for breast screening with MRI as an adjunct to mammography. CA Cancer J Clin. 2007;57:75–89.
3. Sardanelli F, Boetes C, Borisch B, et al. Magnetic resonance imaging of the breast: recommendations from the EUSOMA working group. Eur J Cancer. 2010;46:1296–316.
4. Evans DG, Kesavan N, Lim Y, et al. MRI breast screening in high-risk women: cancer detection and survival analysis. Breast Cancer Res Treat. 2014;145:663–72.
5. Morris EA. Diagnostic breast MR imaging: current status and future directions. Radiol Clin North Am. 2007;45:863–80.
6. Gierach GL, Ichikawa L, Kerlikowske K, et al. Relationship between mammographic density and breast cancer death in the Breast Cancer Surveillance Consortium. J Natl Cancer Inst. 2012;104:1218–27.

7. King V, Brooks JD, Bernstein JL, Reiner AS, Pike MC, Morris EA. Background parenchymal enhancement at breast MR imaging and breast cancer risk. Radiology. 2011;260:50–60.
8. Lee NA, Rusinek H, Weinreb J, et al. Fatty and fibroglandular tissue volumes in the breasts of women 20-83 years old: comparison of X-ray mammography and computer-assisted MR imaging. AJR Am J Roentgenol. 1997;168:501–6.
9. Wang L, Chitiboi T, Meine H, Gunther M, Hahn HK. Principles and methods for automatic and semi-automatic tissue segmentation in MRI data. MAGMA. 2016;29:95–110.
10. Uematsu T, Kasami M, Watanabe J. Should breast MRI be performed with adjustment for the phase in patients' menstrual cycle? Correlation between mammographic density, age, and background enhancement on breast MRI without adjusting for the phase in patients' menstrual cycle. Eur J Radiol. 2012;81:1539–42.
11. Jansen SA, Lin VC, Giger ML, Li H, Karczmar GS, Newstead GM. Normal parenchymal enhancement patterns in women undergoing MR screening of the breast. Eur Radiol. 2011; 21:1374–82.
12. Ha R, Mema E, Guo X, et al. Three-dimensional quantitative validation of breast magnetic resonance imaging background parenchymal enhancement assessments. Curr Probl Diagn Radiol. 2016;45(4):297–303. doi:10.1067/j.cpradiol.2016.02.003.
13. Klifa C, Suzuki S, Aliu S, et al. Quantification of background enhancement in breast magnetic resonance imaging. J Magn Reson Imaging. 2011;33:1229–34.
14. Chen JH, Yu HJ, Hsu C, Mehta RS, Carpenter PM, Su MY. Background parenchymal enhancement of the contralateral nNormal breast: association with tumor response in breast cancer patients receiving neoadjuvant chemotherapy. Transl Oncol. 2015;8:204–9.
15. van der Velden BH, Dmitriev I, Loo CE, Pijnappel RM, Gilhuijs KG. Association between parenchymal enhancement of the contralateral breast in dynamic contrast-enhanced MR imaging and outcome of patients with unilateral invasive breast cancer. Radiology. 2015;276: 675–85.
16. American College of Radiology. (2014) ACR practice parameter for the performance of screening and diagnostic mammography. http://www.acr.org/~/media/5d883e5f6a694c8b8186378b76398837.pdf. Accessed 2 June 2016.
17. Society of Breast Imaging. (2015) ACR and SBI continue to recommend regular mammography starting at age 40. https://www.sbi-online.org/Portals/0/ACR-SBI%20press%20release%20ACS%20FINAL%20for%20web.pdf. Accessed 2 June 2016.
18. Perou CM, Sorlie T, Eisen MB, et al. Molecular portraits of human breast tumours. Nature. 2000;406:747–52.
19. Nguyen PL, Taghian AG, Katz MS, et al. Breast cancer subtype approximated by estrogen receptor, progesterone receptor, and HER-2 is associated with local and distant recurrence after breast-conserving therapy. J Clin Oncol. 2008;26:2373–8.
20. Harris L, Fritsche H, Mennel R, et al. American Society of Clinical Oncology 2007 update of recommendations for the use of tumor markers in breast cancer. J Clin Oncol. 2007;25: 5287–312.
21. Paik S, Shak S, Tang G, et al. A multigene assay to predict recurrence of tamoxifen-treated, node-negative breast cancer. N Engl J Med. 2004;351:2817–26.
22. Morrow M, Waters J, Morris E. MRI for breast cancer screening, diagnosis, and treatment. Lancet. 2011;378:1804–11.
23. Boisserie-Lacroix M, Hurtevent-Labrot G, Ferron S, Lippa N, Bonnefoi H, Mac Grogan G. Correlation between imaging and molecular classification of breast cancers. Diagn Interv Imaging. 2013;94:1069–80.
24. Bhooshan N, Giger ML, Jansen SA, Li H, Lan L, Newstead GM. Cancerous breast lesions on dynamic contrast-enhanced MR images: computerized characterization for image-based prognostic markers. Radiology. 2010;254:680–90.
25. Grimm LJ. Breast MRI radiogenomics: current status and research implications. J Magn Reson Imaging. 2016;43:1269–78.
26. Sutton EJ, Dashevsky BZ, Oh JH, et al. Breast cancer molecular subtype classifier that incorporates MRI features. J Magn Reson Imaging. 2016;44(1):122–9. doi:10.1002/jmri.25119.

27. Grimm LJ, Zhang J, Mazurowski MA. Computational approach to radiogenomics of breast cancer: luminal A and luminal B molecular subtypes are associated with imaging features on routine breast MRI extracted using computer vision algorithms. J Magn Reson Imaging. 2015; 42:902–7.
28. Zhu Y, Li H, Guo W, et al. Deciphering genomic underpinnings of quantitative MRI-based radiomic phenotypes of invasive breast carcinoma. Sci Rep. 2015;5:17787.
29. Li H, Zhu Y, Burnside ES et al MR imaging radiomics signatures for predicting the risk of breast cancer recurrence as given by research versions of MammaPrint, Oncotype DX, and PAM50 gene assays. Radiology. 2016;152110. doi:10.1148/radiol.
30. Sutton EJ, Oh JH, Dashevsky BZ, et al. Breast cancer subtype intertumor heterogeneity: MRI-based features predict results of a genomic assay. J Magn Reson Imaging. 2015;42: 1398–406.
31. Clark K, Vendt B, Smith K, et al. The Cancer Imaging Archive (TCIA): maintaining and operating a public information repository. J Digit Imaging. 2013;26:1045–57.
32. Mamounas EP. Impact of neoadjuvant chemotherapy on locoregional surgical treatment of breast cancer. Ann Surg Oncol. 2015;22:1425–33.
33. Rastogi P, Anderson SJ, Bear HD, et al. Preoperative chemotherapy: updates of National Surgical Adjuvant Breast and Bowel Project Protocols B-18 and B-27. J Clin Oncol. 2008; 26:778–85.
34. Kaufmann M, von Minckwitz G, Mamounas EP, et al. Recommendations from an international consensus conference on the current status and future of neoadjuvant systemic therapy in primary breast cancer. Ann Surg Oncol. 2012;19:1508–16.
35. Bear HD, Anderson S, Smith RE, et al. Sequential preoperative or postoperative docetaxel added to preoperative doxorubicin plus cyclophosphamide for operable breast cancer: National Surgical Adjuvant Breast and Bowel Project Protocol B-27. J Clin Oncol. 2006;24:2019–27.
36. Boughey JC, McCall LM, Ballman KV, et al. Tumor biology correlates with rates of breast-conserving surgery and pathologic complete response after neoadjuvant chemotherapy for breast cancer: findings from the ACOSOG Z1071 (Alliance) Prospective Multicenter Clinical Trial. Ann Surg. 2014;260:608–14 .discussion 614-606
37. Dialani V, Chadashvili T, Slanetz PJ. Role of imaging in neoadjuvant therapy for breast cancer. Ann Surg Oncol. 2015;22:1416–24.
38. Dialani V, Chadashvili T, Slanetz PJ. Role of imaging in neoadjuvant therapy for breast cancer. Ann Surg Oncol. 2015;22(5):1416–24. doi:10.1245/s10434-015-4403-9.
39. Cho N, Im SA, Park IA, et al. Breast cancer: early prediction of response to neoadjuvant chemotherapy using parametric response maps for MR imaging. Radiology. 2014;272:385–96.
40. Pinker K, Bogner W, Baltzer P, et al. Improved diagnostic accuracy with multiparametric magnetic resonance imaging of the breast using dynamic contrast-enhanced magnetic resonance imaging, diffusion-weighted imaging, and 3-dimensional proton magnetic resonance spectroscopic imaging. Invest Radiol. 2014;49:421–30.
41. Pickles MD, Gibbs P, Lowry M, Turnbull LW. Diffusion changes precede size reduction in neoadjuvant treatment of breast cancer. Magn Reson Imaging. 2006;24:843–7.
42. Iwasa H, Kubota K, Hamada N, Nogami M, Nishioka A. Early prediction of response to neoadjuvant chemotherapy in patients with breast cancer using diffusion-weighted imaging and gray-scale ultrasonography. Oncol Rep. 2014;31:1555–60.
43. Lobbes MB, Prevos R, Smidt M, et al. The role of magnetic resonance imaging in assessing residual disease and pathologic complete response in breast cancer patients receiving neoadjuvant chemotherapy: a systematic review. Insights Imaging. 2013;4:163–75.
44. Tofts PS. Modeling tracer kinetics in dynamic Gd-DTPA MR imaging. J Magn Reson Imaging. 1997;7:91–101.
45. Wu J, Gong G, Cui Y, Li R Intratumor partitioning and texture analysis of dynamic contrast-enhanced (DCE)-MRI identifies relevant tumor subregions to predict pathological response of breast cancer to neoadjuvant chemotherapy. J Magn Reson Imaging. 2016; doi:10.1002/jmri.25279. [Epud ahead of print].

Index

A
Abbreviated protocol
  American Cancer Society, 321
  application, 333
  breast density, 332
  cost benefit analysis, 328
  definition of, 323
  DWI, 331–332
  early postcontrast phase, 329
  interpretation times, 328
  kinetic curves, 329
  Kuhl study, 323, 325–327
  limitations, 332–333
  literature, 323, 324
  MIP, 322, 328
  optimization, 323, 325
  sensitivity and specificity, 323, 326
  supplemental screening, 332
  TWIST, 330–331
Adenoid cystic carcinoma (ACC)
  histology and presentation, 211–212
  imaging, 212
ADH. *See* Atypical ductal hyperplasia (ADH)
Apparent diffusion coefficient (ADC), 112, 135, 136, 191–192, 271–272, 347
ATEC®, 237
Atypical ductal hyperplasia (ADH), 182

B
Background parenchymal enhancement (BPE)
  asymmetric, 29, 30
  breast cancer risk, 339–340
  with heterogeneous FGT, 28, 29
  level, 28, 30
  symmetric, 28–29
  variations, 278–279
Back-patch sign, 129
Bannayan-Riley-Ruvalcaba syndrome, 50, 338
BCT. *See* Breast conservation therapy (BCT)
Bilateral 2D axial short tau inversion recovery sequence, 127
Bilateral 2D axial T2-weighted turbo spin-echo sequence, 126
Biopsy
  accuracy, 244–246
  background and indications, 233–235
  benign
    adequate communication, 254
    BI-RADS® assessment, 254
    correlation, 255
    determination, 252–254
    discordance rates, 256
    histopathology, 255
    management recommendations, 258–262
    MRI utilization, 252
    percutaneous biopsy, 252
    practice guidelines, 255–256
    preoperative wire localization, 256–258
  pitfalls and limitations, 242–244
  procedure
    biopsy related hematoma, 240–241, 243
    efficiency and speed, 237
    grid localisation system, 238, 239
    introducer replacement, 238–240
    magnet and initial contrast enhanced image, 238, 239
    multiple lesions, 241–242
    patient positioning, 238
    pre-biopsy image, 240, 241

S.L. Heller, L. Moy (eds.), *Breast Oncology: Techniques, Indications, and Interpretation*, DOI 10.1007/978-3-319-42563-4

Biopsy (*cont.*)
technical aspects
ATEC®, 237
CAD, 236
coils, 235
EnCorTM, 237
initial and then dynamic images, 236
internal access, 235
Mammotome®, 237
open MRI scanners, 235
Vacora®, 237
Blood oxygen level–dependent (BOLD) MRI, 300–301
BPE. *See* Background parenchymal enhancement (BPE)
Breast cancer surveillance, 170
Breast conservation therapy (BCT)
asymmetric left breast skin thickening, 169
fat necrosis, 167, 168
hyperdense oval mass, 165
mammographic findings, 164, 165
moderate skin thickening and breast edema, 165–166
patient selection, 164
pleomorphic calcifications, 169
post lumpectomy scar tissue, 167, 168
postoperative collections, 165
post surgical seroma, 166, 167
recurrence *vs.* scarring, 149–150
seroma, 166, 167
thick walled complex fluid collection, 165–166
Breast imaging reporting and data system (BI-RADS®), 27
amount of FGT, 26, 28
assessment, 254
associated features, 39, 42
BI-RADS 3
BPE, variations of, 278–279
clinical indication, 272–273
fibroadenomata, 271–272
foci, 274, 276, 277
frequency, MRI and malignancy rate, 268, 269
mammography, 268
masses on, 273–275
morphologic features, 270–271
MR-directed ultrasound, 269
NME, 276, 278
short-interval follow-up MRI, 268
traditional definition, 267–268
BPE
asymmetric, 29–30
with heterogeneous FGT, 28, 29
level of, 28, 30
symmetric, 28–30
invasive carcinomas
kinetic features, 202
morphologic features, 201–202
kinetic curve assessment, 42–43
masses
circumscribed margin, 31–32, 34
dark internal septations, 35, 37
heterogeneous enhancement, 33, 35
homogeneous enhancement, 33, 36
irregular margin, 32, 34
rim enhancement, 34, 36
shape, 31–33
spiculated margin, 32–34
NME
diffuse, 39, 41
focal, 37, 38
internal enhancement, 38–39, 41
linear, 37, 38
multiple regions, 37, 39, 40
regional, 37, 39, 40
segmental, 37, 39
reporting system, 43
benign, 44
highly suggestive of malignancy, 44–45
incomplete, 43–44
known biopsy-proven malignancy, 45
negative, 44
probably benign, 44
suspicious, 44–45
Breast MRI. *See* Magnetic resonance imaging (MRI)
Breast-specific gamma imaging (BSGI), 302

C

Cancer Genome Atlas (TCGA), 343
Chemical exchange saturation transfer (CEST), 300
Clear-PEM system, 303–304
Computed tomography (CT), 302–304
Computer aided detection software (CAD), 236
Computer algorithms, 340
Cowden syndrome, 50
C-sign, 129

D

Dark internal septations, 35, 37
DCE-MRI. *See* Dynamic contrast-enhanced MRI (DCE-MRI)
DCIS. *See* Ductal carcinoma in situ (DCIS)

Delayed enhancement phase, 189
Deoxyhemoglobin, 300–301
Diffusion tensor imaging (DTI), 291–292
Diffusion-weighted imaging (DWI)
abbreviated protocol, 331–332
DCE-MRI
biomarker, 290
diagnosis, 289
DKI, 291
DTI, 291–292
IDC, 289, 290
IVIM, 291
detection and characterization, 21
diagnose breast cancer, 135
features, 192
NAC, 111–113
in situ disease, 191–192
Diffusion-weighted kurtosis (DKI), 291
Dixon methods, 13
DTI. *See* Diffusion tensor imaging (DTI)
Ductal carcinoma in situ (DCIS)
ADH, 182
classification, 182
DWI, 191–192
efficacy, 51–52
heterogeneous nature, 183
imaging modalities, 183–184
MRI features
clumped internal enhancement, 185
clustered ring, 184, 185
3D space, mass, 185–186, 188
focus, morphologic appearance, 186, 188–189
kinetic pattern, 189–191
NME, 184
occult invasion, 192–193
segmental distribution, 184–185, 187
significance, 189
1.5 T *vs.* 3 T, 191
overdiagnosis, 182
pathology, 181–182
treatment, 183
Dutch MRI screening study, 53
DWI. *See* Diffusion-weighted imaging (DWI)
Dynamic contrast-enhanced MRI (DCE-MRI)
combined application, 284
DWI
biomarker, 290
diagnosis, 289
DKI, 291
DTI, 291–292
IDC, 289, 290
IVIM, 291
high-resolution high-field and ultra-high-field, 288, 289
multiparametric
concept of, 295, 297
diagnostic accuracy, 295
functional parameters, 294
ROC curves, 295–297
7 T DCE-MR, 297, 298
proton MR spectroscopy, 292–294
quantitative
cancer development, 285
kinetic enhancement analysis, 285–286
NAC, 287
pharmacokinetic modeling, 287
semi-quantitative enhancement curve assessment, 287–288
Tofts Two-Compartment model, 286

E
EnCorTM, 237
Equivocal lesions
focal asymmetry, 145, 146
lumpectomy and questionable subtle asymmetry, 145, 147
questionable associated distortion, 146–149
screen recalled asymmetry, 145
Estrogen receptor (ER), 198
Extracapsular rupture, 130–132

F
Fat suppression methods, 12–13
Fat-water separation techniques, 12–13
[^{18}F]Fluorodeoxyglucose ([^{18}F]), 302–303
[^{18}F]Fluoromisonidazole ([^{18}F]FMISO), 305, 307
FGT. *See* Fibroglandular tissue (FGT)
Fibroadenomata, 271–272
Fibroglandular tissue (FGT), 26, 28, 339
Field-of-view (FOV), 7, 18
Focus, 29, 31
Fractional anisotropy (FA), 291, 292
Fully collapsed intracapsular implant rupture, 129–130
Functional MRI assessment, 111–113

H
Hangnoose sign, 129
Her2 enriched breast cancer, 199, 200
High-resolution high-field DCE-MRI, | 288, 289

Human epidermal growth factor receptor (HER) 2–positive breast cancer, 105
Hyperpolarized MRI (HP MRI), 301–302
Hypoxia, 300–301

I

IBC. *See* Inflammatory breast cancer (IBC)
IDC. *See* Invasive ductal carcinoma (IDC)
IDC-NOS. *See* Invasive ductal carcinoma not otherwise specified (IDC-NOS)
ILC. *See* Invasive lobular carcinoma (ILC)
Imaging artifacts
  aliasing/phase wrap, 18–19
  inhomogeneous fat suppression, 16–17
  metallic/susceptibility, 17–18
  misregistration, 15–16
  motion, 15, 16
Imaging-histopathologic correlation, 229, 230
IMPCa. *See* Invasive micropapillary carcinoma (IMPCa)
Implants
  anaplastic large cell lymphoma, 136–138
  bilateral 2D axial short tau inversion recovery sequence, 127
  bilateral 2D axial T2-weighted turbo spin-echo sequence, 126
  breast cancer detection, 133, 135–137
  history, 121–122
  implant rupture, 125–126
  integrity/complications, 127–130
  mammography, 124, 125
  ruptured silicone implant, 133–135
  saline implants, 130–135
  scout sequence, 126
  single *vs.* double lumen implant, 133
  types, 122–123
  ultrasound, 124, 125
Inflammatory breast cancer (IBC)
  diagnosis of, 110, 111
  preoperative staging, 75, 77–78, 85–86
  skin changes, 156, 157
Inhomogeneous fat suppression, 16–17
Initial enhancement phase, 42, 189
Intact®, 235
Internal enhancement patterns
  masses
    dark internal septations, 35, 37
    heterogeneous, 33, 35
    homogeneous, 33, 36
    rim, 34, 36
  NME
    clumped, 39, 41
    clustered ring, 39, 41
    heterogeneous, 39
    homogeneous, 38, 39
Intracapsular implant rupture, 125, 128–131
Intravoxel incoherent motion (IVIM), 291
Intrinsic susceptibility-weighted imaging. *See* Blood oxygen level–dependent (BOLD) MRI
Invasive breast cancer
  categorization of, 198
  molecular classification, 198–199
    Her2 enriched, 199, 200
    luminal A/luminal B, 199, 200
    triple negative/basal, 199–201
  MRI, 197
    DWI, 202
    MR-BI-RADS and descriptors, 201–202
    MR proton spectroscopy, 202–204
  radiologic-pathologic correlation
    ACC, 211–212
    IDC NOS, 204–205
    ILC, 212–214
    IMPCa, 206–207
    medullary carcinoma, 207–208
    metaplastic carcinoma, 215
    mucinous carcinoma, 208–210
    phyllodes tumors, 215–216
    tubular carcinoma, 210–211
    tumor types and MRI appearance, 204
Invasive ductal carcinoma (IDC), 290
Invasive ductal carcinoma not otherwise specified (IDC-NOS), 204–205
Invasive lobular carcinoma (ILC), 84
  histology and presentation, 212–213
  imaging, 213–214
Invasive micropapillary carcinoma (IMPCa)
  histology and presentation, 206
  imaging, 206–207
Inverted-loop sign, 129
Investigation of serial studies to predict your therapeutic response with imaging and molecular analysis (I-SPY trials), 113–114
I-SPY 1 TRIAL/ACRIN 6657 trial schema, 11

K

Keyhole sign, 129
Kinetic curve assessment, 42–43

L

Li-Fraumeni syndrome, 50
Linguine sign, 125, 130

Luminal A/B breast cancer, 199, 200
Lumpectomy. *See* Breast conservation therapy (BCT)

M

Magnetic resonance imaging (MRI)
abbreviated protocol (*see* Abbreviated protocol)
artifacts
aliasing/phase wrap, 18–19
inhomogeneous fat suppression, 16–17
metallic/susceptibility, 17–18
misregistration, 15–16
motion, 15, 16
bilateral imaging, 7
BI-RADS® (*see* Breast imaging reporting and data system (BI-RADS®))
BOLD, 300–301
breast biopsy (*see* Biopsy)
for breast cancer detection, 3
breast cancer risk, 338–339
BPE, 339–340
fibroglandular tissue, 339
CEST, 300
coils, 5–6
contrast agent, 6
DCIS (*see* Ductal carcinoma in situ (DCIS))
DWI, 21
fat suppression method, 12–13
FOV, 7
genetics, 341–343
high spatial and temporal resolution, 11–12
HP MRI, 301–302
implants (*see* Implants)
invasive breast cancer, 197
DWI, 202
MR-BI-RADS and descriptors, 201–202
MR proton spectroscopy, 202–204
magnetic field strength, 5
molecular imaging
fibroadenomatous hyperplasia, 305, 306
invasive ductal carcinoma G3, 305, 307
multiparametric criteria, 305
non-parametric Pearson's correlation coefficient matrix, 305, 308
proliferation, 308
receptor status, 308–309
tumor hypoxia, 305, 307
MPRs, 13, 14
MRS, 21
NAC (*see* Neoadjuvant chemotherapy (NAC))
^{23}Na MRI, 297–299
patient positioning and comfort, 4–5
^{31}P MRS, 299
preoperative staging (*see* Preoperative staging)
primary acquisition plane, 6–7
problem solving (*see* Problem solving MRI)
protocol sequences and sequence timings, 15
pulse sequences, 8
multi-phase T1-weighted sequence, 9–11
non-fat suppressed T1-weighted sequence, 9
scout/three-plane localizer, 8
silicone implants, 10–11
T2-weighted sequence, 9
screening (*see* Screening)
subtraction MIP, 13, 14
3 T, 17, 19–20
therapy
ADC, 347
NAC, 344
pathologic complete response, 344
post-processing techniques, 345, 346
targeted systemic therapy, 343
Magnetic resonance imaging (MRI)-directed ultrasound (US)
evidence-based findings
histology, 228
lesion type, 226–227
size, 227–228
sonographic correlate, frequency of, 225–226
suspicion and kinetics level, 228
imaging-histopathologic correlation, 229, 230
potential limitations, 228–229
techniques
3D reconstructions, 222, 223
known cancer, 224–226
nipple, 224, 225
prone position, 222–224
shape, size and contours, 225, 227
Magnetic resonance spectroscopy (MRS), 21, 292–293
Mammography, 51
equivocal lesions, 144–149
palpable findings, 153–155
positive predictive value, 142
probably benign lesions, 144
recurrence *vs.* scarring, 149–150
suspicious lesions, 142–144

Mammotome®, 237
Masses
  circumscribed margin, 31–32, 34
  dark internal septations, 35, 37
  internal enhancement, 33, 35–36
  irregular margin, 32, 34
  rim enhancement, 34, 36
  shape, 31–33
  spiculated margin, 32–34
Mastectomy
  biopsy, 171
  MRM, 170
  NSM, 172
  seromas, 171
  SSM, 170–171
  TRAM reconstruction, 172
Maximum intensity projection (MIP), 322, 328
Mean diffusivity (MD), 291
Medullary carcinoma
  histology and presentation, 207–208
  imaging, 208
Metallic/susceptibility artifacts, 17–18
Metaplastic carcinoma, 215
Minimally collapsed intracapsular implant rupture, 129
MIP. *See* Maximum intensity projection (MIP)
Misregistration artifacts, 15–16
Modified radical mastectomy (MRM), 170
Molecular imaging
  fibroadenomatous hyperplasia, 305, 306
  invasive ductal carcinoma G3, 305, 307
  multiparametric criteria, 305
  non-parametric Pearson's correlation coefficient matrix, 305, 308
  proliferation, 308
  receptor status, 308–309
  tumor hypoxia, 305, 307
Motion artifacts, 15, 16, 243
MRI-guided vacuum-assisted biopsy, 244
MR proton spectroscopy (^{1}H-MRS), 202–204
^{99}mTc-sestamibi scintigraphic mammography (^{99}mTc-MIBI-SM), 302
Mucinous carcinoma
  histology and presentation, 208–209
  imaging, 209–210
Multicentric disease, 73, 74
Multifocal disease, 73
Multiparametric MRI
  concept of, 295, 297
  diagnostic accuracy, 295
  functional parameters, 294
  ROC curves, 295–297
  7 T DCE-MR, 297, 298
Multi-planar reformats (MPRs), 13, 14

N
NAC. *See* Neoadjuvant chemotherapy (NAC)
Na^{+}/K^{+} ATPase pump, 298
Neoadjuvant chemotherapy (NAC), 90, 287, 344
  assess response
    mammography, 106
    physical exam, 106
    sonography, 107
    triple negative invasive ductal carcinoma, 106
  diffusion-weighted MRI, 111–113
  I-SPY trials, 113–114
  MRI assessment
    tumor enhancement, 110–111
    tumor size, 109–110
  MRI *vs.* modalities, 106–109
Nipple-areolar complex (NAC), 79
Nipple discharge
  benign etiology, 150
  bloody nipple discharge, 151
  breast retraction, 151
  direct *vs.* conventional MR-galactography, 152
  ductal system evaluation, 151
  MRI utility, 152
  negative predictive value, 150, 152
  nipple retraction, 151
  outcomes, 152
  positive predictive value, 150, 152
  pre-operative MRI, 152–153
Nipple-sparing mastectomy (NSM), 85, 172
Non-mass enhancement (NME), 184
  BI-RADS 3, 276, 278
  diffuse, 39, 41
  focal, 37, 38
  internal enhancement, 38–39, 41
  linear, 37, 38
  multiple regions, 37, 39, 40
  regional, 37, 39, 40
  segmental, 37, 39
Nuclear imaging
  ^{99}mTc-MIBI-SM and BSGI, 302
  PET/CT and PEM, 302–304

O
Oncotype DX 12-gene assay (DCIS Score), 183

P
Paget's disease, 88
Papillary carcinoma
  histology and presentation, 205

imaging, 20
Partial breast irradiation (PBI), 85
Partially collapsed intracapsular implant rupture, 129
Pathological complete response to therapy (pCR), 105, 113, 114
PET mammography (PEM), 302–304
Phase wrap artifacts, 18–19
Phosphorus spectroscopy (^{31}P MRS), 299
Phyllodes tumors
histology and presentation, 215–216
imaging, 216
Positive predictive value (PPV), 74
Positron emission tomography (PET), 302–304
Preoperative staging
anatomic stage/prognostic groups, 66, 69
biologic markers, 66
BPE, 76
clinical utility
bilateral disease, 90
clinical examination and imaging modalities, 70, 90
IBC, 75, 77–78, 85–86
metastatic axillary lymphadenopathy, 81, 87–88
neoadjuvant chemotherapy, 90
Paget's disease, 88
positive surgical margins, 89, 90
diffuse erythema, right breast, 74, 75
distant metastases (M), 66, 68
multicentric disease, 73, 74, 90
multifocal disease, 73, 74, 90
newly diagnosis breast cancer
definitive therapy, 91
dense breast tissue, 84
genetic alterations, 84
high grade DCIS/invasive cancer, 85
ILC, 84
increased mastectomy rates, 92–93
long-term survival impact, 93–94
NSM, 85
PBI, 85
posterior breast cancer, 85
re-excision rate, 91–92
pectoral muscle and chest wall involvement
left breast mass and nipple retraction, 76, 79
posteriorly located invasive ductal carcinoma, 76, 77
triple-negative invasive ductal carcinoma, 76, 78
positive predictive value, 74
primary tumor (T), 66, 67
regional lymph nodes (N)
axillary nodes, 80–83
clinical staging, 66, 68, 69, 80
internal mammary nodes, 80, 82
interpectoral node, 80, 82
ipsilateral intramammary node, 80
nodal metastasis, 83
perifocal edema, 83
rim enhancement, 83
supraclavicular nodes, 80
size and extent
extensive ductal carcinoma in-situ, 69, 72
extensive intraductal component, 69, 71–72
multicentric right breast cancer, 69, 72
nipple involvement, 69, 72
palpable mass, 67, 70
skin and nipple involvement, 67–69, 71–72, 75, 77–80
Problem solving MRI
clinical findings, 150–153
focal/diffuse pain, 155
mammographic and ultrasound findings
equivocal lesions, 144–149
palpable findings, 153–155
positive predictive value, 142
probably benign lesions, 144
recurrence *vs.* scarring, 149–150
suspicious lesions, 142–144
skin changes, 155–157
Proton MR spectroscopy (^{1}H-MRS), 292–294

Q

Quantitative DCE-MRI
cancer development, hallmark of, 285
kinetic enhancement analysis, 285–286
NAC, 287
pharmacokinetic modeling, 287
semi-quantitative enhancement curve assessment, 287–288
Tofts Two-Compartment model, 286

R

Radiofrequency excisional biopsy devices, 235
Reconstruction techniques
free flaps, 173–174
imaging findings, 175–176
implant, 174–175
nipple, 176
pedicled flaps, 172–173

Recurrence Score, 342
Regional lymph nodes (N)
axillary nodes, 80–83
clinical staging, 66, 68, 69, 80
internal mammary nodes, 80, 82
interpectoral node, 80, 82
ipsilateral intramammary node, 80
nodal metastasis, 83
perifocal edema, 83
rim enhancement, 83
supraclavicular nodes, 80
Residual cancer burden (RCB), 113, 114
Rim enhancement, 34, 36

S
Screening
clinical history, 50
efficacy, 51–53
epidemiological factors, 50
equipment and protocols, 56
family history assessment, 50
genetic testing, 50
high risk, 54–55
limitations, 59
low risk, 54
management options, 50–51
moderate risk, 54
reporting and image interpretation, 56–58
very high risk, 55
Skin sparing mastectomy (SSM), 170–171
Snowstorm pattern, 126
Sodium imaging (^{23}Na MRI), 297–299
Spatiotemporally encoded (SPEN), 135
Specific absorption rate (SAR), 20
Stage 0 breast cancer. *See* Ductal carcinoma in situ (DCIS)
Subcapsular line, 129
Subtraction maximum intensity projection (MIP), 13, 14
Subtraction reformats, 13

T
Targeted ultrasound. *See* Magnetic resonance imaging (MRI)-directed ultrasound (US)
Teardrop sign, 129
Time-resolved angiography with stochastic trajectories (TWIST) technique, 330–331
TNBC. *See* Triple negative breast cancer (TNBC)
Tofts Two-Compartment model, 286
Trastuzumab, 309
Triple negative breast cancer (TNBC), 105, 199–201
Tubular carcinoma
histology and presentation, 210
imaging, 211
Tumor hypoxia, 305, 307
Tumor recurrence, 170
TWIST technique. *See* Time-resolved angiography with stochastic trajectories (TWIST) technique

U
Ultra-high-field MRI, 288, 289
Ultrasound, 51
equivocal lesions, 144–149
palpable findings, 153–155
positive predictive value, 142
probably benign lesions, 144
recurrence vs. scarring, 149–150
suspicious lesions, 142–144
Uncollapsed/very early implant rupture, 129

V
Vacora®, 237

W
Wavy-line sign, 130
Wire localisation, 245

MIX
Papier aus verantwortungsvollen Quellen
Paper from responsible sources
FSC® C105338

If you have any concerns about our products,
you can contact us on
ProductSafety@springernature.com

In case Publisher is established outside the EU,
the EU authorized representative is:
Springer Nature Customer Service Center GmbH
Europaplatz 3, 69115 Heidelberg, Germany

Printed by Libri Plureos GmbH
in Hamburg, Germany